GENE THERAPY IMMUNOLOGY

GENE THERAPY IMMUNOLOGY

Edited by

ROLAND HERZOG, Ph.D.
Department of Pediatrics
University of Florida

WILEY-BLACKWELL

A JOHN WILEY & SONS, INC., PUBLICATION

Wiley-Blackwell is an imprint of John Wiley & Sons, formed by the merger of Wiley's global Scientific, Technical, and Medical business with Blackwell Publishing.

Published by John Wiley & Sons, Inc., Hoboken, New Jersey.
Published simultaneously in Canada.

Library of Congress Cataloging-in-Publication Data:

Gene therapy immunology / [edited by] Roland Herzog.
p. ; cm.
Includes bibliographical references.
ISBN 978-0-470-13406-1 (cloth)
1. Gene therapy. 2. Immunology. I. Herzog, Roland, Ph. D.
[DNLM: 1. Gene Therapy. 2. Gene Transfer Techniques. 3. Immune Tolerance. 4. Immunity, Natural. 5. Transplantation Immunology. QZ 52 I33 2008]
RB155.8.I46 2008
616′.042—dc22

2008040291

Printed in the United States of America

10 9 8 7 6 5 4 3 2 1

CONTENTS

CONTRIBUTORS

Shizuo Akira, M.D., Ph.D., Research Institute for Microbial Diseases, Osaka University, Osaka, Japan

Valder R. Arruda, M.D., Ph.D., Department of Pediatrics, University of Pennsylvania School of Medicine, The Children's Hospital of Philadelphia, Philadelphia, Pennsylvania

Jessamyn Bagley, Ph.D., Transplantation Research Center, Renal Division, Brigham and Women's Hospital, and Children's Hospital, Harvard Medical School, Boston, Massachusetts

Jorge Boucas, M.S., Clinic I for Internal Medicine, University of Cologne, Cologne, Germany

Suzanne M.K. Buckley, Ph.D., Department of Haematology, Haemophilia Centre and Haemostasis Unit, Royal Free and University College Medical School, London, UK

Hildegard Büning, Ph.D., Clinic I for Internal Medicine and Center for Molecular Medicine, University of Cologne, Cologne, Germany

Maria G. Castro, Ph.D., Gene Therapeutics Research Institute, Cedars-Sinai Medical Center, and Departments of Medicine, and Molecular and Medical Pharmacology, David Geffen School of Medicine, University of California–Los Angeles, Los Angeles, California

Lung-Ji Chang, Ph.D., Department of Molecular Genetics and Microbiology, University of Florida, Gainesville, Florida

Charles Coutelle, M.D., Ph.D., Faculty of Medicine, Imperial College London, London, UK

Oliver Coutelle, M.D., Ph.D., Clinic I for Internal Medicine and Center for Molecular Medicine, University of Cologne, Cologne, Germany

Nelson C. Di Paolo, Ph.D., Division of Medical Genetics, Department of Medicine, University of Washington, Seattle, Washington

Hildegund Ertl, M.D., The Wistar Institute, University of Pennsylvania, Philadelphia, Pennsylvania

Terence R. Flotte, M.D., Department of Pediatrics, University of Massacchusetts Medical School, Worcester, Massachusetts

Soosan Ghazizadeh, Ph.D., Departments of Oral Biology and Pathology, and Dermatology, Stony Brook University, Stony Brook, New York

Nick Giannoukakis, Ph.D., Diabetes Institute, Rangos Research Center, Children's Hospital of Pittsburgh, and Department of Pathology, University of Pittsburgh School of Medicine, Pittsburgh, Pennsylvania

Michael Hallek, M.D., Clinic I for Internal Medicine and Center for Molecular Medicine, University of Cologne, Cologne, Germany

Roland W. Herzog, Ph.D., Department of Pediatrics, University of Florida, Gainesville, Florida

Brad E. Hoffman, Ph.D., Department of Pediatrics, University of Florida, Gainesville, Florida

John Iacomini, Ph.D., Transplantation Research Center, Renal Division, Brigham and Women's Hospital, and Children's Hospital, Harvard Medical School, Boston, Massachusetts

Ken J. Ishii, M.D., Ph.D., Research Institute for Microbial Diseases, Osaka University, Osaka, Japan

Shohei Koyama, M.D., Research Institute for Microbial Diseases, Osaka University, Osaka, Japan

Kurt Kroeger, M.S., Gene Therapeutics Research Institute, Cedars-Sinai Medical Center, and Departments of Medicine, and Molecular and Medical Pharmacology, David Geffen School of Medicine, University of California–Los Angeles, Los Angeles, California

David Lillicrap, M.D., Department of Pathology and Molecular Medicine, Richardson Laboratory, Queen's University, Kingston, Ontario, Canada

Shih-Wen Lin, Ph.D., The Wistar Institute, University of Pennsylvania, Philadelphia, Pennsylvania

Pedro R. Lowenstein, M.D., Ph.D., Gene Therapeutics Research Institute, Cedars-Sinai Medical Center, and Departments of Medicine, and Molecular and Medical Pharmacology, David Geffen School of Medicine, University of California–Los Angeles, Los Angeles, California

Jay Lozier, M.D., Ph.D., Department of Laboratory Medicine, NIH Clinical Center, Bethesda, Maryland

Ronald J. Mandel, Ph.D., Department of Neuroscience, Powell Gene Therapy Center, McKnight Brain Institute, University of Florida College of Medicine, Gainesville, Florida

Christian Müller, Ph.D., Department of Pediatrics, University of Massachusetts Medical School, Worcester, Massachusetts

Daniel A. Muruve, M.D., Department of Medicine, University of Calgary, Calgary, Alberta, Canada

Megha S. Nivsarkar, Ph.D., Faculty of Medicine, Imperial College London, London, UK

Luca Perabo, Ph.D., Clinic I for Internal Medicine, University of Cologne, Cologne, Germany

Waseem Qasim, M.D., Ph.D., Centre for Immunodeficiency, Institute of Child Health, and Great Ormond Street Hospital NHS Trust, London, UK

Paul D. Robbins, Ph.D., Department of Molecular Genetics and Biochemistry, University of Pittsburgh School of Medicine, Pittsburgh, Pennsylvania

Mark E. Seamone, B.S., Department of Medicine, University of Calgary, Calgary, Alberta, Canada

Dmitry M. Shayakhmetov, Ph.D., Division of Medical Genetics, Department of Medicine, University of Washington, Seattle, Washington

Adrian Thrasher, M.D., Ph.D., Centre for Immunodeficiency, Institute of Child Health, and Great Ormond Street Hospital NHS Trust, London, UK

Chaorui Tian, M.D., Transplantation Research Center, Renal Division, Brigham and Women's Hospital, and Children's Hospital, Harvard Medical School, Boston, Massachusetts

Massimo M. Trucco, M.D., Diabetes Institute, Rangos Research Center, Children's Hospital of Pittsburgh, and Department of Pediatrics, University of Pittsburgh School of Medicine, Pittsburgh, Pennsylvania

Simon N. Waddington, Ph.D., Department of Haematology, Haemophilia Centre and Haemostasis Unit, Royal Free and University College Medical School, London, UK

Braden Waters, B.S., Department of Pathology and Molecular Medicine, Richardson Laboratory, Queen's University, Kingston, Ontario, Canada

Wei-Dong Xiong, M.D., Ph.D., Gene Therapeutics Research Institute, Cedars-Sinai Medical Center and Departments of Medicine, and Molecular and Medical Pharmacology, David Geffen School of Medicine, University of California–Los Angeles, Los Angeles, California

PREFACE

Gene therapy for genetic diseases is based on a simple concept: transfer of a functional gene to replace the endogenous defective gene. This novel form of molecular medicine was made possible by advances in molecular genetics made in the 1980s, including the discovery of genetic defects and the cloning of human genes. Subsequently, development of animal models of human disease led to numerous preclinical studies on gene-based treatments. The initial quest was to create potent vectors (gene transfer vehicles) and routes of delivery to obtain therapeutic expression. Because viruses have evolved to infect cells efficiently, substantial improvements in gene transfer were achieved through virology research. More than 1300 clinical trials in gene therapy have been conducted since the first trial in 1990. The first clear successes have been documented, in particular for severe immune deficiencies. In addition, multiple successes in animals validate the concept of gene therapy and establish a strong foundation for this young field to move forward.

Over the past decade, it has become clear that immune responses are the next big hurdle for gene therapy. In other words, we have to coax the immune system into tolerating rather than rejecting the donated gene. After all, the immune system has evolved to fight off pathogens such as viruses. In particular, the invading nucleic acid may be sensed by the innate immune system, while the novel protein expressed from the therapeutic gene or proteins derived from the vector (such as viral proteins) may be subject to antigen-specific adaptive responses. Innate immunity can have serious complications resulting from inflammatory reactions. Antibody and cytotoxic responses against vectors and transgene products can negate therapy, hinder readministration of vector, and may interfere with other treatments, such as protein replacement therapies. Certainly, we can learn from transplantation surgeons, who have developed methodologies for stable engraftment of donated cells and organs. However, there are gene therapy–specific immunological aspects, such as vector-derived activation signals, presence of memory lymphocytes in patients from natural infection with parent viruses of vectors, and immune regulation. Moreover, immune responses differ substantially depending on vector, target organ, and details of the protocol. It is now clear that any student or scientist entering the gene therapy arena needs to know immunology and appreciate the complex interactions between the immune system and gene transfer. The authors of this book provide a wealth of information and a comprehensive coverage of this complex topic, which should be an integral part of any gene therapy class.

ROLAND W. HERZOG

1

THE IMMUNOLOGY OF GENE TRANSFER: AN OVERVIEW

BRADEN WATERS, B.S., AND DAVID LILLICRAP, M.D.

Department of Pathology and Molecular Medicine, Richardson Laboratory, Queen's University, Kingston, Ontario, Canada

Gene Therapy Immunology, Edited by Roland Herzog

1.1 INTRODUCTION

As the science of gene transfer has progressed over the past two decades it has become apparent that certain obstacles to the success of this therapeutic approach are substantial in nature. Attaining clinical benefits from gene transfer requires the effective delivery of a therapeutic transgene to cells of the host and the establishment of levels of transgene expression that are sufficient in both magnitude and duration to result in a therapeutic benefit. Although these objectives are straightforward in principle, their attainment has required the interaction of life scientists from a variety of backgrounds to optimize each of the many steps involved in a gene transfer protocol [Anson and Fletcher 2007; Cardone 2007; Pierce et al. 2007].

While the development of efficient transgene delivery systems and transgene expression cassettes has occupied a considerable amount of time during the evolution of gene transfer protocols, it has long been clear that the host immune response to gene transfer will present a formidable obstacle to the attainment of therapeutic goals. The aim of this introductory chapter is to summarize the current status of knowledge pertaining to the immunological challenges facing gene transfer and to illustrate specific aspects of this challenge with examples from the gene transfer literature. Detailed discussions of various subject areas follow in the succeeding chapters.

1.2 COMPONENTS OF THE IMMUNE RESPONSE TO GENE TRANSFER

There is very good evidence that recipients of gene transfer develop responses that involve the full spectrum of innate and adaptive immunity. Initial responses to transgene delivery can be seen within hours of administration, depending on the means and route of delivery. These early responses involve mechanisms that include the detection of pathogen-associated molecular patterns (PAMPs) present on the transgene particle (i.e., viral structural proteins or nucleic acids) by pattern recognition receptors (PRRs) on cells of the innate immune system (i.e., macrophages and dendritic cells) and the subsequent elaboration of pro-inflammatory cytokines that can up-regulate later adaptive immune responses. These adaptive responses can include the generation of antibodies to the transgene delivery vehicle and to the transgene product, as well as cell-mediated responses to these entities. Overall, depending on the context of the gene transfer protocol and a variety of factors pertaining to the details of the protocol, the host immune system can elicit adverse reactions that can span an interval from within hours of vector administration to months after gene transfer.

1.3 THE CONCEPT OF IMMUNOLOGICAL DANGER AND GENE TRANSFER

Two nonexclusive theories of immunologic responsiveness have emerged in the past few decades. The first of these is the *self–nonself theory*, which predicts that adaptive immune responses will be generated against any antigen to which the organism has not been exposed during early development [Janeway 1992]. In this instance, self-antigens presented in the thymus to T cells that are reactive to these self-antigens are selected for elimination by apoptosis. This form of centrally mediated immunological tolerance accounts for the limitation of autoreactive immune responses in normal physiology. However, the self–nonself theory of immune reactivity does not explain how self-neoantigens, which can be expressed within an organism after the development of initial central tolerance, are preserved without evoking a nonself adaptive response. This situation is best exemplified by the appearance of self-neoantigens, at the time of puberty and in pregnancy, that do not routinely generate adaptive immune reactions. To explain how these new nonself antigens are tolerated, the *theory of immunological danger* has been proposed and is now widely accepted as a complementary principle for the development of adaptive immunity [Matzinger 1994]. According to the danger theory of immune reactivity, antigens are tolerated unless they are presented to immune cells in the context of "dangerous," inflammatory signals. The coexistence of these signals at the time of antigen presentation alters the maturation state of the antigen-presenting cell and predisposes the generation of effector cell responses rather than the acquisition of immunologic tolerance [Gallucci et al. 1999].

It has become clear that many aspects of gene transfer protocols result in the presentation of antigens in the context of inflammatory danger signals, and thus the likelihood that immunogenic responses are generated to the delivery vehicle and/or transgene product is enhanced significantly [Brown and Lillicrap 2002]. Various factors relating to the mode of transgene delivery, the nature of the delivery vehicle, and the way in which the delivery process affects host cells have all been implicated in the generation of inflammatory microenvironments, scenarios in which effector cell responses are readily generated.

1.4 TARGETS OF THE IMMUNOLOGIC RESPONSE TO GENE TRANSFER

Delivery of transgenes through a variety of means can result in immune responses to several components of the gene transfer system. These responses can take the following forms:

- Innate immunity
    - Fever

- Thrombocytopenia
- Systemic cytokine elevations
- Multiorgan inflammation leading to death
- Activation of the adaptive immune response

- Adaptive immunity
  - Antibodies to the vector, compromising vector readministration
  - Antibodies to the transgene product, nullifying transgene expression
  - Cytotoxicity to vector and/or transgene product, leading to loss of transduced cells

Although the efficiency of nonviral delivery protocols continues to be inferior to viral vector–mediated approaches to transgene delivery, there are still instances where nonviral delivery may prove efficacious. In these cases, immune responses may be generated to the transgene nucleic acid depending on how and where this is delivered and the nature of the nucleotide sequence. In particular, unmethylated CpG sequences, which are found more frequently in prokaryotic genomes (i.e., plasmid backbones), can incite innate immune responses through interaction with Toll-like receptor (TLR) 9 [Verthelyi 2006].

In contrast to nonviral delivery protocols, viral-mediated gene transfer offers the potential for a significantly wider array of immunological responses. While the various forms of disabled viruses used for this purpose are unable to replicate, the delivery to host cells utilizes very large numbers of viral particles to optimize the delivery efficiency [Lowenstein 2003]. The result of these high-multiplicity-of-infection protocols on the immune system are twofold: The large viral load is a potent stimulus for PRR signaling, and there is good evidence that receptors such as TLR7 are activated by exposure to engineered viral genomes. Furthermore, once inside the transduced host cells, the viral proteins are disassembled and presented on the cell surface in the context of MHC class I molecules and can incite potent $CD8^+$ cytotoxic T-lymphocyte (CTL) responses that will, in turn, eliminate the transduced cells. Peptides derived from the viral vector will also be presented after uptake by antigen-presenting cells in the context of MHC class II molecules, and effector $CD4^+$ T-cell responses will ultimately lead to the generation of antibodies to the vector that will limit vector readministration.

Aside from immune responses to the delivery vehicle and the transgene particle, in gene transfer protocols for the replacement of proteins in monogenic inherited deficiencies (e.g., lysosomal storage diseases, hemophilia), the transgene product may be recognized as a neoantigen, and adaptive immune responses may be generated to the protein [Lillicrap 2000]. These can either target destruction of the cell of synthesis through a CTL-mediated response or, more often, result in the formation of antibodies through a $CD4^+$ T-cell-facilitated mechanism. In either instance it is clear that the beneficial effects of the gene transfer protocol will be compromised significantly by the host's adaptive immune response.

1.5 FACTORS AFFECTING THE IMMUNE RESPONSE TO GENE TRANSFER

1.5.1 Host Influences

Not surprisingly, factors inherent to the host can have a profound influence on the nature and extent of the immune response to gene transfer. Both genetic and acquired factors, such as the following, can significantly alter the innate and adaptive responses to various forms of gene therapy:

- Host factors
  - Recipient immunogenotype
  - Prior exposure to virus
  - Prior exposure to transgene product
  - Maturity of immune system at time of transfer
  - Coexistent inflammation
  - Coexistent immunosuppression
- Gene transfer protocol factors
  - Route of transgene delivery
  - Type of delivery system
- Transgene delivery vehicle factors
  - Type of viral vector
  - Vector dose
  - Pseudotype of vector particle
  - Type of transgene promoter
  - Presence of vector preparation contaminants

As one would anticipate, these influences can best be dissected in inbred strains of laboratory animals, where genetic homogeneity enhances the contributions of genetic loci involved either directly or indirectly in generation of the immune response [Rawle et al. 2004]. Thus, testing the immunogenic potential of a particular gene transfer protocol should take into account the inherent immunogenic phenotype of the test animals so that immunogenicity is neither significantly under- or overestimated. In outbred species such as humans, the analysis of genetic factors influencing immunity (the immunogenotype) is considerably more complex and may rely on indirect evidence of immune dysregulation obtained through personal or family histories of disorders with immune contributions. The situation is somewhat less complicated in the case of the adaptive immune response to newly delivered proteins in inherited protein-deficient states (e.g., hemophilia). In these circumstances, there is an incidence of antibody development to the protein neoantigen, even with standard protein replacement therapy. This complication is especially likely in patients in whom the underlying genetic defect results in a null phenotype [Schwaab et al. 1995], although this risk can be reduced by prior tolerance induction to the protein in question.

In contrast to the complexity of the immunogenic phenotype and its variable influence on gene transfer outcomes, there is strong evidence to indicate that acquired coexistent pathologies (e.g., infection), which can act as inflammatory adjuvants at the time of gene transfer, may significantly enhance the host immune response, with occasionally catastrophic consequences [Raper et al. 2003]. Thus, the administration of any form of gene transfer to recipients in whom inflammatory pathologies coexist, or in whom the immune response is being manipulated, should be approached with caution.

1.5.2 Influence of Mode and Route of Transgene Delivery

The mode and route of transgene administration can influence transgene immunity through a number of mechanisms. As one distinct example, certain anatomical sites in the body, such as the anterior chamber of the eye, experience only attenuated immunologic responses to newly introduced antigens [Kaplan and Niederkorn 2007]. Thus, the delivery of transgenes to the eye through a variety of approaches may be significantly less complicated by immune compromise than delivery to many other sites. Similarly, transgene delivery to sites of mucosal uptake, such as the nasal and gut epithelium, may also predispose to the generation of a tolerogenic as opposed to an immunogenic outcome [Faria and Weiner 2006].

In contrast, systemic delivery of transgenes through the circulation will inevitably result in the involvement of cells of both the innate and adaptive immune systems at various sites. This problem can be overcome to some extent by directing delivery through means such as organ-specific vascular injections (e.g., hepatic artery injection) or through delivery directly into specific tissues (e.g., intramuscular injection). An additional level of tissue specificity for transgene expression can be achieved through the use of a targeted transcriptional regulatory element. In selected anatomical sites, different subsets of immune cells may be involved that may result in significantly different immunological outcomes. As one important example, limiting transgene expression to the liver by a combination of local vascular injection and the use of a liver-specific transgene promoter has recently been shown to promote the generation of tolerance to a secreted transgene product through the expansion of antigen-specific regulatory T cells [Cao et al. 2007].

In addition to regulating immunogenicity through altering the route of administration, the mode of transgene delivery also influences the host response. Thus, while viral vector–mediated delivery to skeletal muscle may be relatively nonimmunogenic, potent host responses can be elicited if high vector doses are delivered to single sites [Arruda et al. 2004]. Similarly, while nonviral vector transgene delivery is generally better tolerated by the immune system, protocols such as hydrodynamic injection, which result in perivascular tissue trauma, are often associated with adaptive immune responses to the transgene product, due, at least in part, to the inflammatory environment in which the transgene is expressed [Miao et al. 2006].

1.5.3 Vector Influences

Viruses have evolved over millions of years to deliver nucleic acids efficiently to host cells, and thus represent ideal transgene delivery vehicles [Kay et al. 2001]. To date, despite intensive investigation, gene transfer scientists employing strategies that utilize components of the viral delivery system have not come close to emulating the efficiency of viral transduction. Nevertheless, despite their efficiency as delivery vehicles, all disabled viruses suffer from the inevitable consequence of being viewed as "foreign" and "dangerous" by the host immune system. Fortunately, the degree to which this immunologic limitation exists appears to vary significantly between types of viral vector.

A number of vector-related variables merit general comment prior to a more detailed consideration of each viral vector type. First is the issue of vector production and the potential for delivering immunogenic contaminants of the production system along with the vector itself. Viral vectors are generated through protocols that provide access to essential viral structural components that are deleted from the viral genome through their expression *in trans* from helper constructs in the producer cell lines. These helper constructs may be delivered through transient transfection or, in instances where larger vector yields are desired, through the generation of stably transfected cell lines in which helper proteins are usually under the control of inducible promoter elements. Whatever the details of helper protein expression, a potential consequence of the presence of these proteins is that they may be co-purified with the vector and can elicit independent innate and adaptive responses following gene transfer. During vector production, depending on the transgene promoter used, expression of the transgene product can occur from the producer cell line. Thus, in addition to the co-purification of viral structural helper proteins, vector isolation may also be complicated by the presence of contaminating transgene protein that will be co-administered at the time of transgene delivery and may elicit an adaptive immune response.

Upon delivery to the gene transfer recipient, the immunological consequence of viral vector exposure will depend on a variety of factors, including the history of prior contact with the virus, the route and mode of vector delivery, the vector dose, and the presence of any coexistent conditions within the recipient that might influence the ability to generate an immune response. Viruses possess structural elements, PAMPs, that will be recognized by receptors, PRRs, on cells of the recipient's innate immune system. To date, most of our knowledge related to these interactions involves the family of Toll-like receptors (TLRs), which are expressed on the surface and within endocytic compartments of cells of the innate immune system [Seth et al. 2006]. Thus, the activation of TLR signaling pathways by a variety of ligands involved in gene transfer protocols, such as viral double (TLR3) and single (TLR7 and TLR8)-stranded RNA, envelope glycoproteins (TLR2 and TLR4), and unmethylated CpG nucleotides (TLR9), all have the potential to mediate downstream inflammatory cytokine and chemokine synthesis and release. Even though viral vectors have been engineered to remove many of their intrinsic structural elements, the vector particles will still possess peptide sequences that facilitate cell entry but at the same time signal to the cell that it has been invaded by a potential pathogen. Removal or manipulation of these sequences may reduce innate immunogenicity but will probably also reduce transduction efficiency. Overall, the early interaction of viral vector elements with components of the innate immune system remains a major obstacle to the attainment of efficient delivery and long-term persistence of the transgene.

The ability of viral vectors to transduce cells varies significantly for different viruses and cell types. This variable has profound effects on the immunogenic potential of a particular vector type. More specifically, the transduction of and expression within professional antigen-presenting cells (APCs: e.g., dendritic cells) will generate situations in which vector particles and the transgene product are processed and presented on MHC class I molecules to cognate CTLs. In circumstances in which there is a coincident expression of co-stimulatory molecules by the APCs, an adverse CTL response will result in the potential of cytotoxicity for any host cell presenting the appropriate vector or transgene-derived peptide. Thus, the use of vectors that are inherently less inclined to transduce APCs or can be targeted away from APCs represent strategies that will very likely reduce cellular adaptive immunity.

Once inside the cell, the vector particle must gain entry to the nucleus and disassemble the protein elements that have facilitated entry into the cell. In many instances, the details of where, when, and over what duration of time this event occurs are still vague [Thomas et al. 2004], but the subsequent presentation of these vector-derived peptides on the surface of the transduced cell in the context of MHC class I receptors represents a significant limitation to vector-mediated gene transfer [Arruda and Xiao 2007]. Once presented at the transduced cell surface, the subsequent host response will depend on prior exposure to the virus (i.e., the potential presence of immunologic memory) and whether the presentation is occurring from an APC, in which co-stimulatory molecule expression can result in cognate CTL activation. In cases where the virus has been seen previously by the host immune system and an adaptive memory response has been generated, expansion of vector-specific CTLs and subsequent destruction of transduced host cells may ensue.

1.6 IMMUNOLOGIC CONSIDERATIONS FOR SPECIFIC VIRAL VECTORS

1.6.1 Adenoviral Gene Transfer

Although adenoviral vectors provide a very efficient transgene delivery system for most cell types, their excellent ability to transduce cells is matched by limitations imposed by the host immune response. Cellular entry by these vectors is mediated by an interaction of the viral capsid with several cell surface receptors, including the coxsackie and adenovirus receptor (CAR) and the family of α_v integrins. However, studies in which these interactions have been ablated suggest that the viral capsid can still promote associations with cells of the innate immune system through other, as yet unidentified mechanisms.

Although preexistent adaptive immunity to adenovirus will compromise vector administration and potentially result in targeted cytotoxicity of transduced host cells, it is the effects of adenoviral vectors on innate immunity that have limited the recent development of systemic adenoviral transgene delivery [Muruve 2004]. Systemic adenovector delivery is associated with avid uptake by Kupffer cells in the liver and the interaction and uptake by other cells of the innate immune system. This effect has two consequences: First, there is a threshold effect for adenoviral vector dosing such that when the innate immune cell "sink" has been saturated, rapid increments in parenchymal cell transduction can be achieved with minimal vector dose escalation. Second, and of major importance for the safety of in vivo systemic gene transfer employing adenovectors, is the fact that the interaction of these vectors with innate immune cells signals the expression and release of an array of pro-inflammatory cytokines and chemokines, including IL-1, IL-6, TNF-α, macrophage inhibitory protein-2, and RANTES. This effect results in a complex constellation of inflammatory manifestations within 3 to 4 hours of vector administration. These include fever, thrombocytopenia, and other signs of systemic inflammation. Although the extent of this pro-inflammatory cascade can be predicted to some extent based on variables such as vector dose, past clinical experience with adenovectors indicates that the inflammatory response may sometimes far exceed expectations and lead to catastrophic clinical outcomes [Raper et al. 2003].

There is strong evidence to indicate that the innate response against adenovectors is mediated to components of the viral capsid and their interaction with innate immune cells. Thus, while adaptive immunity against these vectors has been reduced substantially through the development of helper-dependent adenovectors that contain no adenoviral genes, the problems with innate responsiveness have remained unchanged [Muruve et al. 2004]. Although the innate immune response to systemically delivered adenovectors has significantly limited further development of gene substitution trials, this phenomenon has been beneficial for vaccine development and for cancer immunotherapy with this vector system. Indeed, the first commercially available gene transfer product, Gendicine, employs an adenoviral vector expressing p53 for the treatment of various forms of neoplasia [Peng 2005].

1.6.2 Adeno-Associated Viral Gene Transfer

Adeno-associated viruses (AAVs) are widely regarded as excellent vehicles for gene transfer. Their preferred selection as gene transfer vectors is due at least in part to the fact that they appear to be minimally provocative to the host immune system. While adenovectors efficiently transduce APCs and elicit rapid and significant pro-inflammatory responses from the innate immune system, the AAV serotypes that have been studied to date do not seem to transduce APCs effectively and do not generate innate immune reactivity [Sarukhan et al. 2001; Zaiss and Muruve 2005]. Thus, acute immunologic consequences of AAV gene transfer have been negligible.

However, while the interaction of AAVs with the innate immune system seems inconsequential, there are significant problems relating to the adaptive immune response to this vector. Natural, asymptomatic AAV infection in humans is common, and estimates of up to 80% of human populations possess neutralizing antibodies to some AAV serotypes [Moskalenko et al. 2000]. Furthermore, strong conservation of immunodominant capsid epitopes suggests that changing serotypes may meet with only partial success in attempting to evade existing anti-AAV immunity. The presence of anti-AAV antibodies will compromise vector delivery and adversely influence transduction efficiency.

Whereas the incidence of humoral immune responses to AAVs is relatively well documented, far less is known about the frequency with which cell-mediated reactivity to the vector is generated. Unfortunately, there does not appear to be a useful correlation between the finding of humoral responses to AAVs and the presence of a cell-mediated response. However, there is now strong evidence from the evaluation of AAV gene transfer in human clinical trials that CTL responses to AAV capsid antigens can result in significant cytotoxicity and the loss of cells that have been transduced by the vector [High et al. 2003; Manno et al. 2006; Mingozzi et al. 2007]. Whether these adverse CTL responses can be predicted from an analysis of circulating cells prior to gene transfer seems unlikely. Nevertheless, the result of these cytotoxic responses remains a critical obstacle to persistent AAV-mediated gene transfer, and the outcome of trials of immunosuppression administered around the time of transgene delivery is eagerly awaited [Herzog et al. 2001; Jiang et al. 2006].

1.6.3 Retroviral Gene Transfer

Recent efforts to utilize recombinant retroviruses as a means of transgene delivery have been complicated principally by concerns relating to their propensity to cause insertional mutagenesis. Detailed studies have now documented what may be important differences between the sites of insertion for onco-retroviral and lentiviral genomes [Bushman 2007]. However, aside from these complications, recent evidence has been presented to suggest that these vectors may also have immunologic consequences that were previously overlooked. Persistent high-level lentiviral-mediated transgene expression following in vivo delivery has been difficult to achieve and appears to be due, at least in part, to the fact that lentiviral particles pseudotyped with commonly used envelopes such as VSV-G transduce and activate APCs more efficiently than they transduce parenchymal cells. This propensity results in subsequent activation of the adaptive immune system and the frequent generation of humoral and cell-mediated responses to the transgene product [Follenzi et al. 2004]. As a further result of this predilection, lentivectors show the same type of threshold dosing effect seen with adenovirus. Saturation of reticuloendothelial cell "sinks" such as the Kupffer cell population will then allow significant increments in parenchymal cell transduction with relatively small increases in vector dose [van Til et al. 2005]. However, in addition to acting as a sink for lentivector distribution, the transduction of these innate immune cells also generates a type I interferon response (i.e., IFN-α and IFN-β) [Brown et al. 2007]. These events have several adverse effects on the persistence of lentivector gene transfer. First, lentivector transduction of APCs activates these cells and thus establishes an environment in which expression and presentation of the transgene product (in the context of either MHC class I or II) will preferentially result in immunogenic as opposed to tolerogenic T-cell responses. As a result, lentivector delivery is often associated with the generation of a humoral response to the transgene product and the production of CTLs that act to remove the transduced parenchymal cells. In addition to the effects secondary to APC maturation, the elicitation of IFN-αβ further inhibits transduction of parenchymal cells and stimulates the cytotoxic clearance of cells that have already been transduced. In response to these interactions with the innate immune system, future studies of in vivo lentivector delivery will need to find ways in which these early adverse events are abrogated or minimized.

1.7 PRECLINICAL MODELING OF GENE TRANSFER IMMUNOLOGY

While the challenges of the host immune response to gene transfer are now very well appreciated, developing preclinical strategies to determine the mechanisms underlying these responses and to evaluate potential means to circumvent them are not straightforward. Most in vivo gene transfer studies begin in laboratory mice. These animals offer significant advantages in that mouse immunology has been very well studied and reagents to assess immune responses in the mouse are abundant. However, the commonly used inbred mouse strains also have the disadvantage of generating immune reactions that are relatively homogeneous and to some extent predetermined by the particular immunophenotype of the inbred strain. As just one example, Balb/c mice have a much greater tendency to generate Th2 polarized responses than do C57BL/6 mice, in which Th1 responses are predominant [Rawle et al. 2004]. As a result of these differences, the prediction of immunological outcomes of gene transfer strategies in outbred species such as humans should be approached with caution.

The second complicating issue with the use of animals for preclinical testing of the immune responses to gene transfer is the separation of responses that are prompted by exposure to heterologous transgene products from those responses that are inherent to the gene transfer strategy itself. Even in animals with null mutations for specific proteins, the choice of a species-matched transgene replacement may prove essential to prevent a humoral response to the transgenic protein and limit the potential to assess long-term persistence of transgene expression [Connelly et al. 1996].

Finally, the natural infectivity of animal models with viruses that are now being used as candidate vectors for human studies is sometimes limiting. As a result, memory responses of humoral and cell-mediated adaptive immunity to the vector are difficult to assess [Herzog 2007]. This important limitation can be addressed by various approaches involving passive immunization in which either immunoglobulin preparations possessing antivector activity are administered [Scallan et al. 2006] or adoptive transfer of cytotoxic memory T cells can be delivered prior to trials of gene transfer. However, all of these strategies are complex, and none of them recapitulate the details of the memory response in the naturally infected host.

1.8 APPROACHES TO ABROGATING THE IMMUNE RESPONSE TO GENE TRANSFER

As alluded to at the start of this overview, there is now a realization that the host immune response to various components of the gene transfer protocol represents the most challenging obstacle to the clinical implementation of this therapeutic paradigm. Therefore, the development of strategies such as the following, used to abrogate or at least minimize these responses, is essential for the future translation of gene transfer benefits:

- Reducing innate immunity
  - Utilizing an ex vivo transgene delivery approach
  - Minimizing the vector dose
  - Avoiding coexisting inflammation in the host
  - Using AAV vectors for in vivo delivery
- Reducing adaptive immunity
  - Delivery to prenatal and neonatal immune systems
  - Avoiding antigen-presenting cell transduction
  - Blocking co-stimulatory molecule interactions
  - Peri-gene transfer immunosuppression
  - Delivery to immunoprivileged sites (e.g., eye)
  - Delivery to the liver
  - Delivery to mucosal epithelium

Of course, as mentioned previously, immune reactivity can, in some instances, be a desirable effect of gene transfer, and thus studies aimed at using this approach for vaccination or immunotherapy of cancer have used this effect to their advantage [Li et al. 2005; Xue and Stauss 2007].

From the discussion above it is clear that both innate and adaptive immune responsiveness need to be taken into consideration in terms of gene transfer protocols. The activation of either arm of the immune system can result in a failure to express the transgene for therapeutically relevant periods of time and can, in extreme circumstances, result in systemic inflammatory states that can have catastrophic outcomes.

1.8.1 Strategies to Limit Innate Immune Responses

One obvious option to limit innate responses to the transfer process is to deliver the transgene via an ex vivo approach. Here, there can be exclusive targeting of the vector to cells isolated ex vivo, and the exposure of the host innate immune system to the vector is negligible. However, adaptive humoral and cell-mediated responses to the transgene product and cell-mediated cytotoxicity to the disassembled vector can still ensue upon reintroduction of the transduced cells.

As indicated above, innate immune responses to adenovectors and, to a lesser extent, lentivectors are both significant. In both instances, keeping the vector dose to the minimum required to achieve a therapeutic response will limit innate responses, as will the transient depletion of reticuloendothelial cells. Efforts to target these vectors away from interacting with cells of the innate immune system have been attempted with strategies such as conjugation with polyethylene glycol and have shown some success in reducing the acute cytokine increments and thrombocytopenia [De et al. 2005]. Overall, and at the current time, the well-studied serotypes of AAV vectors seem to offer the best option in terms of minimizing innate immunity in the context of gene transfer.

1.8.2 Strategies to Limit Immune Responses to the Transgene Vector

Adaptive immune responses to the transgene vector compromise vector delivery through interaction with antivector antibodies in the circulation and limit the persistence of transgene expression through cytotoxic clearance of transduced cells by vector-specific CTLs. Both mechanisms are significant obstacles to achieving long-term gene transfer. Circumventing the memory humoral response to the vector is difficult, and while increasing the vector dose or attempting to reduce antivector antibodies transiently through strategies such as plasma exchange might facilitate vector delivery, this obstacle may always reduce transduction efficiency. Similarly, efforts to abolish or at least minimize the memory CTL response to vector epitopes presented at the transduced cell surface following capsid disassembly have not yet been explored adequately. There is some evidence, with certain vectors, to suggest that these capsid proteins may persist for several weeks following vector administration. In this context, the delivery of a T-cell immunosuppressive regimen for a period of time following vector exposure (i.e., for two to four months) may significantly reduce the loss of transduced cells. This type of approach requires systematic evaluation in clinical trials where memory T-cell responses are anticipated.

1.8.3 Strategies to Limit Immune Responses to the Transgene Product

The final area of concern relating to adaptive immune reactivity involves the potential for humoral and cell-mediated responses to the transgene product. In some instances, the gene transfer recipient may already have been exposed to the transgene product and have preexisting tolerance to this antigen. In these recipients, the likelihood of an adaptive response developing following gene transfer is reduced significantly unless the transfer protocol involves a strategy that could break tolerance (e.g., an approach that is accompanied by inflammation). Thus, in most gene transfer recipients, in contrast to the adaptive responses to vector epitopes, memory cells specific for the transgene product will not be present and the immune response will be primary in nature. With this in mind, there is an opportunity to utilize gene transfer to establish tolerance to the transgene product. With existing knowledge concerning tolerance mechanisms, the goal would appear to be the attainment of peripheral tolerance through the induction of T regulatory cells. To facilitate this outcome, the transgene product must be presented to antigen-specific T cells in the context of a tolerogenic environment, in which the expression of co-stimulatory molecules on APCs is minimized, with the consequence that the likelihood of activating effector T cells is reduced markedly.

One strategy that appears to reduce adaptive responses to the transgene product is to target expression of the transgene away from APCs. Interestingly, while this approach would be expected to minimize $CD8^+$ effector T-cell activation and subsequent cytotoxic responses to the transgene product, the avoidance of APC transgene expression also reduces humoral responses to the transgene protein, even though the protein will be presented on MHC class II molecules after uptake of extracellular material [Follenzi et al., 2004]. Thus, the effect of targeting transgene expression away from APCs on minimizing humoral responses suggests that there may be mechanisms through which proteins synthesized within APCs can somehow be presented on MCH class II molecules and interact with $CD4^+$ effector T cells. Targeting transgene expression away from APCs can be achieved by a variety of approaches, including the following: through the use of a type of vector that transduces APCs inefficiently (e.g., an AAV); through pseudotyping the vector particle to avoid APC transduction; through the use of a tissue-specific transgene promoter that minimizes expression within APCs (this will still occur through "promoter trapping" with integrating vectors); and finally, through the use of a miRNA-based approach in which the $3'$ end of the transgene transcript contains binding sites for miRNAs expressed exclusively in hematopoietic cells [Brown et al. 2006]. The latter, elegant strategy targets transgene mRNA for degradation or blocks translation of the transcript through the binding of the hematopoietic miRNA to their cognate sequences in the mRNA.

Administration of immunosuppressive therapy at the time of transgene delivery may also eliminate the adaptive response to the newly expressed protein. However, the type of immunomodulatory agent, the degree of immunosuppression required, and the duration of treatment are details that require much further study.

In general, additional strategies for attaining tolerance to the transgene product involve expression of the protein in a tolerogenic context with the subsequent expansion of regulatory T-cell populations. There appear to be a number of approaches to achieving this objective. One strategy that has been tested successfully in animal models is to deliver the transgene during fetal or neonatal development, when the effector arm of the immune system is still relatively underdeveloped and at a time when central tolerance mechanisms may still be invoked [Waddington et al. 2004; Xu et al. 2007]. Central tolerance to the transgene product can also be achieved by direct intrathymic delivery of vector [Marodon et al. 2006]. Nevertheless, given the significant differences between the time of maturation of the mouse and human immune systems, it is not easy to see how these approaches could be translated into clinical practice.

Aside from changing the stage of development at which the transgene is delivered, other approaches can be utilized to bias the tolerogenic expression of the transgene. Synthesis and presentation of the transgene product in the presence of co-stimulatory blockade will be successful in some instances [Haegel-Kronenberger et al. 2004; Jiang et al. 2004], although how long the blockade needs to be maintained and how complete the blockade should be remain unanswered questions. Finally, expression of the transgene within specific organs or at specific anatomical locations seems predictive of tolerogenic presentation of the protein to the adaptive immune system. Thus, AAV-mediated gene transfer to the liver has been associated with the generation of $CD4^+CD25^+FoxP3^+$ transgene-specific regulatory T cells [Mingozzi et al. 2003; Cao et al. 2007]. Similarly, delivery of transgenes to cells of the nasal and gut mucosa also predisposes to a tolerogenic response to the transgene product through mechanisms that may involve generation of several regulatory T-cell populations, including TGF-β- and IL-10-producing cells [Cao et al. 2006].

1.9 CONCLUSIONS

In concluding this overview, it should be apparent that the immunological challenges to successful gene transfer are many and varied. In particular, the use of viral vectors for transgene delivery provides a significant provocation to the innate and adaptive immune systems that can result in major safety concerns and eliminate the potential for long-term benefit from the gene transfer process. Nevertheless, substantial progress has been made in the past decade in elucidating details of the immune response to gene transfer, and some advances have been achieved in developing approaches to circumvent or minimize these responses. Perhaps most important, substantial coincident advances have been made in our understanding of certain basic aspects of immunology, such as the evolving details of T-cell tolerance. Just as scientists and physicians in transplantation medicine have learned to manipulate the immune system to achieve cell and solid organ transplants, the gene therapy field is defining strategies to prevent immune-mediated rejection of vectors and therapeutic genes.

There is realistic optimism that gene transfer will provide clinical benefits within the foreseeable future. If these successes are to be achieved, strategies to minimize adverse immune responses to gene transfer protocols must be established. In the remainder of the book, details of our current knowledge are provided, together with future perspectives of this biologically fascinating and clinically important topic.

REFERENCES

Anson DS and Fletcher JM. 2007. Gene therapy for disorders affecting children: progress and potential. *J Paediatr Child Health* 43:323–330.

Arruda VR and Xiao W. 2007. It's all about the clothing: capsid domination in the adeno-associated viral vector world. *J Thromb Haemost* 5:12–15.

Arruda VR, Schuettrumpf J, Herzog RW, et al. 2004. Safety and efficacy of factor IX gene transfer to skeletal muscle in murine and canine hemophilia B models by adeno-associated viral vector serotype 1. *Blood* 103:85–92.

Brown BD and Lillicrap D. 2002. Dangerous liaisons: the role of "danger" signals in the immune response to gene therapy. *Blood* 100:1133–1140.

Brown BD, Venneri MA, Zingale A, Sergi SL, and Naldini L. 2006. Endogenous microRNA regulation suppresses transgene expression in hematopoietic lineages and enables stable gene transfer. *Nat Med* 12:585–591.

Brown BD, Sitia G, Annoni A, et al. 2007. In vivo administration of lentiviral vectors triggers a type I interferon response that restricts hepatocyte gene transfer and promotes vector clearance. *Blood* 109:2797–2805.

Bushman FD. 2007. Retroviral integration and human gene therapy. *J Clin Invest* 117:2083–2086.

Cao O, Armstrong E, Schlachterman A, et al. 2006. Immune deviation by mucosal antigen administration suppresses gene-transfer-induced inhibitor formation to factor IX. *Blood* 108:480–486.

Cao O, Dobrzynski E, Wang L, et al. 2007. Induction and role of regulatory $CD4^{+}CD25^{+}$ T cells in tolerance to the transgene product following hepatic in vivo gene transfer. *Blood* 110:1132–1140.

Cardone M. 2007. Prospects for gene therapy in inherited neurodegenerative diseases. *Curr Opin Neurol* 20:151–158.

Connelly S, Mount J, Mauser A, et al. 1996. Complete short-term correction of canine hemophilia A by in vivo gene therapy. *Blood* 88:3846–3853.

De GB, Snoeys J, Van LS, Lievens J, and Collen D. 2005. Elimination of innate immune responses and liver inflammation by PEGylation of adenoviral vectors and methylprednisolone. *Hum Gene Ther* 16:1439–1451.

Faria AM and Weiner HL. 2006. Oral tolerance: therapeutic implications for autoimmune diseases. *Clin Dev Immunol* 13:143–157.

Follenzi A, Battaglia M, Lombardo A, Annoni A, Roncarolo MG, and Naldini L. 2004. Targeting lentiviral vector expression to hepatocytes limits transgene-specific immune response and establishes long-term expression of human antihemophilic factor IX in mice. *Blood* 103:3700–3709.

Gallucci S, Lolkema M, and Matzinger P. 1999. Natural adjuvants: endogenous activators of dendritic cells. *Nat Med* 5:1249–1255.

Haegel-Kronenberger H, Haanstra K, Ziller-Remy C, et al. 2004. Inhibition of costimulation allows for repeated systemic administration of adenoviral vector in rhesus monkeys. *Gene Ther* 11:241–252.

Herzog RW. 2007. Immune responses to AAV capsid: Are mice not humans after all? *Mol Ther* 15:649–650.

Herzog RW, Mount JD, Arruda VR, High KA, and Lothrop CD Jr. 2001. Muscle-directed gene transfer and transient immune suppression result in sustained partial correction of canine hemophilia B caused by a null mutation. *Mol Ther* 4:192–200.

High KA, Manno CS, Sabatino DE, et al. 2003. Immune responses to AAV and to factor IX in a phase I study of AAV-mediated, liver-directed gene transfer for hemophilia B. *Blood* 102: abstract 532.

Janeway CA Jr. 1992. The immune system evolved to discriminate infectious nonself from noninfectious self. *Immunol Today* 13:11–16.

Jiang H, Couto LB, Patarroyo-White S, et al. 2006. Effects of transient immunosuppression on adenoassociated, virus-mediated, liver-directed gene transfer in rhesus macaques and implications for human gene therapy. *Blood* 108:3321–3328.

Jiang Z, Schiedner G, Van RN, Liu CC, Kochanek S, and Clemens PR. 2004. Sustained muscle expression of dystrophin from a high-capacity adenoviral vector with systemic gene transfer of T cell costimulatory blockade. *Mol Ther* 10:688–696.

Kaplan HJ and Niederkorn JY. 2007 Regional immunity and immune privilege. *Chem Immunol Allergy* 92:11–26.

Kay MA, Glorioso JC, and Naldini L. 2001. Viral vectors for gene therapy: the art of turning infectious agents into vehicles of therapeutics. *Nat Med* 7:33–40.

Li CY, Huang Q, and Kung HF. 2005. Cytokine and immuno-gene therapy for solid tumors. *Cell Mol Immunol* 2:81–91.

Lillicrap D. 2000. Hemophilia treatment. Gene therapy, factor VIII antibodies and immune tolerance: hopes and concerns. *Haematologica* 85:108–111.

Lowenstein PR. 2003. Virology and immunology of gene therapy, or virology and immunology of high MOI infection with defective viruses. *Gene Ther* 10:933–934.

Manno CS, Pierce GF, Arruda VR, et al. 2006. Successful transduction of liver in hemophilia by AAV-factor IX and limitations imposed by the host immune response. *Nat Med* 12:342–347.

Marodon G, Fisson S, Levacher B, Fabre M, Salomon BL, and Klatzmann D. 2006. Induction of antigen-specific tolerance by intrathymic injection of lentiviral vectors. *Blood* 108:2972–2978.

Matzinger P. 1994. Tolerance, danger and the extended family. *Annu Rev Immunol* 12:991–1045.

Miao CH, Ye P, Thompson AR, Rawlings DJ, and Ochs HD. 2006. Immunomodulation of transgene responses following naked DNA transfer of human factor VIII into hemophilia A mice. *Blood* 108:19–27.

Mingozzi F, Liu YL, Dobrzynski E, et al. 2003. Induction of immune tolerance to coagulation factor IX antigen by in vivo hepatic gene transfer. *J Clin Invest* 111:1347–1356.

Mingozzi F, Maus MV, Hui DJ, et al. 2007. $CD8^+$ T-cell responses to adeno-associated virus capsid in humans. *Nat Med* 13:419–422.

Moskalenko M, Chen L, van Roey M, et al. 2000. Epitope mapping of human anti-adeno-associated virus type 2 neutralizing antibodies: implications for gene therapy and virus structure. *J Virol* 74:1761–1766.

Muruve DA. 2004. The innate immune response to adenovirus vectors. *Hum Gene Ther* 15:1157–1166.

Muruve DA, Cotter MJ, Zaiss AK, et al. 2004. Helper-dependent adenovirus vectors elicit intact innate but attenuated adaptive host immune responses in vivo. *J Virol* 78:5966–5972.

Peng Z. 2005. Current status of gendicine in China: recombinant human Ad-p53 agent for treatment of cancers. *Hum Gene Ther* 16:1016–1027.

Pierce GF, Lillicrap D, Pipe SW, and VandenDriessche T. 2007. Gene therapy, bioengineered clotting factors and novel technologies for hemophilia treatment. *J Thromb Haemost* 5:901–906.

Raper SE, Chirmule N, Lee FS, et al. 2003. Fatal systemic inflammatory response syndrome in a ornithine transcarbamylase deficient patient following adenoviral gene transfer. *Mol Genet Metab* 80:148–158.

Rawle FE, Shi CX, Brown B, et al. 2004. Heterogeneity of the immune response to adenovirus-mediated factor VIII gene therapy in different inbred hemophilic mouse strains. *J Gene Med* 6:1358–1368.

Sarukhan A, Camugli S, Gjata B, von Boehmer H, Danos O, and Jooss K. 2001. Successful interference with cellular immune responses to immunogenic proteins encoded by recombinant viral vectors. *J Virol* 75:269–277.

Scallan CD, Jiang H, Liu T, et al. 2006. Human immunoglobulin inhibits liver transduction by AAV vectors at low AAV2 neutralizing titers in SCID mice. *Blood* 107:1810–1817.

Schwaab R, Brackman HH, Meyer C, et al. 1995. Haemophilia A: mutation type determines risk of inhibitor formation. *Thromb Haemost* 74:1402–1406.

Seth RB, Sun L, and Chen ZJ. 2006. Antiviral innate immunity pathways. *Cell Res* 16:141–147.

Thomas CE, Storm TA, Huang Z, and Kay MA. 2004. Rapid uncoating of vector genomes is the key to efficient liver transduction with pseudotyped adeno-associated virus vectors. *J Virol* 78:3110–3122.

van Til NP, Markusic DM, van der Rijt R, et al. 2005. Kupffer cells and not liver sinusoidal endothelial cells prevent lentiviral transduction of hepatocytes. *Mol Ther* 11:26–34.

Verthelyi D. 2006. Adjuvant properties of CpG oligonucleotides in primates. *Methods Mol Med* 127:139–158.

Waddington SN, Nivsarkar MS, Mistry AR, et al. 2004. Permanent phenotypic correction of hemophilia B in immunocompetent mice by prenatal gene therapy. *Blood* 104:2714–2721.

Xu L, Mei M, Haskins ME, et al. 2007. Immune response after neonatal transfer of a human factor IX–expressing retroviral vector in dogs, cats, and mice. *Thromb Res* 120:269–280.

Xue SA and Stauss HJ. 2007. Enhancing immune responses for cancer therapy. *Cell Mol Immunol* 4:173–184.

Zaiss AK and Muruve DA. 2005. Immune responses to adeno-associated virus vectors. *Curr Gene Ther* 5:323–331.

2

INNATE IMMUNE RESPONSES TO NUCLEIC ACIDS

KEN J. ISHII, M.D., PH.D, SHOHEI KOYAMA, M.D., AND SHIZUO AKIRA, M.D., PH.D.

Research Institute for Microbial Diseases, Osaka University, Osaka, Japan

2.1 INTRODUCTION

All living organisms are exposed continuously to foreign entities such as food, microorganisms, and unnecessary self-metabolites. Therefore, there is a need to be able to discriminate dangerous nonself from safe self, particularly in the case of life-threatening microorganisms invading the body. Recent studies have shown that the innate immune system has a greater degree of specificity than previously

Gene Therapy Immunology, Edited by Roland Herzog

thought and that it is highly developed in its ability to discriminate between self and nonself entities, such as microorganisms and unnecessary self-molecules, including not only proteins and lipids but also nucleic acids.

Although nucleic acids such as DNA and RNA are essential components of all living organisms, recent advances in research on innate immunity have revealed that these nucleic acids are no longer exempt from the human immune system. This discrimination relies, to a great extent, on pattern recognition receptors (PRRs), including Toll-like receptors (TLRs) and the recently described RIG-I-like receptors (RLRs), which play crucial roles in early host defenses against invading pathogens [Akira et al. 2006; Ishii and Akira 2006; Medzhitov 2007] (Fig. 2-1).

In this chapter we provide an overview of recent advances in our understanding of innate immune recognition of nucleic acids, especially in light of the discrimination between self and nonself nucleic acids by recently described innate immune sensors, including TLRs and RLRs. This new understanding of innate immune recognition of and regulation by nucleic acids should be translatable into clinical settings and used not only to maximize the innate immune activations by nucleic acids for immunotherapeutic applications against infectious allergic diseases and cancer, but also to minimize undesired immune responses

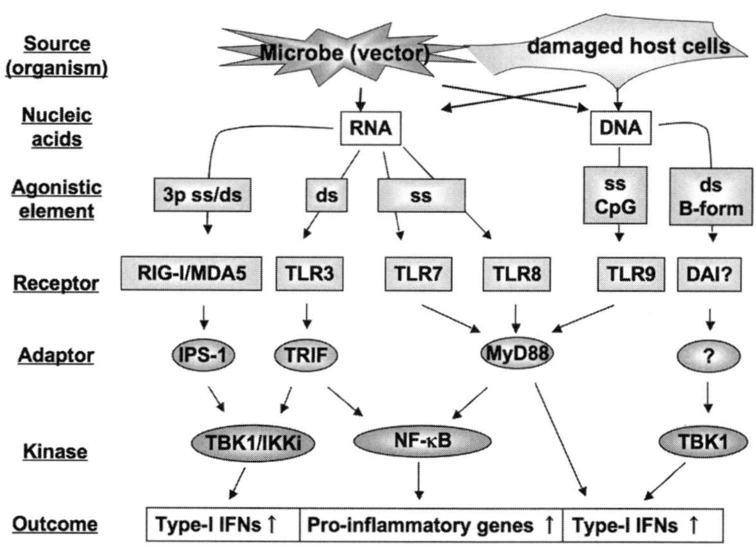

Figure 2-1 Nucleic acids (DNA or RNA) are normally sequestered but can be released from pathogens or damaged host cells. TLR-dependent and TLR-independent recognition of RNA as well as DNA have been described. Currently known innate recognitions are shown, including receptors, adaptors, signal transductions, and transcriptions. An unknown but predicted molecule and pathway are shown as question marks. (Modified from Ishii and Akira 2005b.)

in efficient gene therapies as well as in autoimmune disorders against nucleic acids such as systemic lupus erythematosus (SLE).

2.2 INNATE IMMUNE RECOGNITION OF RNA

RNA is abundant in cells and possesses a variety of functions in biological processes. Host RNA is supposed to be inert to the immune system. However, during invasion of pathogens, unusual RNA structures, such as double-stranded (ds) RNA, are created and recognized by the host immune system. It has long been known that many types of viral infection generate dsRNA during viral replication [Carter and De Clercq 1974]. For example, positive-stranded RNA viruses such as encephalomyocarditis virus (EMCV) generate dsRNA as a by-product of viral replication. Since dsRNA is not normally found in the human body, dsRNA has been considered to be a viral signature that the innate immune system recognizes as a foreign molecule. In fact, dsRNA has been shown to trigger innate immune activation, as evaluated by its strong induction of type I interferons (IFNs). For the last few decades, synthetic dsRNA analogs such as poly(I:C) have been widely used as IFN inducers in many experimental and clinical applications.

2.2.1 PKR

For decades, protein kinase receptor (PKR) [Williams 1999] has been investigated extensively as a potential or sole receptor for dsRNA. However, accumulating evidence suggests that other innate immune sensors, including TLR3 [Alexopoulou et al. 2001], retinoic acid–inducible gene (RIG)-I [Yoneyama et al. 2004], and melanoma differentiation–associated gene (MDA) 5 [Yoneyama et al. 2005], are also engaged in sensing dsRNA. Furthermore, TANK-binding kinase 1 (TBK-1) and IKK-i complexes [Fitzgerald et al. 2003; Sharma et al. 2003] and subsequently, interferon regulatory factor (IRF) 3 or 7 phosphorylation [Honda et al. 2005] are thought to play important roles in both TLR- and RLR-dependent innate immune activation in viral infection as well as poly(I:C) (Fig. 2-1).

In contrast to dsRNA, single-stranded (ss) RNA is abundant not only in pathogens but also in host cells. Therefore, it is essential for the host to be able to detect and discriminate foreign ssRNA from self-ssRNA. It has been shown that ssRNA released from viral particles (envelopes), such as influenza virus and HIV, is engulfed by endosomes in immune cells such as dendritic cells (DCs), while host RNA is not recognized by TLR7 and TLR8 [Diebold et al. 2004; Heil et al. 2004], possibly by discriminating its methylation state and/or other factors, including specific sequences [Crozat and Beutler 2004; Ishii and Akira 2005b; Kariko et al. 2005]. In addition, ssRNA recognition by TLR7 and TLR8 is restricted to certain cell types and/or the intracellular localization of RNA. For example, in addition to TLR7/8-mediated recognition of ssRNA in endosomes, ssRNA generated or introduced into the cytoplasm was found to be recognized by RIG-I via the 5′-triphosphate of the RNA [Hornung et al. 2006; Pichlmair et al. 2006].

Thus, regardless of whether RNA molecules are dsRNA, ssRNA, inside cells, or on cells, they are no longer inert to the human innate immune system, and instead, play important roles in the host defense during infection, and sometimes in the pathogenesis of immunological disorders such as SLE. Avoiding such innate immune recognition of RNA would be beneficial for gene therapies, including RNA interference (RNAi)-based therapies.

2.2.2 TLR3

TLR3 is an unusual member of the TLR family that does not have an apparent transmembrane domain, although it is expressed both on the cell surface and within endosomes. Although the precise structure of TLR3 has recently been resolved [Choe et al. 2005], the true molecular mechanism by which TLR3 interacts with dsRNA remains to be elucidated. The TLR3-N-terminal ectodomain (TLR3-ECD) resembles a horseshoe-shaped solenoid of 23 leucine-rich repeats that are largely covered by carbohydrates. The TLR3-ECD contains a glycan-free face with two patches of positively charged residues. Mutational analyses revealed that this region contains the binding site for negatively charged phosphate-containing dsRNA [Bell et al. 2006]. As a result of this binding, and possibly after some conformational changes and/or homodimerization, TLR3 mediates dsRNA-induced innate immune activation that requires the adaptor protein Toll/IL-1R domain-containing adaptor inducing IFN-β (TRIF) and induces pro-inflammatory cytokine production and type I IFN responses via activation of nuclear factor-kappaB (NF-κB) and IRF3.

TLR3 is highly expressed on myeloid cells, such as monocytes, macrophages, and myeloid DCs. It is also highly inducible in most tissues, and up-regulated by type I IFNs, lipopolysaccharide (LPS), and other cytokines [Alexopoulou et al. 2001]. This may be why a clinical trial for poly(I:C) had to be abandoned due to systemic toxicity [Robinson et al. 1976], despite it being one of the first therapeutic nucleic acid–based agents used to treat HIV and leukemia patients. Several studies have been undertaken to reduce the toxicity of poly(I:C), and there are clinical trials against breast cancer and ovarian cancer [Adams et al. 2003]. To date, there have been few studies investigating the possible involvement of TLR3 in the pathophysiology of human diseases, including anti-HSV-1 immunity in the central nervous system and type I diabetes [Pirie et al. 2005; Zhang et al. 2007].

2.2.3 TLR7 and TLR8

In contrast to dsRNA, ssRNA is an abundant molecule for the host immune system, since a variety of RNA molecules reside and function within cells in almost all tissues of the body. Two closely related TLRs, TLR7 and TLR8, have recently been shown to be innate immune sensors for ssRNA. TLR7 is highly expressed in plasmacytoid DCs (pDCs), B cells, and macrophages, whereas TLR8 is expressed in myeloid DCs and monocytes but not in pDCs. Previous studies have shown that ssRNA genomes, oligonucleotides derived from HIV or influenza virus, some ds short interfering (si) RNAs developed for RNAi, and small synthetic compounds known as imidazoquinolines are recognized by TLR7 in mice and by both TLR7 and TLR8 in humans, leading to activation of various immune cells that elicit type I IFN production and cellular immune responses [Hemmi et al. 2002; Diebold et al. 2004; Heil et al. 2004].

TLR7 and possibly TLR8 utilize myeloid differentiation primary response gene 88 (MyD88) as an essential adaptor for downstream signaling pathways. Due to the ability of TLR7 to stimulate type I IFN production, several TLR7 agonists have been approved for clinical use in various viral infections. The TLR7 agonist imiquimod has been shown to be effective for external genital warts, basal cell carcinoma, and actinic keratosis and is in phase I clinical trials against human papillomavirus [Hoffman et al. 2005]. Several other synthetic TLR7 agonists are in phase I or phase II trials against hepatitis B virus, hepatitis C virus, and cancer.

The physiological importance of TLR7/8-mediated ssRNA recognition has been implicated in host defenses against viral infection as well as autoimmunity. Many viruses with an ssRNA genome have been found to activate TLR7. TLR7 recognizes genomic ssRNA and/or ssRNA generated during replication. Moreover, TLR7-mediated recognition and the subsequent innate immune activations were found to be important for adaptive immune responses to viral infections as well as to host tissues. For example, although both TLR7 and RIG-I detect and respond to influenza A virus (IAV) infection, the TLR7-mediated, but not RIG-I-mediated signaling pathway is required for subsequent protective immunity, which is characterized by B- and T-cell responses to the dominant antigens (HA and NP) [Koyama et al. 2007]. Other studies have shown that TLR7 and TLR8 are activated not only by pathogen-derived ssRNA but also by endogenous ssRNA [Lau et al. 2005], and that TLR7 participates in the recognition of RNA-containing auto antigens [Vollmer et al. 2005; Pisitkun et al. 2006; Subramanian et al. 2006] and production of anti-RNA autoantibodies [Berland et al. 2006; Christensen et al. 2006; Subramanian et al. 2006].

RNAi is a recently discovered biological process in which dsRNA silences endogenous gene expression in a sequence-specific manner [Fire et al. 1998]. Small 21- nucleotide dsRNAs, known as siRNAs, can induce effective RNAi responses in mammalian cells [Elbashir et al. 2001]. A previous study suggested that siRNAs form dsRNAs with no sequence preferences and activate pDCs via TLR7 [Hornung et al. 2005]. In contrast, another study suggested that siRNAs and short hairpin RNAs (shRNAs) induce type I IFN and cytokine production through TLR3 and that these effects are also sequence independent [Kariko et al. 2004]. These results may not be conflicting if different cell types have distinct recognition mechanisms: namely, that pDCs utilize TLR7 to recognize ssRNA or short single-stranded portions of dsRNA while myeloid (conventional) DCs utilize TLR3 to recognize a double-stranded portion of long ssRNA. Thus, it appears that TLR-mediated RNA recognition is mediated by TLR3, TLR7, and TLR8, and that the specificity of their ligands may not be just dsRNA or ssRNA, but further defined by specific cell types or even the intracellular localization of RNA.

2.2.4 RIG-I and MDA5

Recently, three homologous DExD/H box RNA helicases, designated RLRs, were identified as cytoplasmic sensors of viral infection via RNA detection. Two family members, RIG-I (also known as DDX58) and MDA5 (also known as Helicard), share two N-terminal caspase activation and recruitment domains (CARDs) followed by an RNA helicase domain [Yoneyama et al. 2004]. RIG-I, but not MDA5, was found to mount antiviral responses against the positive-strand ssRNA Japanese encephalitis virus, and a set of negative-strand ssRNA viruses, including Newcastle disease virus, vesicular stomatitis virus, Sendai virus, and influenza virus. In contrast, MDA5 senses the presence of the positive-strand ssRNA picornavirus EMCV [Kato et al. 2006]. The protein LGP2 also shares homology with RIG-I in the helicase domain, but lacks a CARD. LGP2 has been suggested to act as a negative regulator of RIG-I/MDA5 signaling.

RNA is abundant in the cytoplasm, and the mechanisms for how RIG-I and MDA5 specifically recognize nonself RNA have remained unsolved issues. Recent studies demonstrated the presence of different features between foreign (nonself) and host (self) RNA recognized by RIG-I [Hornung et al. 2006; Pichlmair et al. 2006]. Specifically, type I IFN production was triggered by RIG-I through its recognition of a 5′-triphosphate moiety of viral ssRNA or ssRNA synthesized in vitro, but RIG-I did not recognize 5′-capping or base modification of this 5′-triphosphate on host RNA.

Self-RNAs undergo several processing steps to remove or mask their 5′-triphosphate group. Briefly, messenger (m) RNA is modified by the addition of a 7-methyl guanosine cap structure at its 5′ end, transfer (t) RNA is cleaved at the 5′ end and decorated with a series of nucleotide base modifications, and ribosomal (r) RNAs associate with ribosomal proteins [Kariko and Weissman 2007]. It is likely that additional features of the viral 5′-triphosphate on ssRNA are also important for RNA recognition by RIG-I, since some host RNAs present in the cytosol do contain 5′-triphosphate ends (e.g., 7SL RNA, an abundant cytoplasmic RNA that functions in protein secretion as a component of the signal recognition particle), but are not recognized by RIG-I [Bowie and Fitzgerald 2007].

Recently, a protein harboring an N-terminal CARD resembling those in MDA5 and RIG-I was cloned as a critical signaling adaptor for RIG-I/MDA5, and designated IFN-β-promoter stimulator 1 (IPS1; also known as MAVS, VISA, or CARDIF) [Kawai et al. 2005; Meylan et al. 2005; Seth et al. 2005; Xu et al. 2005]. When expressed in cells, this protein has the ability to induce activation of the type I IFN promoter as well as NF-κB. Genetic and RNAi-based gene silencing studies have demonstrated that IPS-1 plays an essential role in RIG-I/MDA5 signaling. Interestingly, this protein is present in the outer mitochondrial membrane, suggesting that mitochondria may be important for IFN responses in addition to their roles in metabolism and cell death. Downstream of RIG-I-IPS-1, noncanonical IKKs, including TBK1 (TRAF-family-member-associated NF-κB activator-binding kinase 1) and IKKi, are activated and phosphorylate IRF3 and IRF7, indicating that the signaling pathways triggered by TLR stimulation and RIG-I converge at the level of TBK1/IKKi.

2.2.5 Other RNA Receptors

A third helicase gene, Lgp2, which is homologous to RIG-I and MDA5 but lacks a CARD, was reported to function as a negative regulator of RIG-I and MDA5 activities [Yoneyama et al. 2005]. On the other hand, a recent study showed that LGP2 was not the primary negative regulator of type I IFN production and that LGP2-deficient mice exhibited resistance to vesicular stomatitis virus, which induces type I IFN responses via a RIG-I-dependent pathway [Venkataraman et al. 2007]. However, these mice exhibited a defect in type I IFN production in response to EMCV, which activates MDA5-dependent innate immune responses [Venkataraman et al. 2007].

Production of the inflammatory cytokines interleukin (IL)-1β and IL-18 through activation of caspase-1 is also an antiviral immune response. Poly(I:C), viral dsRNA, and Sendai virus all activate caspase-1 through the nucleotide oligomerization domainlike receptor protein Nalp3 (also known as cryopyrin) [Kanneganti et al. 2006]. Nalp3 belongs to a family of cytosolic nucleotide-binding and oligomerization domain-like receptors (NLRs), which mediate caspase-1 activation in response to a wide variety of bacterial ligands, imidazoquinolines, and dsRNA, as well as the endogenous danger signal uric acid, and are linked genetically to human autoinflammatory disorders [Kanneganti et al. 2007].

2.3 INNATE IMMUNE RECOGNITION OF DNA

Compared to RNA, DNA is much longer and more stable, and its intracellular location is more restricted to the cell nucleus and mitochondria in eukaryotes. Normally, DNA is tightly packed within the cell and sequestered from the host immune system. However, in cases of microbial infection or failure of host DNA clearance, DNA can be released from pathogens or damaged host cells and become exposed to the host innate immune system. Accumulating evidence suggests that the human innate immune system can recognize and respond to such DNA [Ishii and Akira 2005a, 2006; Nagata 2005; Wagner and Bauer 2006] (Fig. 2-1).

DNA rich in unmethylated CpG dinucleotides (CpG motifs), such as microbial DNA, activates TLR9 to mount immune responses. In fact, TLR9 is the only well-known receptor [Hemmi et al. 2000; Krieg 2002; Wagner 2004] for DNA detection. TLR9 activation by CpG oligodeoxynucleotides (ODNs) has been demonstrated by many groups and is now under clinical trials for many therapeutic applications, including vaccine adjuvants against infectious diseases, allergic disorders, and cancer [Klinman 2004; Krieg 2006]. TLR9, together with TLR7, has been implicated in the pathogenesis of some autoimmune diseases [Marshak-Rothstein and Rifkin 2007], although there are controversial results among research groups and experimental models [Christensen et al. 2006; Lartigue et al. 2006; Wu and Peng 2006].

Recently, the issue of what TLR9 recognizes has been revisited. Although CpG ODNs are quite potent agonists for TLR9, ODNs that do not contain CpG motifs stimulate macrophages and DCs in a TLR9-dependent manner [Roberts et al. 2005]. Moreover, the heme-polymer hemozoin, which is generated from red blood cell hemoglobin during malaria infection, was found to activate the innate immune system via TLR9 [Coban et al. 2005, 2007], although another group claimed that crude hemozoin had a synergistic effect with malarial DNA for TLR9 activation [Parroche et al. 2007].

Moreover, dsDNA derived not only from microbes but also from host cells activates the innate immune system in a sequence-independent manner when introduced into the cytosol [Suzuki et al. 1999; Ishii et al. 2001] or when its homeostatic clearance is hampered [Kawane et al. 2003]. The activation is not mediated by TLR9. Instead, it occurs via undefined DNA recognition machinery that activates both immune and nonimmune cells to produce type I IFNs, cytokines, and chemokines as well as up-regulating co-stimulatory molecules [Okabe et al. 2005; Yasuda et al. 2005; Cortez-Gonzalez et al. 2006; Ishii et al. 2006; Martin and Elkon 2006; Shirota et al. 2006; Stetson and Medzhitov 2006]. One candidate cytosolic dsDNA sensor that has recently emerged is the IFN-inducible protein DLM-1 (also known as Z-DNA-binding protein 1), which has now been renamed DNA-dependent activator of IFN-regulatory factors (DAI) [Takaoka et al. 2007], although confirmation of its effects awaits data from DAI-knockout mice.

2.3.1 TLR9 and CpG DNA

Unmethylated CpG dinucleotides are prevalent in bacterial and viral DNA but not in mammalian DNA. The innate immune system detects and responds to such DNA-containing CpG motifs via TLR9. CpG DNA bound to immune cells is taken up by the endocytic pathway and co-accumulates with TLR9 in phagosomelike vesicles. PI3 kinase controls this process [Ishii et al. 2002; Kuo et al. 2006]. Upon ligation with CpG DNA, TLR9 recruits the adaptor protein MyD88 to its cytoplasmic TIR domain, which culminates in the activation of NF-κB and mitogen-activated protein (MAP) kinase, thereby leading to pro-inflammatory cytokine production as well as IRF7-dependent type I IFN responses [Kawai and Akira 2006]. This CpG DNA-mediated activation of the innate immune system also induces B-cell proliferation, DC maturation, and natural killer cell activation, followed by strong Th1-type adaptive immune responses. Hence, a large number of clinical trials are under way for CpG DNA as an adjuvant, antiallergy, and anticancer agent [Krieg 2002; Klinman 2004].

There are at least three distinct classes of immune stimulatory CpG ODNs: D-type (also known as A-class), K-type (also known as B-class), and C-class ODNs. D/A-type CpG ODNs induce high IFN-α production by pDCs but are weak stimulators of TLR9-dependent NF-κB signaling and B-cell activation. In contrast, K/B-type CpG ODNs strongly activate B cells, but stimulate pDCs to secrete only low levels of IFN-α. C-class CpG ODNs show a combination of the characteristics of D/A and K/B ODNs, and stimulate strong IFN-α production and B-cell activation. D/A-type CpG ODNs owe their activities to phosphodiester palindromic CpG motifs, while a poly-G tail at their 3′ ends is important for self-assembly into higher-order tertiary structures through G-tetrad formation [Gursel et al. 2002; Kerkmann et al. 2005]. K/B-type ODNs owe their activities to a phosphorothioate backbone and possibly maintain a linear ss form. The immune stimulatory effects of all three ODN classes require TLR9 [Hemmi et al. 2003].

2.3.2 TLR9 and Self-DNA

TLR9 was originally believed to recognize bacterial or viral DNA uniquely, but it is now appreciated that TLR9 can recognize a variety of other DNA molecules, including mammalian DNA [Barton et al. 2006; Ishii and Akira 2006; Wagner and Bauer 2006]. Although the immunostimulatory activities of non-CpG DNA derived from mammalian DNA or those derived during synthesis are weaker than those induced by synthetic phosphorothioate CpG ODNs, they can be augmented to the equivalent immunostimulatory activity by wrapping in a transfection reagent such as DOTAP [Roberts et al. 2005; Yasuda et al. 2005], anti-DNA antibodies [Vallin et al. 1999; Leadbetter et al. 2002; Means et al. 2005] or certain carrier proteins, such as high-mobility group box1 (HMGB1) [Ivanov et al. 2007; Tian et al. 2007]. These results suggest that to discriminate self from nonself, TLR9 may have developed the ability to detect not only unmethylated CpG motifs distinctive for pathogens but also abnormal compositions, structures, or chemical features of any type of DNA.

Conceivably, self DNA-containing immune complexes can activate pDCs and B cells and contribute to immune dysregulation in disorders such as SLE. In particular, a recent report demonstrated that HMGB1-D/A-type CpG ODN complexes activated pDCs and augmented IFN-α production through a TLR9–Myd88 pathway involving the multivalent receptor for advanced glycation end products (RAGE) and found further that HMGB1 was a key factor in immune complex–triggered activation of autoreactive B cells and the induction of type 1 IFN genes after stimulation with self-DNA containing immune complexes dependent on RAGE engagement [Tian et al. 2007]. It will be of interest to create HMGB1-mediated DNA carrier proteins to improve immunotherapies further using DNA, intervene in DNA-mediated immune disorders, or improve the efficiency of gene therapy by reducing unnecessary immune responses to DNA.

2.3.3 TLR9 and Suppressive DNA

The inflammation after infection or tissue injury must be controlled and ended smoothly by a negative feedback system through competitive and/or inhibitory signals, so that the outcome of the innate immune response is not deleterious for the host. Recent evidence suggests that host DNA contains some antagonistic elements against immunostimulatory effects of DNA or pathogen-derived CpG-rich DNA that possibly suppress DNA-driven immunostimulation [Ishii et al. 2004; Klinman 2004]. Neutralizing or suppressive motifs can selectively block CpG-mediated immune stimulation [Krieg et al. 1998; Lenert et al. 2001; Yamada et al. 2004]. Suppressive motifs are rich in poly-G or GC sequences, and the optimal motifs are surprisingly identical to telomere sequences (with a repeat of TTAGGG) that are present in mammalian DNA but not in bacterial DNA [Gursel et al. 2003]. Suppressive ODNs blocked either TLR9 binding or assembly of CpG DNA or the signaling cascade initiated by CpG DNA [Lenert et al. 2001; Yamada et al. 2002; Shirota et al. 2005]. This effect of suppressive ODNs was confirmed in lung and articular inflammation induced by CpG ODNs [Zeuner et al. 2002; Yamada et al. 2004].

2.3.4 TLR9-Independent Recognition of DNA

Besides TLR9, both pathogens and host genomic DNA appear to be detected by unknown receptors. Transfection of thyroid cells with mammalian or bacterial dsDNA, but not ssDNA, and exposure of cells to necrotic cell–derived genomic DNA trigger the activation of macrophages and DCs, leading to up-regulation of co-stimulatory markers and activation of IFN-inducible genes [Suzuki et al. 1999; Ishii et al. 2001]. Curiously, during analyses of DNase II–knockout mice, which lack the ability to digest DNA from dead cells in the phagosome, a large amount of IFN-β was produced [Yoshida et al. 2005]. In DNase II–deficient mice lacking TLR9- or MyD88-mediated signaling, IFN-β production by macrophages and survival were not altered in each double-knockout mouse, suggesting that there is another DNA recognition machinery in the innate immune system [Okabe et al. 2005]. Further direct evidence of TLR-independent DNA recognition and its innate immune signaling pathway in both stromal and immune cells is the large amount of IFN-β production and activation of other IFN-inducible genes induced by transfection with genomic DNA isolated from bacteria, viruses, or mammals [Yasuda et al. 2005; Cortez-Gonzalez et al. 2006; Ishii et al. 2006; Martin and Elkon 2006; Shirota et al. 2006]. Interestingly, these IFN-inducible activities of DNA were attributed to dsDNA with a right-handed helical B-form rather than the unusual left-handed helical Z-form or ssDNA, which activated mouse and human stromal cells and DCs and induced their production of type I IFNs and chemokines [Ishii et al. 2006]. Furthermore, the activation of human embryonic kidney cells (HEK-293) to produce type I IFNs by B-DNA was as strong as that induced by poly(I:C), a well-known IFN-inducing dsRNA.

DNA-activated type I IFN induction was mediated via activation of TBK1, noncanonical IκB-kinase and IRF3, which are shared with TLR-independent

RNA-mediated type I IFN induction [Ishii et al. 2006; Stetson and Medzhitov 2006]. IPS-1, an essential adaptor molecule for RIG-I and MDA5-mediated RNA-activated type I IFN induction, appeared to play a critical role in DNA-activated type I IFN induction in human cells [Ishii et al. 2006; Opitz et al. 2006; Cheng et al. 2007], but was not essential for DNA-activated type I IFN induction in mouse cells [Kumar et al. 2006; Sun et al. 2006]. DNA-transfected cells exhibited strong resistance against RNA (vesicular stomatitis virus) and DNA (modified vaccinia Ankara virus) viral infections, suggesting that this effect may be involved in antiviral responses under physiological conditions [Ishii et al. 2006]. A similar phenomenon was indicated in macrophages infected with the intracellular bacteria *Listeria monocytogenes* and *Legionella pneumophila* [Stetson and Medzhitov 2006].

Recently, DAI (also known as ZBP-1 or DLM-1, and previously known as Z-DNA-binding protein) has emerged as a candidate for a cytosolic DNA sensor [Takaoka et al. 2007]. Binding of DAI to dsDNA increases its ability to interact with TBK-1 and IRF3, while DAI overexpression enhances the response to DNA and endogenous DAI knockdown decreases the response by half [Takaoka et al. 2007]. Confirmation of these findings in vivo using DAI-knockout mice will be of interest.

2.4 CONCLUSIONS

Taken together, accumulating evidence, only part of which has been presented above, clearly suggests that DNA and RNA as essential parts of gene therapies are no longer inert in the immune system. Elucidating the molecular and cellular mechanisms underlying these immune recognition machineries is essential and will be of interest not only to immunologists but also to microbiologists who want to know the virulence factors for avoiding such effects, and of course, researchers who are developing novel methods and/or technologies to enhance the efficiency of gene therapies.

REFERENCES

Adams M, Navabi H, Jasani B, et al. 2003. Dendritic cell (DC) based therapy for cervical cancer: use of DC pulsed with tumour lysate and matured with a novel synthetic clinically non-toxic double stranded RNA analogue poly [I]:poly [C12U] (Ampligen®). *Vaccine* 21:787–790.

Akira S, Uematsu S, and Takeuchi O. 2006. Pathogen recognition and innate immunity. *Cell* 124:783–801.

Alexopoulou L, Holt AC, Medzhitov R, and Flavell RA. 2001. Recognition of double-stranded RNA and activation of NF-kappaB by Toll-like receptor 3. *Nature* 413:732–738.

Barton GM, Kagan JC, and Medzhitov R. 2006. Intracellular localization of Toll-like receptor 9 prevents recognition of self DNA but facilitates access to viral DNA. *Nat Immunol* 7:49–56.

Bell JK, Botos I, Hall PR, et al. 2006. The molecular structure of the TLR3 extracellular domain. *J Endotoxin Res* 12:375–378.

Berland R, Fernandez L, Kari E, et al. 2006. Toll-like receptor 7–dependent loss of B cell tolerance in pathogenic autoantibody knockin mice. *Immunity* 25:429–440.

Bowie AG and Fitzgerald KA. 2007. RIG-I: tri-ing to discriminate between self and non-self RNA. *Trends Immunol* 28:147–150.

Carter WA and De Clercq E. 1974. Viral infection and host defense. *Science* 186:1172–1178.

Cheng G, Zhong J, Chung J, and Chisari FV. 2007. Double-stranded DNA and double-stranded RNA induce a common antiviral signaling pathway in human cells. *Proc Natl Acad Sci U S A* 104:9035–9040.

Choe J, Kelker MS, and Wilson IA. 2005. Crystal structure of human Toll-like receptor 3 TLR3 ectodomain. *Science* 309:581–585.

Christensen SR, Shupe J, Nickerson K, Kashgarian M, Flavell RA, and Shlomchik MJ. 2006. Toll-like receptor 7 and TLR9 dictate autoantibody specificity and have opposing inflammatory and regulatory roles in a murine model of lupus. *Immunity* 25:417–428.

Coban C, Ishii KJ, Kawai T, et al. 2005. Toll-like receptor 9 mediates innate immune activation by the malaria pigment hemozoin. *J Exp Med* 201:19–25.

Coban C, Ishii KJ, Horii T, and Akira S. 2007. Manipulation of host innate immune responses by the malaria parasite. *Trends Microbiol* 15:271–278.

Cortez-Gonzalez X, Pellicciotta I, Gerloni M, et al. 2006. TLR9-independent activation of B lymphocytes by bacterial DNA. *DNA Cell Biol* 25:253–261.

Crozat K and Beutler B. 2004. TLR7: a new sensor of viral infection. *Proc Natl Acad Sci U S A* 101:6835–6836.

Diebold SS, Kaisho T, Hemmi H, Akira S, and Reis e Sousa C. 2004. Innate antiviral responses by means of TLR7-mediated recognition of single-stranded RNA. *Science* 303:1529–1531.

Elbashir SM, Lendeckel W, and Tuschl T. 2001. RNA interference is mediated by 21- and 22-nucleotide RNAs. *Genes Dev* 15:188–200.

Fire A, Xu S, Montgomery MK, Kostas SA, Driver SE, and Mello CC. 1998. Potent and specific genetic interference by double-stranded RNA in *Caenorhabditis elegans*. *Nature* 391:806–811.

Fitzgerald KA, McWhirter SM, Faia KL, et al. 2003. IKKepsilon and TBK1 are essential components of the IRF3 signaling pathway. *Nat Immunol* 4:491–496.

Gursel I, Gursel M, Yamada H, Ishii KJ, Takeshita F, and Klinman DM. 2003. Repetitive elements in mammalian telomeres suppress bacterial DNA-induced immune activation. *J Immunol* 171:1393–1400.

Gursel M, Verthelyi D, and Klinman DM. 2002. CpG oligodeoxynucleotides induce human monocytes to mature into functional dendritic cells. *Eur J Immunol* 32:2617–2622.

Heil F, Hemmi H, Hochrein H, et al. 2004. Species-specific recognition of single-stranded RNA via Toll-like receptor 7 and 8. *Science* 303:1526–1529.

Hemmi H, Takeuchi O, Kawai T, et al. 2000. A Toll-like receptor recognizes bacterial DNA. *Nature* 408:740–745.

Hemmi H, Kaisho T, Takeuchi O, et al. 2002. Small anti-viral compounds activate immune cells via the TLR7 MyD88–dependent signaling pathway. *Nat Immunol* 3:196–200.

Hemmi H, Kaisho T, Takeda K, and Akira S. 2003. The roles of Toll-like receptor 9, MyD88, and DNA-dependent protein kinase catalytic subunit in the effects of two distinct CpG DNAs on dendritic cell subsets. *J Immunol* 170:3059–3064.

Hoffman ES, Smith RE, and Renaud RC Jr. 2005. From the analyst's couch: TLR-targeted therapeutics. *Nat Rev Drug Discov* 4:879–880.

Honda K, Yanai H, Negishi H, et al. 2005. IRF-7 is the master regulator of type-I interferon-dependent immune responses. *Nature* 434:772–777.

Hornung V, Guenthner-Biller M, Bourquin C, et al. 2005. Sequence-specific potent induction of IFN-alpha by short interfering RNA in plasmacytoid dendritic cells through TLR7. *Nat Med* 11:263–270.

Hornung V, Ellegast J, Kim S, et al. 2006. 5′-Triphosphate RNA is the ligand for RIG-I. *Science* 314:994–997.

Ishii KJ and Akira S. 2005a. Innate immune recognition of nucleic acids: beyond Toll-like receptors. *Int J Cancer* 117:517–523.

Ishii KJ and Akira S. 2005b. TLR ignores methylated RNA? *Immunity* 23:111–113.

Ishii KJ and Akira S. 2006. Innate immune recognition of, and regulation by, DNA. *Trends Immunol* 27:525–532.

Ishii KJ, Suzuki K, Coban C, et al. 2001 Genomic DNA released by dying cells induces the maturation of APCs. *J Immunol* 167:2602–2607.

Ishii KJ, Takeshita F, Gursel I, et al. 2002. Potential role of phosphatidylinositol 3 kinase, rather than DNA-dependent protein kinase, in CpG DNA-induced immune activation *J Exp Med* 196:269–274.

Ishii KJ, Gursel I, Gursel M, and Klinman DM. 2004. Immunotherapeutic utility of stimulatory and suppressive oligodeoxynucleotides. *Curr Opin Mol Ther* 6:166–174.

Ishii KJ, Coban C, Kato H, et al. 2006. A Toll-like receptor-independent antiviral response induced by double-stranded B-form DNA. *Nat Immunol* 7:40–48.

Ivanov S, Dragoi AM, Wang X, et al. 2007. A novel role for HMGB1 in TLR9-mediated inflammatory responses to CpG-DNA. *Blood* 110:1970–1981.

Kanneganti TD, Body-Malapel M, Amer A, et al. 2006. Critical role for Cryopyrin/Nalp3 in activation of caspase-1 in response to viral infection and double-stranded RNA. *J Biol Chem* 281:36560–36568.

Kanneganti TD, Lamkanfi M, and Nunez G. 2007. Intracellular NOD-like receptors in host defense and disease. *Immunity* 27:549–559.

Kariko K and Weissman D. 2007. Naturally occurring nucleoside modifications suppress the immunostimulatory activity of RNA: implication for therapeutic RNA development. *Curr Opin Drug Discov Dev* 10:523–532.

Kariko K, Bhuyan P, Capodici J, and Weissman D. 2004. Small interfering RNAs mediate sequence-independent gene suppression and induce immune activation by signaling through Toll-like receptor 3. *J Immunol* 172:6545–6549.

Kariko K, Buckstein M, Ni H, and Weissman D. 2005. Suppression of RNA recognition by Toll-like receptors: the impact of nucleoside modification and the evolutionary origin of RNA. *Immunity* 23:111–113.

Kato H, Takeuchi O, Sato S, et al. 2006. Differential roles of MDA5 and RIG-I helicases in the recognition of RNA viruses. *Nature* 441:101–105.

Kawai T and Akira S. 2006. TLR signaling. *Cell Death Differ* 13:816–825.

Kawai T, Takahashi K, Sato S, et al. 2005. IPS-1, an adaptor triggering RIG-I- and MDA5-mediated type I interferon induction. *Nat Immunol* 6:981–988.

Kawane K, Fukuyama H, Yoshida H, et al. 2003 Impaired thymic development in mouse embryos deficient in apoptotic DNA degradation. *Nat Immunol* 4:138–144.

Kerkmann M, Costa LT, Richter C, et al. 2005. Spontaneous formation of nucleic acid–based nanoparticles is responsible for high interferon-alpha induction by CpG-A in plasmacytoid dendritic cells. *J Biol Chem* 280:8086–8093.

Klinman DM. 2004. Immunotherapeutic uses of CpG oligodeoxynucleotides. *Nat Rev Immunol* 4:249–258.

Koyama S, Ishii KJ, Kumar H, et al. 2007. Differential role of TLR- and RLR-signaling in the immune responses to influenza A virus infection and vaccination. *J Immunol* 179:4711–4720.

Krieg AM. 2002. CpG motifs in bacterial DNA and their immune effects. *Annu Rev Immunol* 20:709–760.

Krieg AM. 2006. Therapeutic potential of Toll-like receptor 9 activation. *Nat Rev Drug Discov* 5:471–484.

Krieg AM, Wu T, Weeratna R, et al. 1998. Sequence motifs in adenoviral DNA block immune activation by stimulatory CpG motifs. *Proc Natl Acad Sci U S A* 95:12631–12636.

Kumar H, Kawai T, Kato H, et al. 2006. Essential role of IPS-1 in innate immune responses against RNA viruses. *J Exp Med* 203:1795–1803.

Kuo CC, Lin WT, Liang CM, and Liang SM. 2006. Class I and III phosphatidylinositol 3′-kinase play distinct roles in TLR signaling pathway. *J Immunol* 176:5943–5949.

Lartigue A, Courville P, Auquit I, et al. 2006. Role of TLR9 in anti-nucleosome and anti-DNA antibody production in lpr mutation-induced murine lupus. *J Immunol* 177:1349–1354.

Lau CM, Broughton C, Tabor AS, et al. 2005. RNA-associated autoantigens activate B cells by combined B cell antigen receptor/Toll-like receptor 7 engagement. *J Exp Med* 202:1171–1177.

Leadbetter EA, Rifkin IR, Hohlbaum AM, Beaudette BC, Shlomchik MJ, and Marshak-Rothstein A. 2002. Chromatin–IgG complexes activate B cells by dual engagement of IgM and Toll-like receptors. *Nature* 416:603–607.

Lenert P, Stunz L, Yi AK, Krieg AM, and Ashman RF. 2001. CpG stimulation of primary mouse B cells is blocked by inhibitory oligodeoxyribonucleotides at a site proximal to NF-kappaB activation. *Antisense Nucleic Acid Drug Dev* 11:247–256.

Marshak-Rothstein A and Rifkin IR. 2007. Immunologically active autoantigens: the role of Toll-like receptors in the development of chronic inflammatory disease. *Annu Rev Immunol* 25:419–441.

Martin DA and Elkon KB. 2006. Intracellular mammalian DNA stimulates myeloid dendritic cells to produce type I interferons predominantly through a Toll-like receptor 9-independent pathway. *Arthritis Rheum* 54:951–962.

Means TK, Latz E, Hayashi F, Murali MR, Golenbock DT, and Luster AD. 2005. Human lupus autoantibody–DNA complexes activate DCs through cooperation of CD32 and TLR9. *J Clin Invest* 115:407–417.

Medzhitov R. 2007. Recognition of microorganisms and activation of the immune response. *Nature* 449:819–826.

Meylan E, Curran J, Hofmann K, et al. 2005. Cardif is an adaptor protein in the RIG-I antiviral pathway and is targeted by hepatitis C virus. *Nature* 437:1167–1172.

Nagata S. 2005. DNA degradation in development and programmed cell death. *Annu Rev Immunol* 23:853–875.

Okabe Y, Kawane K, Akira S, Taniguchi T, and Nagata S. 2005. Toll-like receptor-independent gene induction program activated by mammalian DNA escaped from apoptotic DNA degradation. *J Exp Med* 202:1333–1339.

Opitz B, Vinzing M, van Laak V, et al. 2006. Legionella pneumophila induces IFNbeta in lung epithelial cells via IPS-1 and IRF3, which also control bacterial replication. *J Biol Chem* 281:36173–36179.

Parroche P, Lauw FN, Goutagny N, et al. 2007. Malaria hemozoin is immunologically inert but radically enhances innate responses by presenting malaria DNA to Toll-like receptor 9. *Proc Natl Acad Sci U S A* 104:1919–1924.

Pichlmair A, Schulz O, Tan CP, et al. 2006. RIG-I-mediated antiviral responses to single-stranded RNA bearing 5′-phosphates. *Science* 314:997–1001.

Pirie FJ, Pegoraro R, Motala AA, et al. 2005. Toll-like receptor 3 gene polymorphisms in South African blacks with type 1 diabetes. *Tissue Antigens* 66:125–130.

Pisitkun P, Deane JA, Difilippantonio MJ, Tarasenko T, Satterthwaite AB, and Bolland S. 2006. Autoreactive B cell responses to RNA-related antigens due to TLR7 gene duplication. *Science* 312 1669–1672.

Roberts TL, Sweet MJ, Hume DA, and Stacey KJ. 2005. Cutting edge: species-specific TLR9-mediated recognition of CpG and non-CpG phosphorothioate-modified oligonucleotides. *J Immunol* 174:605–608.

Robinson RA, DeVita VT, Levy HB, Baron S, Hubbard SP, and Levine AS. 1976. A phase I–II trial of multiple-dose polyriboinosic–polyribocytidylic acid in patients with leukemia or solid tumors. *J Natl Cancer Inst* 57:599–602.

Seth RB, Sun L, Ea CK, and Chen ZJ 2005. Identification and characterization of MAVS, a mitochondrial antiviral signaling protein that activates NF-kappaB and IRF 3. *Cell* 122:669–682.

Sharma S, tenOever BR, Grandvaux N, Zhou GP, Lin R, and Hiscott J. 2003. Triggering the interferon antiviral response through an IKK-related pathway. *Science* 300:1148–1151.

Shirota H, Gursel I, Gursel M, and Klinman DM. 2005. Suppressive oligodeoxynucleotides protect mice from lethal endotoxic shock. *J Immunol* 174:4579–4583.

Shirota H, Ishii KJ, Takakuwa H, and Klinman DM. 2006. Contribution of interferon-beta to the immune activation induced by double-stranded DNA. *Immunology* 118:302–310.

Stetson DB and Medzhitov R. 2006. Recognition of cytosolic DNA activates an IRF3-dependent innate immune response. *Immunity* 24:93–103.

Subramanian S, Tus K, Li QZ, et al. 2006. A Tlr7 translocation accelerates systemic autoimmunity in murine lupus. *Proc Natl Acad Sci U S A* 103:9970–9975.

Sun Q, Sun L, Liu HH, et al. 2006. The specific and essential role of MAVS in antiviral innate immune responses. *Immunity* 24:633–642.

Suzuki K, Mori A, Ishii KJ, et al. 1999. Activation of target-tissue immune-recognition molecules by double-stranded polynucleotides. *Proc Natl Acad Sci U S A* 96:2285–2290.

Takaoka A, Wang Z, Choi MK, et al. 2007. DAI DLM-1/ZBP1 is a cytosolic DNA sensor and an activator of innate immune response. *Nature* 448:501–505.

Tian J, Avalos AM, Mao SY, et al. 2007. Toll-like receptor 9-dependent activation by DNA-containing immune complexes is mediated by HMGB1 and RAGE. *Nat Immunol* 8:487–496.

Vallin H, Blomberg S, Alm GV, Cederblad B, and Ronnblom L. 1999. Patients with systemic lupus erythematosus SLE have a circulating inducer of interferon-alpha IFN-alpha production acting on leucocytes resembling immature dendritic cells. *Clin Exp Immunol* 115:196–202.

Venkataraman T, Valdes M, Elsby R, et al. 2007. Loss of DExD/H box RNA helicase LGP2 manifests disparate antiviral responses. *J Immunol* 178:6444–6455.

Vollmer J, Tluk S, Schmitz C, et al. 2005. Immune stimulation mediated by autoantigen binding sites within small nuclear RNAs involves Toll-like receptors 7 and 8. *J Exp Med* 202:1575–1585.

Wagner H. 2004. The immunobiology of the TLR9 subfamily. *Trends Immunol* 25:381–386.

Wagner H and Bauer S. 2006. All is not Toll: new pathways in DNA recognition. *J Exp Med* 203:265–268.

Williams BR. 1999. PKR; a sentinel kinase for cellular stress. *Oncogene* 18:6112–6120.

Wu X and Peng SL. 2006. Toll-like receptor 9 signaling protects against murine lupus. *Arthritis Rheum* 54:336–342.

Xu LG, Wang YY, Han KJ, Li LY, Zhai Z, and Shu HB. 2005. VISA is an adapter protein required for virus-triggered IFN-beta signaling. *Mol Cell* 19:727–740.

Yamada H, Gursel I, Takeshita F, et al. 2002. Effect of suppressive DNA on CpG-induced immune activation. *J Immunol* 169:5590–5594.

Yamada H, Ishii KJ, and Klinman DM. 2004. Suppressive oligodeoxynucleotides inhibit CpG-induced inflammation of the mouse lung. *Crit Care Med* 32:2045–2049.

Yasuda K, Yu P, Kirschning CJ, et al. 2005. Endosomal translocation of vertebrate DNA activates dendritic cells via TLR9-dependent and -independent pathways. *J Immunol* 174:6129–6136.

Yoneyama M, Kikuchi M, Natsukawa T, et al. 2004. The RNA helicase RIG-I has an essential function in double-stranded RNA-induced innate antiviral responses. *Nat Immunol* 5:730–737.

Yoneyama M, Kikuchi M, Matsumoto K, et al. 2005. Shared and unique functions of the DExD/H-box helicases RIG-I, MDA5, and LGP2 in antiviral innate immunity. *J Immunol* 175:2851–2858.

Yoshida H, Okabe Y, Kawane K, Fukuyama H, and Nagata S. 2005. Lethal anemia caused by interferon-beta produced in mouse embryos carrying undigested DNA. *Nat Immunol* 6:49–56.

Zeuner RA, Ishii KJ, Lizak MJ, et al. 2002. Reduction of CpG-induced arthritis by suppressive oligodeoxynucleotides. *Arthritis Rheum* 46:2219–2224.

Zhang SY, Jouanguy E, Ugolini S, et al. 2007. TLR3 deficiency in patients with herpes simplex encephalitis. *Science* 317:1522–1527.

3

THE ANTIVIRAL INNATE IMMUNE RESPONSE

MARK E. SEAMONE, B.S., AND DANIEL A. MURUVE, M.D.
Department of Medicine, University of Calgary, Calgary, Alberta, Canada

3.1 INTRODUCTION

In the past 15 years, the field of gene therapy has generated new hope for the treatment of various disorders. Viruses have evolved to gain entry into cells and use host machinery to facilitate their replication. This natural and efficient process of genomic delivery has resulted in the development of viral vectors for gene therapy. As viruses have evolved to infect their hosts, the host itself has also

Gene Therapy Immunology, Edited by Roland Herzog

evolved to defend against these microbes. Similar to wild-type viral infection, viral vectors that are utilized in gene therapy induce host innate and adaptive immune responses, one of the major obstacles in applying these novel therapies in humans. In addition, many of the genes that viruses use to down-regulate the immune response are not present in viral vectors. Therefore, the immune response to viral vectors may, in some instances, be greater than that of a wild-type infection. As gene therapy represents a potentially groundbreaking method for disease treatment, an understanding of the immune system's antiviral response is essential.

The innate immune system is the first line of defense during a viral infection. In gene therapy, the antiviral innate response remains one of the major barriers to successful in vivo gene transfer. Recognition of viruses is facilitated by pattern recognition receptors within the host. These receptors include Toll-like receptors (TLRs) and RNA helicases that trigger the activation of signaling pathways that function to generate an antiviral state. In particular, type I interferons, which include IFN-α and IFN-β, are primary mediators of the innate response to viruses. In this chapter we review the mechanisms utilized by the innate immune system to recognize and respond to viral infection. It is beyond our scope in this chapter to review in depth this rapidly emerging field. We refer the reader to a number of excellent reviews in this area [Grandvaux et al. 2002; Kawai and Akira 2006; Chelbi-Alix and Wietzerbin 2007; Paun and Pitha 2007]. Ultimately, continued research in the field of innate immunity will result in new strategies that will make gene therapy safer and more effective for human disease.

3.2 TOLL-LIKE RECEPTORS

Toll-like receptors (TLRs) represent a valuable line of defense in the innate response to viral infection. Like other pattern recognition receptors (PRRs), TLRs recognize pathogen-associated molecular patterns (PAMPs). With respect to viral infection, TLR3, TLR7/8 (TLR7 exists in the mouse and TLR8 in humans), and TLR9 function to recognize patterns associated with the viral genome. In turn, these receptors facilitate the induction of an antiviral state through the transcription of type I interferons and pro-inflammatory cytokines [Kawai and Akira 2006].

TLR7/8 and TLR9 are found within plasmacytoid dendritic cells (pDCs). These cells resemble dendritic cells with plasmacytoid morphology. They function to produce copious amounts of type I interferons (especially IFN-α) and thus are also referred to as interferon-producing cells [Colonna et al. 2004; Liu 2005]. In comparison to other TLRs, TLR7/8 and TLR9 are located within endosomal compartments rather than on the cell surface. The administration of lysosomal inhibitors such as chloroquine reduces the responsiveness of these receptors when stimulated by the appropriate ligand. Thus, viral nucleic acids delivered to the cell during endocytosis are recognized in endosomal compartments and mediate signal transduction [Lund et al. 2003, 2004; Diebold et al. 2004].

TLR7 recognizes single-stranded RNA and ribonucleic acid homologs. These compounds include imiquimod, resiquimod (R-848), and loxribine. In addition, TLR7 is known to respond to synthetic single-stranded RNA rich in guanine and uradine [Diebold et al. 2004]. Thus, TLR7 is important in combating ssRNA viruses such as the influenza virus and HIV [Hemmi et al. 2002; Diebold et al. 2004; Heil et al. 2004; Lund et al. 2004]. Mice deficient in TLR7 exhibit a marked decrease in the production of IFN-α in response to infection with influenza virus. Similar results are noted upon infection with vesicular stomatitis virus (VSV) [Diebold et al. 2004; Lund et al. 2004].

TLR9 recognizes CpG DNA motifs that can be observed within genomes of DNA viruses. These molecules include unmethylated 2′-deoxyribocytosine–phosphate–guanosine (CpG). Activation of TLR9 by CpG DNA induces a strong type I interferon response from pDCs [Hemmi et al. 2000]. TLR9-knockout mice demonstrate diminished IFN-α production in response to infection with DNA viruses, such as mouse cytomegalovirus, HSV-1, and HSV-2 [Lund et al. 2003; Krug et al. 2004a,b]. In addition, there is a notable difference between the TLR9 recognition system in humans and mice. In human subjects, TLR9 is located exclusively within pDCs, whereas mice also demonstrate expression in conventional dendritic cells (cDCs). Furthermore, experimental data have revealed differences in responsiveness to TLR9 agonists. Human pDCs secrete IFN-α and do not secrete interleukin-12 in response to TLR9 agonists. However, murine pDCs commonly produce both IFN-α and interleukin-12 following TLR9 activation [Kawai and Akira 2006].

During viral replication within host cells, dsRNA is generated. This ligand functions to activate TLR3. Localization of TLR3 varies according to cell type. In cDCs, TLR3 is localized in vesicular compartments. It is believed that TLR_3 in cDCs is found in endosomes since inhibition of endosomal acidification abrogates the response to a synthetic analog of dsRNA, polyinosine–polycytosine [poly(I:C)] that mimics viral infection and induces the production of type I interferons [Alexopoulou et al. 2001; Matsumoto et al. 2003]. Fibroblasts, in contrast, express TLR3 on the cell surface. Despite a clear link between TLR3 and the type I interferon system, the role of TLR3 during viral infection remains unclear. For example, West Nile virus induces a TLR3-dependent inflammatory response that causes a disturbance of the blood–brain barrier leading to dramatic encephalitis. Thus, TLR3-deficient mice demonstrate great resistance to this ssRNA virus [Wang et al. 2004]. In contrast, TLR3-deficient mice are far more susceptible to MCMV as a result of decreased type I interferon levels produced upon infection [Tabeta et al. 2004]. Further studies are required to clarify the exact function of TLR3 in the antiviral immune response.

3.3 TLR SIGNALING–MYD88-DEPENDENT PATHWAYS

The recognition of PAMPs by TLRs is facilitated via extracellular N-terminal regions, which contain leucine-rich repeats. It is the cytosolic Toll-interleukin-1 receptor (TIR) homology domain that is responsible for the induction of intracellular signaling pathways [Akira et al. 2001]. The recognition of PAMPs facilitates the recruitment of a number of TIR-adaptors, including MyD88, TRIF, TIRAP/Mal, and TRAM. All TLRs use MyD88 except for TLR3, which signals in a MyD88-independent fashion via TRIF, as discussed below [Takeda and Akira 2005]. In the classical model of TLR signaling (Fig. 3-1), the recruitment of MyD88 to the TIR domain of TLRs results in the formation of a complex with members from the IL-1 receptor-associated kinase (IRAK) family, including IRAK-1 and IRAK-4 [Akira et al. 2001; Takeda and Akira 2005]. Phosphorylated IRAK-1 interacts with TRAF-6, which in turn activates the TAK-1/TAB1/TAB2 complex via K63-linked ubiquitin E3 ligase activity [Deng et al. 2000; Wang et al. 2001]. TAK-1/TAB1/TAB2 complex mediates signaling via the canonical IκB kinase (IKK) complex, which consists of IKKα, IKKβ, and NEMO (IKKγ). As a result, IκBα is phosphorylated and degraded allowing NF-κB to translocate to the nucleus [Ishitani et al. 2003; Jin et al. 2004]. Another protein, ECSIT (evolutionary conserved signaling intermediate in Toll pathways), has also been described that can bridge TRAF6 to the IKK complex [Kopp et al. 1999]. TAK-1 also phosphorylates two members of the MAP kinase family, MKK3 and MKK6. MKK3/6 function to phosphorylate c-Jun N-terminal kinase (JNK) and p38 MAP kinase, which activate AFT2/c-Jun transcription factors (AP-1) [Sato et al. 2005]. Activation of NF-κB and MAP kinase signaling pathways downstream of TLRs results in the transcription of genes that are essential in the inflammatory response to viral infection. These genes are also important in activation of the adaptive response. Among the genes transcribed as a result of activation of this pathway, IL-6, IL-1β, TNF-α, and IL-12p40 are of the greatest significance [Kawai et al. 1999, 2001; Kaisho et al. 2001].

3.4 TLR7/8, TLR9–MYD88-DEPENDENT PATHWAYS

Although activation of NF-κB and MAP kinases is an essential component of the innate response to viral infection, TLR7/8 and TLR9 function to elicit the transcription of type I interferons in a MyD88-dependent fashion that differs from signaling downstream of most other TLRs (Fig. 3-2). Upon stimulation via the appropriate ligand within the endosome of pDCs, MyD88 generates a molecular complex with the interferon regulatory factor IRF-7 [Honda et al. 2004; Kawai et al. 2004]. IRF-7 is phosphorylated by IRAK-1 and then translocates to the nucleus to mediate the transcription of IFN-α genes [Uematsu et al. 2005]. In this regard, and unlike signaling to NF-κB, IRAK-1 appears to be an essential component in the MyD88 pathway that results in IRF-7 activation. IRAK-1-deficient mice are incapable of activating IRF-7 (but are capable of activating NF-κB, which is dependent primarily on intact IRAK-4) [Honda et al. 2004; Uematsu et al. 2005]. The activation of IRF-7 is also dependent on TRAF6 E3 ubiquitin ligase activity [Kawai et al. 2004]. In addition to IRF-7, MyD88 can also associate

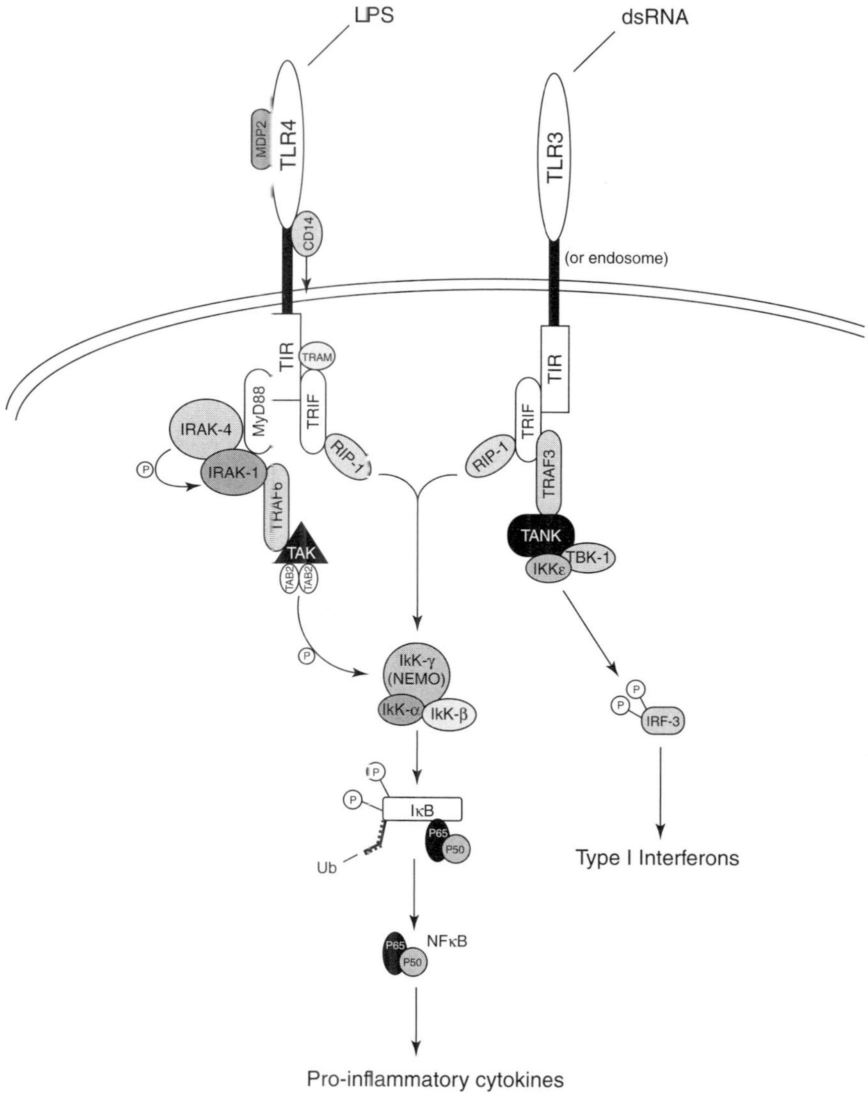

Figure 3-1 Overview of classical MyD88-dependent and MyD88-independent signaling.

with IRF-5 downstream of TLR7/8 and TLR9. Phosphorylated IRF-5 translocates to the nucleus, binds to interferon response elements, and drives the transcription of pro-inflammatory cytokines [Takaoka et al. 2005]. It has been suggested that in humans, IRF-5 selectively participates in the induction of type I interferon rather than pro-inflammatory cytokines. However, the functional differences between human and mouse IRF-5 requires further clarification [Takaoka et al. 2005].

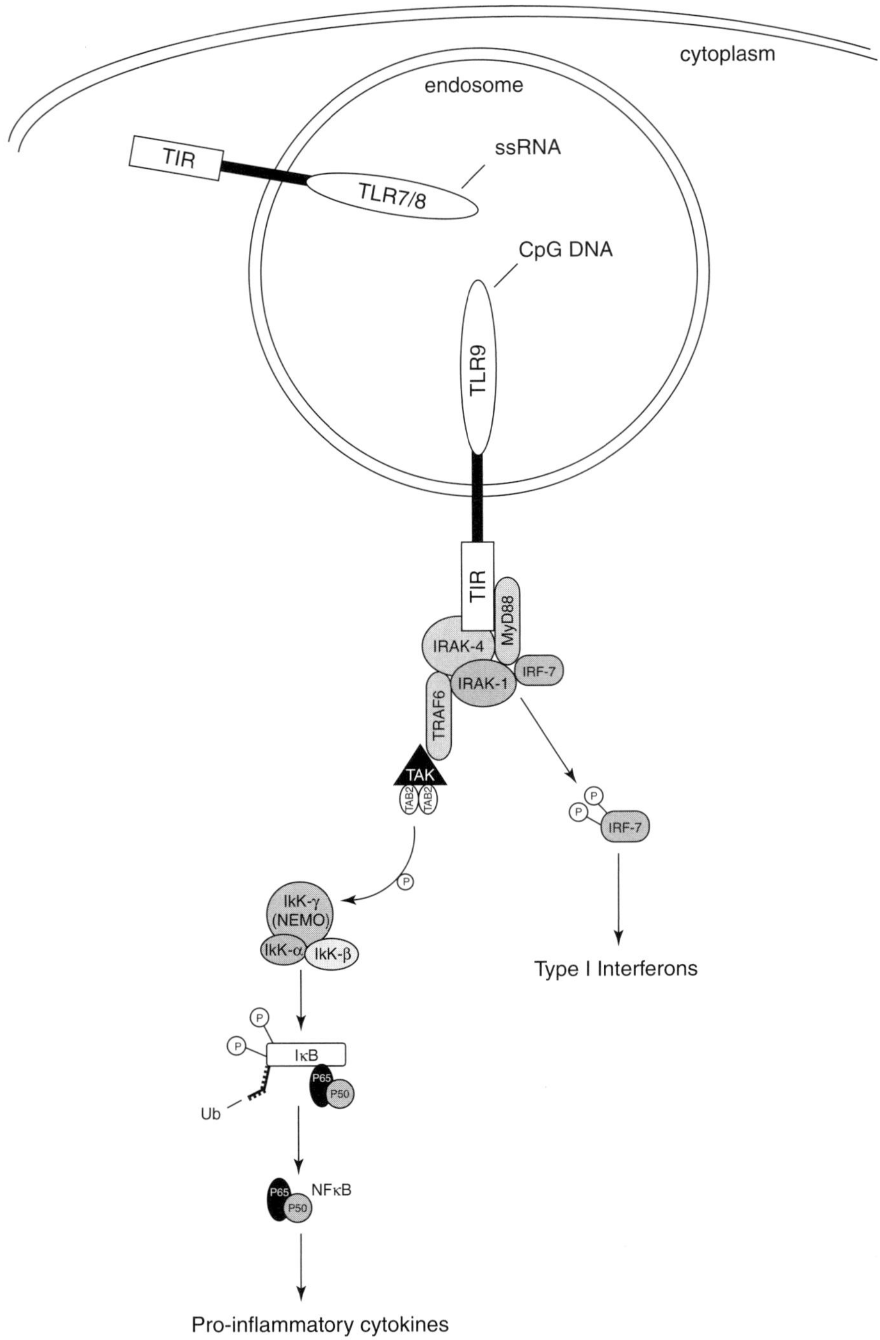

Figure 3-2 MyD88-dependent signaling downstream of TLR7/8 and TLR9.

3.5 TLR3, TLR4–MYD88-INDEPENDENT PATHWAYS

MyD88-independent signaling pathways downstream of TLRs was suggested by the observation of ongoing IRF-3 and delayed NF-κB activation following TLR3 and TLR4 stimulation in MyD88-deficient cells [Takaoka et al. 2005]. In a yeast two-hybrid screen, the adaptor TRIF (TIR-containing adaptor inducing IFN-β) was found to be essential in this pathway [Yamamoto et al. 2002]. Signaling through TLR3 via TRIF causes the activation of IRF-3 that results in the transcription of IFN-3 (Fig. 3-1). Activation of IRF-3 is facilitated via two noncanonical IKKs, TBK-1 and IKKε (IKKi) [Fitzgerald et al. 2003; Sharma et al. 2003]. Thus, ligand association with TLR3 stimulates an interaction between TRIF and TBK-1/IKKe, thereby inducing the phosphorylation of IRF-3. This induction is facilitated via the adaptor protein TANK, which forms a complex with TRAF3 that recruits TBK-1 to the signalosome [Hacker et al. 2006; Oganesyan et al. 2006; Guo and Cheng 2007]. Phosphorylated IRF-3 translocates to the nucleus to transcriptionally activate the IFN-β gene, and also IFN-α4 [Fitzgerald et al. 2003; Sato et al. 2003; Sharma et al. 2003; Perry et al. 2004; McWhirter et al. 2004]. TBK-1/IKKε also play a role in IRF-7 activation and are redundant kinases since a deficiency in both kinases is required to abrogate IRF-3/7 activity and type I interferon production [Takaoka and Taniguchi 2003; Hemmi et al. 2004].

TRIF also plays a role in NF-κB activation downstream of TLR3 and TLR4. Receptor-interacting protein-1 (RIP1) binds to TRIF at the C-terminal RHIM (RIP homotypic interaction motif) domain. Cells deficient in RIP1 show a marked reduction in TRIF-dependent NF-κB activation but maintain normal IRF-3 activity. [Meylan et al. 2004]. TRIF can also interact with TRAF6. This interaction is facilitated via an N-terminal TRAF6 binding motif and contributes to NF-κB activation probably via TAK-1 [Gohda et al. 2004; Ishii et al. 2006].

Taken together, the TLRs play a significant role in the antiviral innate immune response. The activation of TLRs in response to virus-derived PAMPs results in the activation of complex and redundant signaling pathways that result in the expression of NF-κB-dependent genes and type I interferons that are essential in viral eradication.

3.6 ANTIVIRAL RNA HELICASES

It is becoming clear that cells have alternative mechanisms that function in the recognition of and response to viruses. Studies show that TLR3 is dispensable in the host response to viral infection. For example, cDCs and fibroblasts from TLR3-deficient mice exhibit unhindered production of IFN-β upon infection with Sendai virus, vesicular stomatitis virus (VSV), and Newcastle disease virus. Furthermore, the transcription of IFN-β remains prominent in TLR3-deficient mice challenged with poly(I:C) [Hemmi et al. 2003, 2004; Lopez et al. 2004; Yoneyama et al. 2004] and in MyD88-deficient pDCs infected with respiratory syncitial virus [Hornung et al. 2004]. Together, these observations highlight alternative systems present within the host cell that recognize and respond to viral infection [Yoneyama et al. 2004].

Retinonic acid–inducible gene I (RIG-I) participates in viral recognition within the cytosol (Fig. 3-3). RIG-I is a DExD/H helicase and a cytoplasmic receptor for viral double-stranded RNA. This molecule possesses a C-teminal helicase domain and two N-terminal caspase activation and recruitment domains (CARD). The helicase domain of RIG-I is probably responsible for binding dsRNA in an ATP-dependent fashion, although the exact mechanism of this interaction and

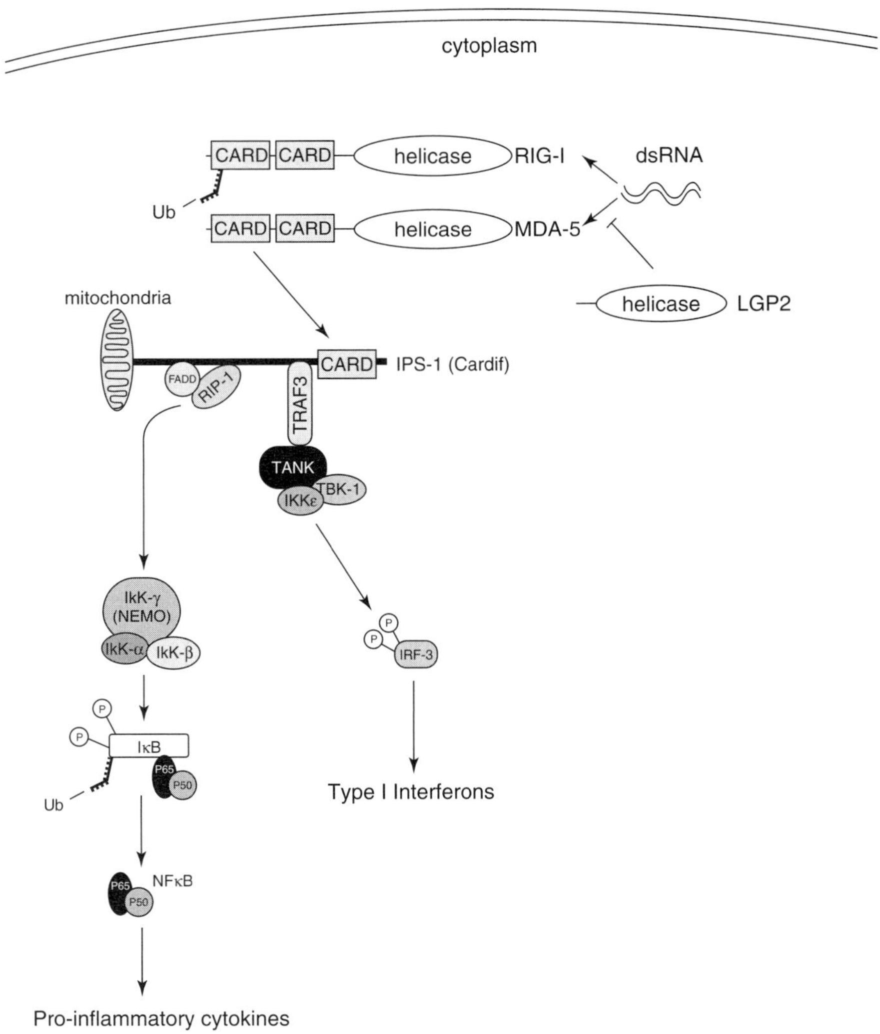

Figure 3-3 Antiviral RNA helicases and signaling.

role of the helicase activity remain unknown. The dsRNA-dependent activation of RIG-I results in the activation of IRF-3 and NF-κB transcription factors [Yoneyama et al. 2004]. Thus, RIG-I-dependent signaling plays an important role in the host response to viral infection since RIG-I deficiency results in impaired type I interferon and pro-inflammatory cytokine production following infection with Newcastle disease virus, Sendai virus, or VSV [Yoneyama et al. 2004; Kato et al. 2005].

Melanoma differentiation-associated gene-5 (MDA5) is a second cytosolic DExD/H helicase with a similar domain structure to RIG-I [Kang et al. 2002; Kovacsovics et al. 2002; Yoneyama et al. 2005; Childs et al. 2007]. MDA5 functions in a manner similar to RIG-I and increases the host response to viruses such as VSV and encephalomyocarditis virus through IRF-3 and NF-κB-dependent gene expression [Yoneyama et al. 2005; Kato et al. 2006]. Finally, Lgp2 is an RNA helicase, which differs from RIG-1 and MDA5 in that it does not contain N-terminal CARD domains. Preliminary studies show that Lgp2 is a negative regulator of MDA5- and RIG-I-dependent signaling [Yoneyama et al. 2005; Childs et al. 2007].

The signaling pathway downstream of the antiviral RNA helicases involves the IKK complex (IKKα/β/γ) and IKKε/TBK-1, which drive the phosphorylation of IκBα and IRF-3/7, respectively (Fig. 3-3). The adaptor linking the RNA helicase to the IKKs was recently identified as a mitochondrial localized protein named IPS-1 (Cardif/MAVS/VISA). IPS-1 consists of a C-terminal effector domain in combination with an N-terminal CARD domain, which mediates a homotypic interaction with RIG-I and MDA5. IPS-1 is essential for mediating IRF-3 and NF-κB activation downstream of the RNA helicases via IKKε/TBK-1 and FADD/RIP1, respectively [Kawai et al. 2005; [Meylan et al. 2005]. Modulation of signaling via RNA helicases is aided by the adaptor protein TANK and TRAF3, similar to the associations observed downstream of TLR3/TRIF [Guo and Cheng 2007].

3.7 TLR-RNA HELICASE-INDEPENDENT ANTIVIRAL RESPONSE

Although many of the signaling pathways that are elicited upon the recognition of viral PAMPs have been characterized, others are still emerging. Recently, a signaling pathway triggered by the intracellular administration of double-stranded B-form DNA has been identified This pathway is distinct from both TLR and RNA helicase-dependent signaling. Activation of this pathway elicits a type I interferon and pro-inflammatory cytokine response via IRF-3 and NF-κB [Ishii et al. 2006]. The receptors and other components of this pathway have yet to be fully identified but represent a novel host defense mechanism that will probably play a significant role during viral infection [Stetson and Medzhitov 2006]. Recently, a novel DNA-binding protein, DAI (DNA-dependent activator of interferon-regulatory factors), has been proposed as the putative receptor [Takaoka et al. 2007].

3.8 TYPE I INTERFERONS: REGULATION OF TRANSCRIPTION

Interferons are named as a result of their ability to interfere with viral replication within the cell [Vilcek 2006]. Interferons are divided into three categories: types I, II, and III. Type I interferons are composed primarily of IFN-α and β, but other members exist, including IFN-ω, κ, and ε [Pestka et al. 2004]. In humans, the IFN-α gene family consists of approximately 13 isoforms, whereas the IFN-β gene is singular. All type I interferon genes are located on chromosome 9 in humans and chromosome 4 in mice. Type I interferons transmit signals though a receptor complex consisting of the two subunits IFNAR-1 and IFNAR-2 [Weissmann and Weber 1986]. Human type II interferon consists of a single IFN-γ gene that is located on chromosome 12. These signal through a different receptor than type I interferons, consisting of IFNGR-1 and IFNGR-2 subunits [Chelbi-Alix and Wietzerbin 2007]. Finally, the type III interferon family includes three homologous proteins, IFN-$\lambda 1-3$. The genes for type III IFNs are located on chromosome 9 in humans [Kotenko et al. 2003] and exhibit some antiviral activity but bind to a distinct membrane receptor complex consisting of IFNLR-1 and IFNLR-2 subunits [Chelbi-Alix and Wietzerbin 2007]. Type I IFN production is transcriptionally regulated. The promoter region of type I interferon genes contains regulatory cis elements, which are known as positive regulatory domains (PRDs). The IFN-β promoter region consists of PRD I–IV. In contrast, the IFN-α promoter consists of PDR I–III-like elements (PDR-LEs) [Ryals et al. 1985; Honda et al. 2006]. With respect to their different numerations, PRD I and III associate with the IRFs, whereas PRD II binds NF-κB, and PRD-IV associate with AP-1 transcription factors. PRD I can also function as a negative regulator of IFN-β via its association with the repressor PDRI-BF1 (Blimp-1 in mice) [Gyory et al. 2004].

Upon the recognition of viral infection by the mechanisms discussed previously (TLRs and RNA helicases), the PRDs create what is known as an *enhanceosome*. The enhanceosome is generated by the recruitment of the IRF family of transcription factors (IRF-3/7), along with NF-κB, AP-1, and finally, the high-mobility-group protein HMG-I(Y) [Honda et al. 2006]. HMG I(Y) functions as an architectural protein that stabilizes the proteins of the enhanceosome and induces conformational changes in DNA. Knockout experiments have shown this protein to be essential in type I interferon transcription [Kim and Maniatis 1997]. Formation of the enhanceosome is essential to mediate type I interferon transcription via the recruitment of histone acetyl transferases (HATs) [Panne et al. 2007]. Of these, it is the general-control-of-amino-acid synthesis 5 or GCN5 and CREB-binding protein (CBP) which are of greatest importance. HATs acetylate lysine residues on histones 3 and 4, which force the nucleosome away from the transcription start site. This displacement allows for the recruitment of a final transcription complex, TFIDD, which initiates the expression of the IFN-β gene [Agalioti et al. 2000; Munshi et al. 2001; Panne et al. 2007].

3.9 THE IRF FAMILY OF TRANSCRIPTION FACTORS

The IRF family of transcription factors consists of nine members [Mamane] et al. 1999. A distinctive characteristic of this family is that they have highly conserved, well-defined N-terminal DNA-binding domains. These regions consist of five tryptophan repeats DNA-binding domains form a helix–turn–helix, which recognizes DNA of similar sequences [Taniguchi et al. 2001]. Analysis of the crystal structure of the DNA-binding domain of IRF-1, which was bound to the PRD I enhancer region of the IFN-β promoter, demonstrated that 5′–GAAA–3′ was the recognition sequence of the helix–turn–helix motif [Escalante et al. 1998].

Although the IRF family consists of nine members, only IRF-1, 3, 5, and 7 are responsible for the positive regulation of type I interferons. It was IRF-1 that was first noted to activate type I interferon gene promoters in overexpression studies [Miyamoto et al. 1988]. However, IRF-1-deficient fibroblasts demonstrate normal type I interferon responses [Matsuyama et al. 1993]. IRF-5 is dispensable for type I interferon production during viral infection, functioning mainly in the expression of pro-inflammatory cytokines such as TNF-α and IL-12 [Takaoka et al. 2005]. As a result of these findings, it can be determined that IRF-3 and IRF-7 are the master regulators of type I interferon expression.

IRF-3 and IRF-7 are homologous in structure. IRF-3 is constitutively expressed and is retained in the cytosol. Upon viral recognition by the host cell, IRF-3 is phosphorylated by TBK-1 and/or IKKε, followed by dimerization and nuclear translocation [Lin et al. 1998; Sato et al. 1998b; Yoneyama et al. 1998]. IRF-3 contains several phosphorylation sites in its C-terminal region, such as serines 385/386, also known as the 2S site. This site is found within the Ser–Ser–Leu motif (SSL motif) of IRF-3's protein structure. Deletion of this site results in the abrogation of IRF-3 phosphorylation and dimerization [Takahasi et al. 2003].

The phosphorylation of the 2S site of IRF-3 allows it to interact with a second IRF-3 molecule or IRF-7 [Takahasi et al. 2003]. It is proposed that IRF-3 N- and C-terminal regions interact to form a hydrophobic structure rendering IRF-3 inactive. The opening of this structure following serine phosphorylation allows for subsequent dimerization [Qin et al. 2003]. IRF-3 homodimers and IRF-3/7 heterodimers then translocate to the nucleus and complex with CBP/p300 to initiate the transcription of type I interferon genes [Lin et al. 1998; Sato et al. 1998b; Yoneyama et al. 1998].

IRF-7 is the essential factor in the transcription of type I interferons, as IRF-3 alone cannot induce optimal interferon gene expression. IRF-7-deficient mice are incapable of producing a type I interferon response, whereas IRF-3 is dispensable in response to CpG DNA, VSV, and HSV-1 infection [Honda et al. 2005]. In this regard, pDCs are central to the host antiviral innate response since they express high levels of IRF-7 and produce copious amounts of IFN-α upon TLR stimulation [Dai et al. 2004]. However, as discussed previously, in TLR signaling,

IRF-7 is not constitutively expressed but is an interferon-inducible gene [Marie et al. 1998; Sato et al. 1998a]. Interferon up-regulates IRF-7, which is then phosphorylated and activated to further increase the expression of type I interferons in a positive feedback loop. Since IRF-3 alone is only capable of activating primarily the transcription of IFN-β, the up-regulation and activation of IRF-7 are essential to drive the expression of all type I interferon genes, including IFN-β and IFN-α [Marie et al. 1998; Sato et al. 1998a]. Interestingly, IRF-7 and IRF-3 have an extremely short half-life, due to rapid ubiquitination and proteosomal degradation. This process is believed to be essential in protecting the host from the potentially harmful effects of excessive type I interferon expression.

3.10 TYPE I INTERFERON: SIGNAL TRANSDUCTION

All of the type I interferon subtypes interact with the same receptor complex, known as the IFN-α/β receptor, consisting of two subunits, IFNAR-1 and IFNAR-2 [Uze et al. 1990; Darnell et al. 1994; Novick et al. 1994; Stark et al. 1998]. The intracellular domains of these two subunits associate with the Janus protein tyrosine kinases (Jak PTKs) Tyk2 and Jak1, respectively. The binding of type I interferons to IFNAR results in the activation of Jak PTKs, which then phosphorylate members of the signal transducers and activators of transcription (STAT) family, including Stat1 and Stat2 [Darnell et al. 1994; Schindler and Darnell 1995; Ihle et al. 1997; Stark et al. 1998]. Phosphorylated Stat1/2 form a complex with IRF-9 known as the interferon-stimulated gene factor 3 (ISGF3), which translocates to the nucleus to bind to the *cis*-acting ISRE motifs present upstream of interferon-inducible genes [Decker et al. 1991; Haque and Williams 1994; Bluyssen et al. 1996].

Jak–Stat signaling, induced by type I interferons, is negatively regulated by two groups of protein families. These families include the suppressor of cytokine signaling (SOCS) and protein inhibitors of activated Stats (PIAS). SOCS1 binds directly to the activation loop of Jak1, thereby acting to inhibit interferon-dependent signaling. In addition, SOCS1 binds directly to the type I interferon receptor IFNAR, thus enduring a suppressive effect on type I interferon signaling [Qing et al. 2005; Fenner et al. 2006]. PIAS1, a member of the PIAS family of proteins, binds to Stat1, therefore preventing the activation of interferon-inducible genes. However, the effect is selective, as PIAS1 inhibits DNA binding in genes that exhibit low affinity for Stat1 complexes [O'Shea and Watford 2004].

3.11 GENERATION OF THE ANTIVIRAL STATE

Activation of the Jak–Stat pathway downstream of the interferon receptor induces the expression of genes (interferon-inducible or interferon-stimulated genes) that establish antiviral activity within the cell (Table 3-1). Some of these antiviral

TABLE 3-1 Summary of Type I Interferon–Induced Antiviral Mechanisms

Interferon-Stimulated Gene	Function	References
Protein kinase R (PKR)	Inhibition of mRNA translation and thus viral replication	de Haro et al. [1996]
2′,5′-Oligoadenylate synthetase/RNase L	Nonspecific degradation of cellular RNA, including viral RNA	Hovanessian et al. [1977], Clarke et al. [2001]
Mx proteins	Disrupts viral nucleocapsid transport and/or blocks viral RNA synthesis; action is dependent on cellular localization of Mx proteins	Haller et al. [1998]
Adenosine deaminase acting on RNA 1 (ADAR1)	Deamination of adenosine to yield inosine leading to the alteration of viral RNA	Bass et al. [1997]
ISG20	3′- to 5′-Endonuclease specific for single-stranded RNA	Espert et al. [2003]
ISG56	Inhibits mRNA translation through binding to p48 (IRF-9)	Guo et al. [2000]
Promyelocytic leukemia protein (PML)	Affects replication of RNA viruses by interfering with viral mRNA and protein synthesis	Regad and Chelbi-Alix [2001]
Apolipoprotein B editing enzyme catalytic subunit 3 (APOBEC3)	Deaminates cytosine to uracil in minus-strand retroviral DNA	Harding et al. [2002], Mangeat et al. [2003], Chiu et al. [2005]

target genes have broad effects. One of the best known antiviral genes is protein kinase R (PKR). PKR is expressed constitutively at a low level and is potently induced by type I interferons. The major enzymatic activity of PKR is located in the C-terminal kinase domain, which is activated via the N-terminal binding to dsRNA [Hurst et al. 1987; de Haro et al. 1996]. The antiviral activity of PKR is facilitated by its ability to inhibit protein synthesis via the phosphorylation and inactivation of the protein synthesis initiation factor eIF2α. Thus, the action of PKR is translational arrest and, in turn, inhibition of viral replication [Hurst et al. 1987; de Haro et al. 1996].

Another example of interferon-induced antiviral genes is the 2′,5′-oligoadenylate synthetase (OAS)/RNase L system [Hovanessian et al. 1977; Clarke et al. 2001]. These are interferon-inducible enzymes which work together in response to viral infection. In this antiviral system, the 2′,5′-OAS proteins are sensors of viral infection, functioning to control the effector, RNase L. 2′,5′-OAS consists of three isoforms, all of which are activated upon the binding of viruses or dsRNA, allowing the conversion of ATP to 2′,5′-oligo(A). Oligomers activate RNase L, which functions in the nonspecific degradation of viral RNA [Hovanessian et al. 1977; Clarke et al. 2001].

Other interferon-inducible genes can function in a virus-specific manner. An excellent example of this is the recent discovery of apolipoprotein B editing enzyme catalytic subunit 3 (APOBEC3) cytosine deaminases. Based on the finding that HIV deficient in virion infectivity factor (VIF) displays limited cellular infectivity, subtractive hybridization was used to determine that the nonpermissive phenotype expressed the cellular factor APOBEC3 [Madani and Kabat 1998; Sheehy et al. 2002]. APOBEC3 is interferon induced and acts to deaminate cytosine to uracil in minus-strand retroviral DNA, thereby generating frequent G-to-A mutations and increased degradation of proviral genomes [Mangeat et al. 2003; Chiu et al. 2005].

We have mentioned a few examples of genes involved in the antiviral state generated by type I interferons. For a more complete discussion, we refer the reader to several excellent reviews in this area [Clarke et al. 2001; Samuel 2001].

3.12 VIRAL EVASION OF THE INNATE RESPONSE

As humans have developed mechanisms to combat viral infection, it seems only logical that viruses themselves would develop strategies to combat the host's defense. There are many examples of viral mechanisms that modulate the host immune response. Viruses can target the innate receptors, downstream signaling, or the regulation and effect of type I interferons. It is beyond the scope of this chapter to review this topic in detail. Rather, we provide a few representative examples and refer the reader to several excellent reviews [Goodbourn et al. 2000; Katze et al. 2002].

A46R is a decoy protein expressed by vaccinia virus early during infection. A46R can potently inhibit multiple TLR pathways important to host signaling [Stack et al. 2005]. To date, A46R is the only identified viral protein with TIR domains. Studies involving A46R have demonstrated that it blocks all signals downstream of the IL-1 receptor, which inhibits in NF-κB and MAP kinase activation. Following the knowledge that TIR domains mediate homotypic interactions, it is likely that A46R sequesters MyD88 in the cell [Adachi et al. 1998; Burns et al. 1998; Jefferies et al. 2001; Janssens and Beyaert 2002].

Another well-studied mechanism of viral evasion is that mediated by hepatitis C virus (HCV). The HCV serine protease NS3/4A blocks activation of IRF-3 and therefore type I interferon production in response to dsRNA. NS3/4A is a noncovalent enzyme complex that exhibits both protease and helicase activity. The inhibition of IRF-3 requires only the protease activity occurring upstream of IRF-3 [Foy et al. 2003; Li et al. 2005]. Recent studies show that HCV NS3/4A specifically cleaves TRIF and IPS-1 downstream of TLR3/TLR4 and the RNA helicases [Foy et al. 2003; Li et al. 2005; Meylan et al. 2005]. The interruption of signaling by NS3/4A via these essential components of the innate immune system exerts a crippling effect on host defense mechanisms. The RNA helicase are targeted by other viral proteins in addition to NS3/4A. MDA5 is a binding target for most paramyxoviruses V-proteins that disrupt interferon activation via the inhibition of its downstream signaling pathways [Childs et al. 2007].

In addition to modulation of innate receptor function and signaling, viruses have evolved to antagonize the expression and function of type I interferons. Adenoviridae are generally poor interferon inducers as a result of E1A proteins synthesized during wild-type infection. The E1A protein can effectively impair the IRF-3-stimulated activation of the IFN-α promoter, probably through interaction with the CH/3 region of CBP/p300 [Juang et al. 1998]. CBP/p300 is involved in the acetylation of specific lysine residues on histones H2A, H2B, H3, and H4, which is essential to initiate interferon gene transcription [Honda et al. 2006]. E1A also directly impairs the induction of ISGs (interferon-stimulated genes) during viral infection via an effect on the formation of ISGF3 complexes and the transcriptional activation of ISG promoters [Reich et al. 1988; Gutch and Reich 1991]. Similarly, human cytomegalovirus and the T antigen of murine polyomavirus disrupt interferon signaling and activation of interferon-stimulated genes via antagonistic effects on Jak1. In addition, the V protein of the paramyxovirus simian virus 5 acts to target Stat1, rendering it susceptible to degradation via the proteosome, thus inhibiting the formation of ISGF3 complexes [Weihua et al. 1998; Didcock et al. 1999a,b; Miller et al. 1999].

Finally, viruses can also directly antagonize antiviral mechanisms in the cell. For example, adenovirus can disrupt the action of PKR. Adenovirus functions to code two RNA–polymerase III-directed small RNAs, designated as virus-associated RNAs (VA-RNA) I and II. These accumulate at high levels at late stages of infection. VAI-RNA is extremely important in viral translation, as it binds to and blocks the activation of PKR [Thimmappaya et al. 1982; Schneider et al. 1985]. VAI-RNA consists of two long, imperfectly base-paired stems of approximately 20 to 22 bp. These are joined at the center by a structurally complex region which contains two loops and a short stem–loop. It is this center region that is important in the binding to PKR and subsequent inhibition of its function [Furtado et al. 1989].

3.13 CONCLUSIONS

The innate response to viral infection represents the front line of host defense against it. Over the past few years, our understanding of this antiviral immune response has increased substantially, revealing a complex relationship between the host and the virus in the early stages of infection. Thus, it is not surprising that the host innate immune response remains a significant barrier to the safe and effective application of viral vectors for human disease. Increasing knowledge in this field will allow scientists to develop new strategies for gene therapy and viral vector design. This will include a combination of strategies to disable deleterious host defense mechanisms and harness viral evasion genes to increase the efficiency and safety of gene therapy.

REFERENCES

Adachi O, Kawai T, et al. 1998. Targeted disruption of the MyD88 gene results in loss of IL-1- and IL-18-mediated function. *Immunity* 9:143–150.

Agalioti T, Lomvardas S, et al. 2000. Ordered recruitment of chromatin modifying and general transcription factors to the IFN-beta promoter. *Cell* 103:667–678.

Akira S, Takeda K, et al. 2001. Toll-like receptors: critical proteins linking innate and acquired immunity. *Nat Immunol* 2:675–680.

Alexopoulou L, Holt AC, et al. 2001. Recognition of double-stranded RNA and activation of NF-kappaB by Toll-like receptor 3. *Nature* 413:732–738.

Bass BL, Nishikura K, et al. 1997. A standardized nomenclature for adenosine deaminases that act on RNA. RNA 3:947–949.

Bluyssen AR, Durbin JE, et al. 1996. ISGF3 gamma p48, a specificity switch for interferon activated transcription factors. *Cytokine Growth Factor Rev* 7:11–17.

Burns K, Martinon F, et al. 1998. MyD88, an adapter protein involved in interleukin-1 signaling. *J Biol Chem* 273:12203–12209.

Chelbi-Alix MK and Wietzerbin J. 2007. Interferon, a growing cytokine family: 50 years of interferon research. *Biochimie* 89:713–718.

Childs K, Stock N, et al. 2007. mda-5, but not RIG-I, is a common target for paramyxovirus V proteins. *Virology* 359:190–200.

Chiu YL, Soros VB, et al. 2005. Cellular APOBEC3G restricts HIV-1 infection in resting $CD4^+$ T cells. *Nature* 435:108–114.

Clarke CJ, Trapani JA, et al. 2001. Mechanisms of interferon mediated anti-viral resistance. *Curr Drug Targets Immune Endocr Metabol Disord* 1:117–130.

Colonna M, Trinchieri G, et al. 2004. Plasmacytoid dendritic cells in immunity. *Nat Immunol* 5:1219–1226.

Dai J, Megjugorac NJ, et al. 2004. Regulation of IFN regulatory factor-7 and IFN-alpha production by enveloped virus and lipopolysaccharide in human plasmacytoid dendritic cells. *J Immunol* 173:1535–1548.

Darnell JE Jr, Kerr IM, et al. 1994. Jak-STAT pathways and transcriptional activation in response to IFNs and other extracellular signaling proteins. *Science* 264:1415–1421.

de Haro C, Mendez R, et al. 1996. The eIF-2alpha kinases and the control of protein synthesis. *FASEB J* 10:1378–1387.

Decker T, Lew DJ, et al. 1991. Two distinct alpha-interferon-dependent signal transduction pathways may contribute to activation of transcription of the guanylate-binding protein gene. *Mol Cell Biol* 11:5147–5153.

Deng L, Wang C, et al. 2000. Activation of the IkappaB kinase complex by TRAF6 requires a dimeric ubiquitin-conjugating enzyme complex and a unique polyubiquitin chain. *Cell* 103:351–361.

Didcock L, Young DF, et al. 1999a. Sendai virus and simian virus 5 block activation of interferon-responsive genes: importance for virus pathogenesis. *J Virol* 73:3125–133.

Didcock L, Young DF, et al. 1999b. The V protein of simian virus 5 inhibits interferon signalling by targeting Stat1 for proteasome-mediated degradation. *J Virol* 73:9928–9933.

Diebold SS, Kaisho T, et al. 2004. Innate antiviral responses by means of TLR7-mediated recognition of single-stranded RNA. *Science* 303:1529–1531.

Escalante CR, Yie J, et al. 1998. Structure of IRF-1 with bound DNA reveals determinants of interferon regulation. *Nature* 391:103–106.

Espert L, Degols G, et al. 2003. ISG20, a new interferon-induced RNase specific for single-stranded RNA, defines an alternative antiviral pathway against RNA genomic viruses. *J Biol Chem* 278:16151–16158.

Fenner JE, Starr R, et al. 2006. Suppressor of cytokine signaling 1 regulates the immune response to infection by a unique inhibition of type I interferon activity. *Nat Immunol* 7:33–39.

Fitzgerald KA, McWhirter SM, et al. 2003. IKKepsilon and TBK1 are essential components of the IRF3 signaling pathway. *Nat Immunol* 4:491–496.

Foy E, Li K, et al. 2003. Regulation of interferon regulatory factor-3 by the hepatitis C virus serine protease. *Science* 300:1145–1148.

Furtado MR, Subramanian S, et al. 1989. Functional dissection of adenovirus VAI RNA. *J Virol* 63:3423–3434.

Gohda J, Matsumura T, et al. 2004. Cutting edge: TNFR-associated factor (TRAF) 6 is essential for MyD88-dependent pathway but not Toll/IL-1 receptor domain-containing adaptor-inducing IFN-beta (TRIF)-dependent pathway in TLR signaling. *J Immunol* 173:2913–2917.

Goodbourn S, Didcock L, et al. 2000. Interferons: cell signalling, immune modulation, antiviral response and virus countermeasures. *J Gen Virol* 81:2341–2364.

Grandvaux N, tenOever BR, et al. 2002. The interferon antiviral response: from viral invasion to evasion. *Curr Opin Infect Dis* 15:259–267.

Guo B and Cheng G. 2007. Modulation of the interferon antiviral response by the TBK1/IKKi adaptor protein TANK. *J Biol Chem* 282:11817–11826.

Guo J, Hui DJ, et al. 2000. A new pathway of translational regulation mediated by eukaryotic initiation factor 3. *EMBO J* 19:6891–6899.

Gutch MJ and Reich NC. 1991. Repression of the interferon signal transduction pathway by the adenovirus E1A oncogene. *Proc Natl Acad Sci U S A* 88:7913–7917.

Gyory I, Wu J, et al. 2004. PRDI-BF1 recruits the histone H3 methyltransferase G9a in transcriptional silencing. *Nat Immunol* 5:299–308.

Hacker H, Redecke V, et al. 2006. Specificity in Toll-like receptor signalling through distinct effector functions of TRAF3 and TRAF6. *Nature* 439:204–207.

Haller O, Frese M, et al. 1998. Mx proteins: mediators of innate resistance to RNA viruses. *Rev Sci Tech* 17:220–230.

Haque SJ and Williams BR. 1994. Identification and characterization of an interferon (IFN)-stimulated response element-IFN-stimulated gene factor 3-independent signaling pathway for IFN-alpha. *J Biol Chem* 269:19523–19529.

Harding HP, Calfon M, et al. 2002. Transcriptional and translational control in the mammalian unfolded protein response. *Annu Rev Cell Dev Biol* 18:575–599.

Heil F, Hemmi H, et al. 2004. Species-specific recognition of single-stranded RNA via Toll-like receptor 7 and 8. *Science* 303:1526–1529.

Hemmi H, Takeuchi O, et al. 2000. A Toll-like receptor recognizes bacterial DNA. *Nature* 408:740–745.

Hemmi H, Kaisho T, et al. 2002. Small anti-viral compounds activate immune cells via the TLR7 MyD88-dependent signaling pathway. *Nat Immunol* 3:196–200.

Hemmi H, Kaisho T, et al. 2003. The roles of Toll-like receptor 9, MyD88, and DNA-dependent protein kinase catalytic subunit in the effects of two distinct CpG DNAs on dendritic cell subsets. *J Immunol* 170:3059–3064.

Hemmi H, Takeuchi O, et al. 2004. The roles of two IkappaB kinase-related kinases in lipopolysaccharide and double stranded RNA signaling and viral infection. *J Exp Med* 199:1641–1650.

Honda K, Takaoka A, et al. 2006. Type I interferon [corrected] gene induction by the interferon regulatory factor family of transcription factors. *Immunity* 25:349–360.

Honda K, Yanai H, et al. 2004. Role of a transductional–transcriptional processor complex involving MyD88 and IRF-7 in Toll-like receptor signaling. *Proc Natl Acad Sci U S A* 101:15416–15421.

Honda K, Yanai H, et al. 2005. IRF-7 is the master regulator of type-I interferon-dependent immune responses. *Nature* 434:772–777.

Hornung V, Schlender J, et al. 2004. Replication-dependent potent IFN-alpha induction in human plasmacytoid dendritic cells by a single-stranded RNA virus. *J Immunol* 173:5935–5943.

Hovanessian AG, Brown RE, et al. 1977. Synthesis of low molecular weight inhibitor of protein synthesis with enzyme from interferon-treated cells. *Nature* 268:537–540.

Hurst R, Schatz JR, et al. 1987. Inhibition of rabbit reticulocyte lysate protein synthesis by heavy metal ions involves the phosphorylation of the alpha-subunit of the eukaryotic initiation factor 2. *J Biol Chem* 262:15939–15945.

Ihle JN, Nosaka T, et al. 1997. Jaks and Stats in cytokine signaling. *Stem Cells* 15(Suppl 1):105–111; discussion, 112.

Ishii KJ, Coban C, et al. 2006. A Toll-like receptor-independent antiviral response induced by double-stranded B-form DNA. *Nat Immunol* 7:40–48.

Ishitani T, Takaesu G, et al. 2003. Role of the TAB2-related protein TAB3 in IL-1 and TNF signaling. *EMBO J* 22:6277–6288.

Janssens S and Beyaert R. 2002. A universal role for MyD88 in TLR/IL-1R-mediated signaling. *Trends Biochem Sci* 27:474–482.

Jefferies C, Bowie A, et al. 2001. Transactivation by the p65 subunit of NF-kappaB in response to interleukin-1 (IL-1) involves MyD88, IL-1 receptor-associated kinase 1, TRAF-6, and Rac1. *Mol Cell Biol* 21:4544–4552.

Jin G, Klika A, et al. 2004. Identification of a human NF-kappaB-activating protein, TAB3. *Proc Natl Acad Sci U S A* 101:2028–2033.

Juang YT, Lowther W, et al. 1998. Primary activation of interferon A and interferon B gene transcription by interferon regulatory factor 3. *Proc Natl Acad Sci U S A* 95:9837–9842.

Kaisho T, Takeuchi O, et al. 2001. Endotoxin-induced maturation of MyD88-deficient dendritic cells. *J Immunol* 166:5688–5694.

Kang DC, Gopalkrishnan RV, et al. 2002. mda-5: an interferon-inducible putative RNA helicase with double-stranded RNA-dependent ATPase activity and melanoma growth-suppressive properties. *Proc Natl Acad Sci U S A* 99:637–642.

Kato H, Sato S, et al. 2005. Cell type-specific involvement of RIG-I in antiviral response. *Immunity* 23:19–28.

Kato H, Takeuchi O, et al. 2006. Differential roles of MDA5 and RIG-I helicases in the recognition of RNA viruses. *Nature* 441:101–105.

Katze MG, He Y, et al. 2002. Viruses and interferon: a fight for supremacy. *Nat Rev Immunol* 2:675–687.

Kawai T and Akira S. 2006. Innate immune recognition of viral infection. *Nat Immunol* 7:131–137.

Kawai T, Adachi O, et al. 1999. Unresponsiveness of MyD88-deficient mice to endotoxin. *Immunity* 11:115–122.

Kawai T, Takeuchi O, et al. 2001. Lipopolysaccharide stimulates the MyD88-independent pathway and results in activation of IFN-regulatory factor 3 and the expression of a subset of lipopolysaccharide-inducible genes. *J Immunol* 167:5887–5894.

Kawai T, Sato S, et al. 2004. Interferon-alpha induction through Toll-like receptors involves a direct interaction of IRF7 with MyD88 and TRAF6. *Nat Immunol* 5:1061–1068.

Kawai T, Takahashi K, et al. 2005. IPS-1, an adaptor triggering RIG-I- and Mda5-mediated type I interferon induction. *Nat Immunol* 6:981–988.

Kim TK and Maniatis T. 1997. The mechanism of transcriptional synergy of an in vitro assembled interferon-beta enhanceosome. *Mol Cell* 1:119–129.

Kopp E, Medzhitov R, et al. 1999. ECSIT is an evolutionarily conserved intermediate in the Toll/IL-1 signal transduction pathway. *Genes Dev* 13:2059–2071.

Kotenko SV, Gallagher G, et al. 2003. IFN-lambdas mediate antiviral protection through a distinct class II cytokine receptor complex. *Nat Immunol* 4:69–77.

Kovacsovics M, Martinon F, et al. 2002. Overexpression of Helicard, a CARD-containing helicase cleaved during apoptosis, accelerates DNA degradation. *Curr Biol* 12:838–843.

Krug A, French AR, et al. 2004a. TLR9-dependent recognition of MCMV by IPC and DC generates coordinated cytokine responses that activate antiviral NK cell function. *Immunity* 21:107–119.

Krug A, Luker GD, et al. 2004b. Herpes simplex virus type 1 activates murine natural interferon-producing cells through Toll-like receptor 9. *Blood* 103:1433–1437.

Li K, Foy E, et al. 2005. Immune evasion by hepatitis C virus NS3/4A protease-mediated cleavage of the Toll-like receptor 3 adaptor protein TRIF. *Proc Natl Acad Sci U S A* 102:2992–2997.

Lin R, Heylbroeck C, et al. 1998. Virus-dependent phosphorylation of the IRF-3 transcription factor regulates nuclear translocation, transactivation potential, and proteasome-mediated degradation. *Mol Cell Biol* 18:2986–2996.

Liu YJ. 2005. IPC: professional type 1 interferon-producing cells and plasmacytoid dendritic cell precursors. *Annu Rev Immunol* 23:275–306.

Lopez CB, Moltedo B, et al. 2004. TLR-independent induction of dendritic cell maturation and adaptive immunity by negative-strand RNA viruses. *J Immunol* 173:6882–6889.

Lund J, Sato A, et al. 2003. Toll-like receptor 9-mediated recognition of herpes simplex virus-2 by plasmacytoid dendritic cells. *J Exp Med* 198:513–520.

Lund JM, Alexopoulou L, et al. 2004. Recognition of single-stranded RNA viruses by Toll-like receptor 7. *Proc Natl Acad Sci U S A* 101:5598–5603.

Madani N and Kabat D. 1998. An endogenous inhibitor of human immunodeficiency virus in human lymphocytes is overcome by the viral Vif protein. *J Virol* 72:10251–10255.

Mamane Y, Heylbroeck C, et al. 1999. Interferon regulatory factors: the next generation. *Gene* 237:1–14.

Mangeat B, Turelli P, et al. 2003. Broad antiretroviral defence by human APOBEC3G through lethal editing of nascent reverse transcripts. *Nature* 424:99–103.

Marie I, Durbin JE, et al. 1998. Differential viral induction of distinct interferon-alpha genes by positive feedback through interferon regulatory factor-7. *EMBO J* 17:6660–6669.

Matsumoto M, Funami K, et al. 2003. Subcellular localization of Toll-like receptor 3 in human dendritic cells. *J Immunol* 171:3154–3162.

Matsuyama T, Kimura T, et al. 1993. Targeted disruption of IRF-1 or IRF-2 results in abnormal type I IFN gene induction and aberrant lymphocyte development. *Cell* 75:83–97.

McWhirter SM, Fitzgerald KA, et al. 2004. IFN-regulatory factor 3–dependent gene expression is defective in Tbk1-deficient mouse embryonic fibroblasts. *Proc Natl Acad Sci U S A* 101:233–238.

Meylan E, Burns K, et al. 2004. RIP1 is an essential mediator of Toll-like receptor 3-induced NF-kappa B activation. *Nat Immunol* 5:503–507.

Meylan E, Curran J, et al. 2005. Cardif is an adaptor protein in the RIG-I antiviral pathway and is targeted by hepatitis C virus. *Nature* 437:1167–1172.

Miller DM, Zhang Y, et al. 1999. Human cytomegalovirus inhibits IFN-alpha-stimulated antiviral and immunoregulatory responses by blocking multiple levels of IFN-alpha signal transduction. *J Immunol* 162:6107–6113.

Miyamoto M, Fujita T, et al. 1988. Regulated expression of a gene encoding a nuclear factor, IRF-1, that specifically binds to IFN-beta gene regulatory elements. *Cell* 54:903–913.

Munshi N, Agalioti T, et al. 2001. Coordination of a transcriptional switch by HMGI(Y) acetylation. *Science* 293:1133–1136.

Novick D, Cohen B, et al. 1994. The human interferon alpha/beta receptor: characterization and molecular cloning. *Cell* 77:391–400.

Oganesyan G, Saha SK, et al. 2006. Critical role of TRAF3 in the Toll-like receptor-dependent and -independent antiviral response. *Nature* 439:208–211.

O'Shea JJ and Watford W. 2004. A peek at PIAS. *Nat Immunol* 5:875–876.

Panne D, Maniatis T, et al. 2007. An atomic model of the interferon-beta enhanceosome. *Cell* 129:1111–1123.

Paun A and Pitha PM. 2007. The IRF family, revisited. *Biochimie* 89:744–753.

Perry AK, Chow EK, et al. 2004. Differential requirement for TANK-binding kinase-1 in type I interferon responses to Toll-like receptor activation and viral infection. *J Exp Med* 199:1651–1658.

Pestka S, Krause CD, et al. 2004. Interferons, interferon-like cytokines, and their receptors. *Immunol Rev* 202:8–32.

Qin BY, Liu C, et al. 2003. Crystal structure of IRF-3 reveals mechanism of autoinhibition and virus-induced phosphoactivation. *Nat Struct Biol* 10:913–921.

Qing Y, Costa-Pereira AP, et al. 2005. Role of tyrosine 441 of interferon-gamma receptor subunit 1 in SOCS-1-mediated attenuation of Stat1 activation. *J Biol Chem* 280:1849–1853.

Regad T and Chelbi-Alix MK. 2001. Role and fate of PML nuclear bodies in response to interferon and viral infections. *Oncogene* 20:7274–7286.

Reich N, Pine R, et al. 1988. Transcription of interferon-stimulated genes is induced by adenovirus particles but is suppressed by E1A gene products. *J Virol* 62:114–119.

Ryals J, Dierks P, et al. 1985. A 46-nucleotide promoter segment from an IFN-alpha gene renders an unrelated promoter inducible by virus. *Cell* 41:497–507.

Samuel CE. 2001. Antiviral actions of interferons. *Clin Microbiol Rev* 14:778–809, table of contents.

Sato M, Hata N, et al. 1998a. Positive feedback regulation of type I IFN genes by the IFN-inducible transcription factor IRF-7. *FEBS Lett* 441:106–110.

Sato M, Tanaka N, et al. 1998b. Involvement of the IRF family transcription factor IRF-3 in virus-induced activation of the IFN-beta gene. *FEBS Lett* 425:112–116.

Sato S, Sugiyama M, et al. 2003. Toll/IL-1 receptor domain-containing adaptor inducing IFN-beta (TRIF) associates with TNF receptor-associated factor 6 and TANK-binding kinase 1, and activates two distinct transcription factors, NF-kappa B and IFN-regulatory factor-3, in the Toll-like receptor signaling. *J Immunol* 171:4304–4310.

Sato S, Sanjo H, et al. 2005. Essential function for the kinase TAK1 in innate and adaptive immune responses. *Nat Immunol* 6:1087–1095.

Schindler C and Darnell JE Jr. 1995. Transcriptional responses to polypeptide ligands: the Jak–Stat pathway. *Annu Rev Biochem* 64:621–651.

Schneider RJ, Safer B, et al. 1985. Adenovirus VAI RNA prevents phosphorylation of the eukaryotic initiation factor 2 alpha subunit subsequent to infection. *Proc Natl Acad Sci U S A* 82:4321–4325.

Sharma S, tenOever BR, et al. 2003. Triggering the interferon antiviral response through an IKK-related pathway. *Science* 300:1148–1151.

Sheehy AM, Gaddis NC, et al. 2002. Isolation of a human gene that inhibits HIV-1 infection and is suppressed by the viral Vif protein. *Nature* 418:646–650.

Stack J, Haga IR, et al. 2005. Vaccinia virus protein A46R targets multiple Toll-like-interleukin-1 receptor adaptors and contributes to virulence. *J Exp Med* 201:1007–1018.

Stark GR, Kerr IM, et al. 1998. How cells respond to interferons. *Annu Rev Biochem* 67:227–264.

Stetson DB and Medzhitov R. 2006. Recognition of cytosolic DNA activates an IRF3-dependent innate immune response. *Immunity* 24:93–103.

Tabeta K, Georgel P, et al. 2004. Toll-like receptors 9 and 3 as essential components of innate immune defense against mouse cytomegalovirus infection. *Proc Natl Acad Sci U S A* 101:3516–3521.

Takahasi K, Suzuki NN, et al. 2003. X-ray crystal structure of IRF-3 and its functional implications. *Nat Struct Biol* 10:922–927.

Takaoka A and Taniguchi T. 2003. New aspects of IFN-alpha/beta signalling in immunity, oncogenesis and bone metabolism. *Cancer Sci* 94:405–411.

Takaoka A, Yanai H, et al. 2005. Integral role of IRF-5 in the gene induction programme activated by Toll-like receptors. *Nature* 434:243–249.

Takaoka A, Wang Z, et al. 2007. DAI (DLM-1/ZBP1) is a cytosolic DNA sensor and an activator of innate immune response. *Nature*. 448:501–505.

Takeda K and Akira S. 2005. Toll-like receptors in innate immunity. *Int Immunol* 17:1–14.

Taniguchi T, Ogasawara K, et al. 2001. IRF family of transcription factors as regulators of host defense. *Annu Rev Immunol* 19:623–655.

Thimmappaya B, Weinberger C, et al. 1982. Adenovirus VAI RNA is required for efficient translation of viral mRNAs at late times after infection. *Cell* 31:543–551.

Uematsu S, Sato S, et al. 2005. Interleukin-1 receptor-associated kinase-1 plays an essential role for Toll-like receptor (TLR)7- and TLR9-mediated interferon-{alpha} induction. *J Exp Med* 201:915–923.

Uze G, Lutfalla G, et al. 1990. Genetic transfer of a functional human interferon alpha receptor into mouse cells: cloning and expression of its cDNA. *Cell* 60:225–234.

Vilcek J. 2006. Fifty years of interferon research: aiming at a moving target. *Immunity* 25:343–348.

Wang C, Deng L, et al. 2001. TAK1 is a ubiquitin-dependent kinase of MKK and IKK. *Nature* 412:346–351.

Wang T, Town T, et al. 2004. Toll-like receptor 3 mediates West Nile virus entry into the brain causing lethal encephalitis. *Nat Med* 10:1366–1373.

Weihua X, Ramanujam S, et al. 1998. The polyoma virus T antigen interferes with interferon-inducible gene expression. *Proc Natl Acad Sci U S A* 95:1085–1090.

Weissmann C and Weber H. 1986. The interferon genes. *Prog Nucleic Acid Res Mol Biol* 33:251–300.

Yamamoto M, Sato S, et al. 2002. Cutting edge: a novel Toll/IL-1 receptor domain-containing adapter that preferentially activates the IFN-beta promoter in the Toll-like receptor signaling. *J Immunol* 169:6668–6672.

Yoneyama M, Suhara W, et al. 1998. Direct triggering of the type I interferon system by virus infection: activation of a transcription factor complex containing IRF-3 and CBP/p300. *EMBO J* 17:1087–1095.

Yoneyama M, Kikuchi M, et al. 2004. The RNA helicase RIG-I has an essential function in double-stranded RNA-induced innate antiviral responses. *Nat Immunol* 5:730–737.

Yoneyama M, Kikuchi M, et al. 2005. Shared and unique functions of the DExD/H-box helicases RIG-I, MDA5, and LGP2 in antiviral innate immunity. *J Immunol* 175:2851–2858.

4

IMMUNE RESPONSES TO ADENOVIRAL VECTORS

NELSON C. DI PAOLO, PH.D., AND
DMITRY M. SHAYAKHMETOV, PH.D.

Division of Medical Genetics, Department of Medicine, University of Washington, Seattle, Washington

Gene Therapy Immunology, Edited by Roland Herzog

4.1 INTRODUCTION

Adenovirus-based vector systems are, to date, the most common vector type used in clinical studies worldwide (www.wiley.co.uk/genmed/clinical), representing 26% of all trials. Transient transfer of therapeutic genes to correct genetic metabolic diseases, treatment of localized and disseminated cancers, and studies of new generations of vaccines are among the most frequent applications for which adenoviral vectors are currently being developed. High efficiency of gene transfer by adenoviral vectors both in vitro and in vivo, relative ease of generation of clinical-grade vector stocks, and a well-studied virus life cycle have made them the vector of choice for many of these gene therapy applications. Adenoviral interactions with host cells, however, inevitably result in the induction of innate immune responses in vitro and in vivo. Natural adenoviral infection and adenoviral vector delivery in vivo both induce robust immune responses, resulting in long-lasting immunity. Three fundamental parameters control the magnitude and consequences of immune responses induced by adenoviral vectors in vivo: the site of vector delivery (local or systemic via the bloodstream), the virus dose delivered, and the immune status of the host (immunocompetent or immunocompromised, naive or previously exposed to the same serotype of virus). While induction of immune responses might be beneficial for some vaccine development strategies, both innate and adaptive antiadenovirus host immune responses impose significant limitations on the utility of adenoviral vectors for application in humans. In this chapter we review recent advances in the understanding of the biology of adenoviral interactions with the host in the light of activation of the innate and adaptive immune systems. We also review new data on adenovirus-based vaccines and strategies to overcome the deleterious effects of antiadenovirus immune responses for successful application of these vectors in humans.

4.2 INNATE IMMUNE RESPONSES TO ADENOVIRAL VECTORS IN VITRO AND IN VIVO

Adenovirus is a nonenveloped virus with a linear double-stranded DNA genome. Adenoviral vectors are developed based on naturally occurring serotypes, which are widespread and have been isolated from vertebrate species ranging from frogs to humans. In humans, multiple serotypes of adenovirus cause a spectrum of illnesses in both normal and immunocompromised hosts [Ruuskanen O 2002; Kojaoghlanian et al. 2003]. Fifty-one human adenovirus serotypes have been identified to date, divided into six species, A to F. This division is based historically on hemagglutination properties, immunological cross-reactivity, and genomic DNA homology. Many of these serotypes exert diverse cell and tissue tropism, which is, at least in part, responsible for the variety of clinical manifestations observed and host responses caused by adenovirus infection. To understand the innate and adaptive responses to adenoviral vectors, it is important to consider the route of vector delivery. For example, upon intranasal, intradermal, or oral delivery, adenoviral vectors will encounter different organ-specific cell types, which will orchestrate the host response depending on their capacity to recognize and confine the infection. Similarly, adenoviral vectors based on different serotypes are likely to utilize different virus attachment receptors to gain cell entry, which, in turn, may induce diverse intracellular downstream signaling events that modulate host responses differentially.

4.2.1 Role of Primary Virus Attachment Receptors in the Induction of Antiadenoviral Responses

According to the currently accepted model, which is based primarily on in vitro data, Adenovirus infects cells in a two-step process (for a review, see Bergelson [1999], Nemerow [2000], Meier and Greber [2003]). The first step involves the fiber coat protein–mediated binding of adenovirus to the primary attachment receptor on the cell surface. Despite diverse natural tissue tropism, the vast majority of human adenoviruses belonging to species A though F, except species B, can utilize the coxsackie and adenovirus receptor (CAR) as a high-affinity primary attachment receptor for cell entry [Bergelson et al. 1997; Tomko et al. 1997; Roelvink et al. 1998, 1999]. We and others have found that the ubiquitously expressed complement regulatory protein CD46 represents a major species B adenovirus receptor on human cells [Gaggar et al. 2003; Segerman et al. 2003]. As CAR lacking its intracellular domain is sufficient to mediate virus infection [Wang and Bergelson 1999], the role of downstream signaling upon adenovirus binding to CAR was considered to be negligible for efficient virus infection. However, in a recent study by Tamanini et al., it was suggested that binding of the Ad5 fiber to CAR is a key pro-inflammatory activation event in epithelial respiratory cells [Tamanini et al. 2006]. Upon infection of A549 cells with an Ad5-based viral vector, the authors found rapid activation of both ERK1/2 and JNK MAPK kinases, and up-regulation of transcription for pro-inflammatory genes, including IL-8, GRO-α, GRO-γ, RANTES, and IP-10. The activation of these genes was found to be dependent on adenovirus fiber binding to CAR, and no activation was observed when cells were exposed to the adenovirus capsid proteins penton or hexon [Tamanini et al. 2006]. After identification of CD46 as a high-affinity attachment receptor for species B adenoviruses, numerous studies investigated the host responses to adenoviral vectors interacting with CD46. Sakurai et al. found that binding of a replication-incompetent Ad35-based vector to CD46 results in long-lasting down-regulation of cell surface CD46 [Sakurai et al. 2007]. Furthermore, in vitro studies demonstrated that human peripheral blood mononuclear cells respond differently depending on whether they are infected with CAR-interacting Ad5-based vectors or CD46-interacting Ad16 and Ad35 [Iacobelli-Martinez et al. 2005]. Infection of PBMCs with Ad35 or Ad16 resulted in significant reduction of mRNA levels for IL-12, IL-1α, IL-1β, IL-1RA, and IL-6, compared to cells infected with Ad5. However, infection of plasmacytoid dendritic cells with CD46 interacting Ad5-based vectors pseudotyped with Ad37, Ad16, or Ad35 fibers, initiated robust production of type I interferon, IFN-α [Iacobelli-Martinez and Nemerow 2007]. In a pioneering study by Rea et al. [2001] it was shown that an Ad5-based vector pseudotyped with the CD46-interacting Ad35 fiber, rAd5F35, is very efficient in transducing human immature dendritic cells. rAd5F35 was 100-fold more efficient, compared to a CAR-ineracting Ad5 vector, in transducing hDCs and inducing their maturation in vitro. It is of interest to note that while human monocyte-derived dendritic cells exhibited rapid maturation (up-regulation of expression of major histocompatibility complex class I/II and CD40, CD80, and CD86 co-stimulatory molecules) even after infection with CAR-interacting Ad5 vectors, these changes were not observed on cell infection with vectors derived from canine adenovirus type 2, CAV-2, which does not use CAR as a primary attachment receptor [Perreau et al. 2007]. Taken together, these data demonstrate that cell exposure to adenovirus inevitably activate genes involved in regulation of the innate and adaptive immune systems. However, the nature of the primary virus attachment receptor may significantly modulate the magnitude and type of cell response observed following infection with adenoviral vectors.

4.2.2 Role of Co-Receptor Binding in Initiation of Innate Antiadenoviral Responses

Following initial attachment, RGD motifs within the adenovirus penton base protein interact with co-receptors, cellular integrins, allowing for the internalization of attached virus particles into the cell [Wickham et al. 1993]. It has been shown that a number of RGD motif-interacting integrins (αvβ1, αvβ3, αvβ5, αvβ6, α5β1) as well as $\alpha_M\beta 2$ and $\alpha_L\beta 2$, can serve as co-receptors, promoting adenovirus internalization into different cell types in vitro [Wickham et al. 1993; Huang et al. 1996; Davison et al. 1997, 2001; Li et al. 2001; Meier and Greber 2003]. Viral interaction with cellular integrins initiates downstream signaling through the activation of two independent but synergistic pathways (for a detailed review, see Liu and Muruve [2003]). The first pathway includes the lipid kinase PI3K, the small G proteins cdc42 and rac1, and p38 kinase MAPK [Li et al. 1998a,b; Suomalainen et al. 2001; Bhat and Fan 2002]. The second pathway involves signal transduction through focal adhesion kinase (FAK), Raf-1, and ERK1/2 protein kinases [Bruder and Kovesdi 1997; Nemerow and Stewart 1999; Li et al. 2000; Tibbles et al. 2002]. Signal transduction through these pathways can induce actin polymerization near the site of virus attachment, triggering endocytosis [Liu and Muruve 2003]. Importantly, the activation of p38 MAPK and ERK1/2 was linked to translocation of NF-κB into the nucleus, and the initiation of pro-inflammatory cytokine and chemokine gene expression [Borgland et al. 2000; Bowen et al. 2002; Liu et al. 2003; Tamanini et al. 2003]. Clearly, binding of adenovirus to integrins, which varies dramatically in different tissues, may contribute to the diverse cellular responses to virus infection. It was previously found that integrins have several activation states, and their adaptor/signal transduction molecules may be involved in activation of the early cellular response genes (e.g., β1-integrin signaling through integrin-linked kinase, ILK, was associated with NF-κB-dependent activation of pro-inflammatory genes, including IL-1

[Yurochko et al. 1992; Roman et al. 1999, 2000; Ritzenthaler and Roman 2001; Brakebusch and Fassler 2003; Tamanini et al. 2003] and TNF-α [Lieber et al. 1997, 1998]. A wealth of information regarding the contribution of integrin signaling in shaping innate immune responses to adenovirus infection was obtained through the analysis of activation of pro-inflammatory genes by adenoviral vectors possessing an RGD motif deletion within the penton base protein. An early study by Liu et al. [2003] demonstrated that adenovirus penton RGD motifs are required for efficient transduction and endothelial cell activation in vivo. The same group later analyzed induction of the CXCL10 (IP-10) chemokine in kidney epithelium-derived REC cells [Liu et al. 2005]. The authors demonstrated that Akt, a downstream effector of integrin signaling, was activated within 10 minutes of cell infection with Ad5 vectors. Inhibition of the Akt pathway by Wortmannin or Ly294002 compounds decreased adenovirus-mediated IP-10 mRNA induction. Importantly, infection of cells with AdL.PB vector, which was unable to bind integrins due to a penton RGD motif deletion, resulted in lack of Akt activation and IP-10 mRNA up-regulation [Liu et al. 2005]. Consistent with these findings, Schoggins and Falk-Pedersen [2006] recently showed that when both fiber and penton-modified vectors were delivered intravenously, the levels of liver transduction was 60- to 80-fold lower for the penton RGD motif-deleted vectors, compared to viruses possessing intact integrin-interacting pentons. The induction of early host inflammatory responses was also reduced dramatically following delivery of penton RGD motif mutated adenoviral vectors compared to unmodified RGD motif possessing counterparts [Schoggins and Falck-Pedersen 2006].

4.2.3 Molecular Sensors of Adenoviral Infection

Although accumulated data suggest that adenovirus binding to primary cellular attachment receptors and integrins can induce intracellular signaling which activates transcription for some pro-inflammatory genes, these known signal transduction events fail to fully explain the rapid and highly complex innate immune and inflammatory responses observed following delivery of adenoviral vectors in vivo. Using microarray technology, it was found that adenovirus infection rapidly dysregulates expression of up to 15% of all mRNA transcripts in mouse liver tissue or in human epithelial A549 cells [Hartman et al. 2007a,b]. In addition to dysregulation of genes involved in endosomal and lysosomal transport, apoptotic pathways, and cell adhesion, a considerable number of genes, which were previously linked to activation of innate immune and inflammatory responses, were highly up-regulated within a few hours after adenovirus infection. These data prompted the search for additional intracellular sensor molecules that might be involved in recognition of adenovirus capsid components that can collectively be called molecular sensors of adenovirus infection.

From earlier studies it was established that expression of genes involved in innate immune and inflammatory responses was significantly up-regulated shortly after adenoviral vector delivery but prior to significant viral gene expression.

In mouse and nonhuman primate models, Wilson and co-workers demonstrated activation of innate responses by transcriptionally defective adenovirus particles [Schnell et al. 2001; Zhang et al. 2001]. Consistent with these findings, severe acute inflammatory response was also observed in a nonhuman primate model after intravenous delivery of a helper-dependent adenoviral vector which lacked all viral genes [Brunetti-Pierri et al. 2004]. These data demonstrate directly that the dose-dependent activation of innate immune and inflammatory responses are mediated primarily by adenovirus particle interaction with host cells and do not require viral gene expression.

In searching for molecular sensors of adenovirus infection, the investigators turned initially to the relatively well studied pathogen detection system, consisting of a specialized family of receptors known as Toll-like receptors (TLRs) [Barton and Medzhitov 2002]. Mammalian TLRs recognize components of bacteria, viruses, fungi, and protozoa, both at the cell surface and within intracellular compartments. Eleven TLRs in mice and 10 TLRs in humans have been discovered to date [Pasare and Medzhitov 2004]. All of them were found to be important proteins in innate immunity, recognizing pathogen-specific products or "molecular patterns" and eliciting host defense responses. Structurally, TLRs are type 1 transmembrane proteins that contain a leucine-rich repeat extracellular domain and an intracellular Toll/IL-1 receptor (TIR) domain [Miggin and O'Neill 2006]. Upon ligand activation of TLRs, cytosolic TIR domain recruits cellular adaptor proteins. Four signaling adaptor proteins have been identified so far; myeloid differentiation factor 88 (MyD88), MyD88 adaptor-like (Mal), TIR domain containing adaptor inducing IFN-β (Trif), and Trif-related adaptor molecule TRAM. MyD88 is recruited by all TLRs except TLR3 and leads to activation of the transcription factor NF-κB [Akira and Takeda 2004]. Mal is required for signaling by the LPS receptor TLR4 and the bacterial lipoprotein receptor TLR2. Trif mediates TLR3 and TLR4 signaling and is involved in activation of the transcription factor IRF-3 [Fitzgerald et al. 2003]. Finally, TRAM mediates only TLR4 signaling, acting as a bridging adapter to recruit Trif to the TLR4 complex. Different TLRs are capable of recognizing very diverse pathogens. Moreover, whereas some TLRs are expressed exclusively on the cell surface (such as TLR2 and TLR4), TLR3 and TLR7-9 are located primarily in cellular endosomal compartments [Hemmi et al. 2000; Alexopoulou et al. 2001]. Individual TLRs exhibit at least some pathogen pattern specificity. For instance, TLR2 recognizes peptidoglycan from gram-positive bacteria and zymosan from yeast call walls. TLR5 can recognize flagellin, TLR3 is activated by double-stranded RNA, and TLR7 and TLR8 are activated by single-stranded RNA. TLR9 is activated by unmethylated CpG DNA motifs present in bacterial DNA and some viruses, such as herpes simplex virus or cytomegalovirus [Hemmi et al. 2000; Krug et al. 2004].

Due to the central role of TLRs in detecting invading pathogens, considerable effort was made in analyzing whether this family of receptors is involved in recognition of adenovirus infection. Recent data suggest that in response to adenovirus infection, plasmacytoid and conventional dendritic cells secrete type I IFN in a

TLR9-dependent manner [Basner-Tschakarjan et al. 2006; Iacobelli-Martinez and Nemerow 2007]. It is of interest to note that human cell lines expressing TLR9, which are permissive to infection by both CAR- and CD46-interacting adenovirus serotypes, showed a preferential activation of TLR9-mediated signaling by CD46-interacting serotypes [Iacobelli-Martinez and Nemerow 2007]. These data are consistent with earlier findings that CD46-interacting adenoviruses select an alternative intracellular trafficking pathway and reside longer in late endosomal compartments than do CAR-interacting serotypes [Shayakhmetov et al. 2003]. Because TLR9 expression is localized to late endosomal compartments, it appears that adenoviral DNA may activate TLR9 and induce type I IFN expression. Using helper-dependent adenoviral vectors, Curello et al. found that the immediate innate immune response, assessed by plasma levels of IL-6 and IL-12, was partially attenuated in TLR9 knockout mice compared to the control group, expressing wild-type levels of TLR9 [Cerullo et al. 2007]. The involvement of TLR-mediated pathways in the induction of antiadenoviral host responses was further analyzed in wild-type and MyD88-knockout mice. These studies provided evidence that type I interferon is induced in response to adenovirus infection in both MyD88-dependent and MyD88-independent ways. For instance, plasmacytoid DCs produced IFN-α/β in a TLR9- and MyD88-dependent manner, however, conventional DCs and macrophages initiated IFN-I production through a MyD88-independent mechanism, which probably involved an as yet unidentified cytosolic sensor of DNA [Zhu et al. 2007a]. In a very thorough study by Nociari et al., the authors provide further evidence that type I interferon expression in response to cell infection with adenoviral vectors occurs in a MyD88-independent manner, also supporting the idea that adenoviral DNA is probably detected by an unidentified sensor of nucleic acids in the cytoplasm [Nociari et al. 2007]. This group provided compelling evidence that the adenovirus genome can induce phosphorylation of interferon regulatory factor IRF-3, which is the key transcription factor in activating the antiviral IFN-type I-mediated signaling pathway. It is worth mentioning that a new cytosolic DNA sensor molecule was described recently by Takaoka et al. [2007]. Their data demonstrate that type I interferon can be activated by cytosolic DNA though DAI (DLM-1/ZBP1, Z-DNA binding protein 1). However, it remains to be shown whether DAI can play a role in detection of adenoviral genomic DNA in infected cells.

4.3 MEDIATORS OF INNATE IMMUNE AND INFLAMMATORY RESPONSES TO ADENOVIRAL INFECTION

Activation of the immune system, and the generation of pro-inflammatory cytokines and chemokines, play a central role in the induction of inflammation, which is the major constituent and the underlying cause of adenovirus-induced tissue damage. The signaling events initiated by the entry of adenovirus into cells clearly contribute to the activation of pro-inflammatory cytokine and chemokine gene expression. Among the most prominent cytokines and chemokines implicated in the induction of antiadenovirus host inflammatory responses are TNF-α, IFN-α and β, IL-1, IL-6, IL-12, and IL-8 in humans, or KC and MIP-2 in mice.

4.3.1 Tumor Necrosis Factor-α

TNF-α was one of the first cytokines found to contribute to adenovirus-induced inflammatory host responses. In an early study by Ginsberg et al. [1991], TNF-α, along with IL-1 and IL-6, was detected in the lung shortly after inoculation of mice with wild-type Ad5 virus. In a later study, Metcalf [1996] demonstrated that the adenovirus E1A 13S protein can directly up-regulate TNF-α gene transcription. Upon intravenous delivery of adenoviral vectors to mice, Lieber et al. [1997] found that liver macrophages, Kupffer cells, are the likely source of plasma TNF-α, which was produced in response to adenovirus injection, and inactivation of Kupffer cells by gadolinium chloride resulted in both reduced adenovirus toxicity and prolonged transgene expression in hepatocytes. These findings were corroborated in a further study by Zhang et al. [1998], who showed that inhibition of TNF-α through administration of a soluble TNF receptor, decreases inflammation significantly and prolongs adenovirus-mediated gene expression in both lung and liver. Finally, adenovirus administration in TNF-α-deficient mice, as well as in TNF-α/LT-α double-knockout mice, resulted in a dramatic reduction of leukocyte infiltration in the liver and alleviation of adenovirus-induced inflammation, which correlated with an improved persistence of vector-encoded trangene expression in vivo [Elkon et al. 1997; Benihoud et al. 1998]. Collectively, these data demonstrates that TNF-α gene transcription and cytokine secretion are rapidly activated in response to adenovirus infection, and that TNF-α plays an essential role in promoting immune-mediated clearance of adenoviral vectors in vivo.

4.3.2 Type I IFN

Type I IFN (IFN-α and IFN-β) was discovered in 1957 as a protein, produced by chick cells infected by influenza virus, possessing potent antiviral activity [Isaacs and Lindenmann 1957]. Although production of high levels of type I IFN was observed in leukocyte cultures following infection with Ad7 [Pitkaranta and Hovi 1993] or in the case of a fatal adenovirus infection in a pediatric patient [Mistchenko et al. 1994], its role in mediating innate immune and inflammatory responses to adenoviral vectors was not clear until recently. Upon in vitro infection of plasmocytoid and conventional DCs with adenoviral vectors, production of high levels of IFN-α was observed [Basner-Tschakarjan et al. 2006]. However, while plasmacytoid DCs appear to induce IFN-α secretion after adenoviral DNA interaction with TLR9 [Basner-Tschakarjan et al. 2006; Iacobelli-Martinez and Nemerow 2007], conventional DCs secret type I IFN in a TLR9-independent manner [Zhu et al. 2007a]. In a very detailed study by Nociari et al. [2007] the adenovirus-mediated activation of type I IFN was linked to phosphorylation of interferon regulatory protein IRF-3 after recognition of adenoviral DNA by an as yet unidentified cytoplasmic sensor. The authors reported that in bone marrow–derived macrophages and DCs, the activation of type I IFN production was TLR independent, and also did not require activation of NF-κB, or the MAPK and AKT kinases [Nociari et al. 2007]. However, production of IFN-α was not observed following adenovirus infection of the same cells derived from IRF-3-knockout mice. Although very insightful, these data were obtained following infection of primary mouse cells with adenoviral vectors at a dose of 25,000 virus particles per cell. Clearly, future studies should show how relevant these findings are to the cellular responses to adenovirus in an in vivo setting, where these high viral doses per cell are unlikely to be achieved. Important evidence regarding the involvement of type I IFN in modulating early immune responses to adenoviral vectors comes from a study by Zhu et al. [2007a], who administered adenoviral vectors into type I IFN-receptor knockout mice. This study showed that plasma levels of IL-6 and IL-12 were markedly reduced in type I IFN receptor knockout mice following administration of adenovirus compared to wild-type control animals. Moreover, it was found that adenovirus-induced type I IFNs were critical for both innate and adaptive immune responses against adenoviral vectors in vivo. Functional blockade of type I IFNs in mice diminished both innate and adaptive immune responses to adenovirus, which resulted in more stable transgene expression and reduction of inflammation in vivo [Zhu et al. 2007a].

4.3.3 IL-1

IL-1 is a major pro-inflammatory cytokine involved in activation of inflammatory host responses. Adenovirus infection activates IL-1 in both mice and humans [Ginsberg et al. 1991; Mistchenko et al. 1998]. Administration of replication-deficient adenoviral vectors into the brain of mice resulted in rapid elevation of body temperature, which was associated with markedly elevated levels of IL-6 and IL-1β (up to 300-fold) [Cartmell et al. 1999]. Importantly, pretreatment of mice with IL-1 receptor antagonist completely abolished adenovirus-induced fever, suggesting that IL-1 is a direct mediator of this response. When adenovirus-induced expression of IL-8 in human A549 cells was analyzed in vitro, IL-8 activation could be also blocked by an IL-1 receptor antagonist [Schwarz et al 1999], suggesting that production of this chemokine depends directly on IL-1 receptor signaling. Local activation of endothelial cells is the key event in virus-induced inflammation. Chang et al. [2002] found that Ad37 infection of respiratory and ocular epithelial cells induced production of IL-1α that could rapidly activate intercellular adhesion molecule 1 (ICAM-1, a prominent marker of endothelial cell activation) on human endothelial cells. These data suggest that epithelial cell-derived IL-1α plays an important role in activation of endothelial cells in Ad37-induced inflammation. The data were further corroborated by a study of Holden et al. [2004], who demonstrated that IL-1 can strongly activate both mRNA and protein expression of ICAM-1 in A549 cells, and that this activation is dependent on NF-κB, but not on p38 or

ERK MAPK signaling. In our own studies of adenovirus-induced inflammatory responses upon intravenous vector delivery, we found that IL-1α was the most prominent cytokine activated in liver tissue within 30 minutes of adenovirus administration [Shayakhmetov et al. 2004, 2005]. Also, administration of adenoviral vectors into IL-1 receptor I–knockout mice revealed drastic reduction in the levels of pro-inflammatory cytokine and chemokine gene activation (MIP-2, TNF-α) in the liver compared to those in control animals. Moreover, preinjection of mice with both anti-IL-1α and IL-1β antibodies ameliorated adenovirus-induced hepatotoxicity, suggesting that IL-1 plays a central role in activation of innate immune and inflammatory host responses to adenoviral vectors in vivo [Shayakhmetov et al. 2005].

4.3.4 IL-6

Interleukin (IL)-6 is a pleiotropic cytokine that has important roles in regulation of the immune response, inflammation, and hematopoiesis. IL-6 is produced by various types of cells, including T cells, B cells, monocytes, fibroblasts, keratinocytes, endothelial cells, mesangial cells, and some tumor cells. IL-6 induces T-cell proliferation and cytotoxic-T-cell differentiation, terminal macrophage differentiation, and megakaryocyte differentiation. In the acute phase of the inflammation reaction, IL-6 stimulates hepatocytes to produce acute-phase proteins such as C-reactive protein, fibrinogen, α1-antitrypsin, and serum amyloid A protein, and simultaneously suppresses albumin production. Overexpression of IL-6 also causes leukocytosis and fever in vivo.

There is abundant literature describing the essential role of IL-6 in adenovirus-induced inflammation, both in animal models of disease and in human clinical trials. Along with IL-1 and TNF-α, IL-6 was described as an early cytokine appearing in lung tissue and plasma of mice inoculated with wild-type Ad5 intranasally [Ginsberg et al. 1991]. Elevated levels of IL-6 were also observed in pediatric patients with moderate to severe respiratory disease caused by wild-type adenovirus infection [Mistchenko et al. 1994]. Importantly, the elevated levels of plasma IL-6 were associated with hypoperfusion, febrile peaks, and septic shock. The first clinical trials with recombinant adenoviral vectors encoding the human CFTR gene showed that when bronchial and nasal [epithelium of cystic fibrosis patients were exposed to adenoviral vector, transient systemic and pulmonary syndrome was observed, which is associated with elevated levels of IL-6 [Crystal et al. 1994; McElvaney and Crystal 1995]. When an adenoviral vector was engineered to express IL-6 in rat lungs following intranasal administration, localized IL-6 expression was associated with profound lymphocytic hyperplasia, characterized by the dramatic expansion of peribronchial lymphoid aggregates and massive lymphocytic infiltration in the pulmonary parenchyma [Xing et al. 1994]. Importantly, all of these pathological changes subsided concomitant with the decrease of IL-6 expression. Direct analysis of the cell types in the lung responsible for activation of IL-6 gene transcription revealed that alveolar macrophages, but not airway epithelial or vascular endothelial cells, rapidly trapped adenovirus particles and up-regulated IL-6 gene transcription [Zsengeller et al. 2000]. Elevated levels of IL-6 were also observed upon adenovirus delivery into the bloodstream [Schnell et al. 2001], or cerebral fluid of rats and nonhuman primates [Driesse et al. 2000]. Accumulated data show that elevated IL-6 levels can serve as a prominent and reliable marker of adenovirus-induced inflammation. Indeed, in numerous reported cases of severe toxicity due to adenovirus vector application in vivo, IL-6 was monitored as the key cytokine, associated with exacerbated inflammatory host responses, and its elevated levels were observed in all animal models as well as human clinical trials [Nemunaitis et al. 2001; Schnell et al. 2001; Zhang et al. 2001; Ben-Gary et al. 2002; Lozier et al. 2002; Morral et al. 2002; Varnavski et al. 2002; Raper et al. 2003]. Although there is a clear correlation with severity of adenovirus-induced inflammation and elevated levels of IL-6, the molecular mechanisms and signaling events leading to IL-6 gene activation remain unclear. While elimination of Kupffer cells in the liver with gadolinium chloride results in a more robust systemic IL-6 release following intravascular adenovirus delivery in mice [Lieber et al. 1997], elimination of splenic DCs and macrophages with clodrinate liposomes resulted in marked reduction in levels of IL-6 and other pro-inflammatory cytokines in response to adenovirus administration [Zhang et al. 2001]. In our studies of toxicity of different capsid-modified adenoviral vectors in mice, we found that although Ad5-based vectors interacting with CAR rapidly induced elevated levels of IL-6 in plasma following intravascular delivery, adenoviral vectors with the Ad35-derived fiber knob domain induced an inflammatory response and hepatotoxicity without significant elevation in plasma IL-6 [Shayakhmetov et al. 2004]. Moreover, upon preadministration of either anti-TNF-α or anti-IL-1 antibodies prior to adenovirus delivery, the plasma levels of IL-6 were markedly reduced compared to animals preinjected with control antibody [Shayakhmetov et al. 2005]. These data suggest that IL-6 gene activation is probably a later step in the cascade of adenovirus-induced inflammation, and depends on earlier activation of either TNF-α or IL-1. In agreement with this hypothesis, data obtained in IL-6-knockout animals demonstrate no differences in leukocyte recruitment into liver in response to intravenous adenovirus delivery compared to wild-type animals [Benihoud et al. 2000, 2007], and only a mild decrease in IgG response, suggesting that the IL-6 induction is likely only a sequale of earlier events of viral recognition by the host innate immune system.

4.3.5 IL-8/MIP-2/KC

CXC chemokines macrophage inflammatory protein (MIP)-2 and KC in mice, and the homologous human chemokine IL-8, are the principal chemokines responsible for recruitment of circulating polymorphonuclear lymphocytes to the sites of inflammation. There is sufficient evidence to suggest that these CXC chemokines are the key mediators of tissue injury upon natural adenovirus infection in humans as well as upon in vivo application of adenovirus-based vectors. In both humans and mice, IL-8 and MIP-2/KC are among the most rapidly activated chemokines found at sites of adenovirus infection [Kajon et al. 2003]. In studies of natural adenovirus infection in pediatric patients, plasma levels of IL-8 correlated directly with the severity of pulmonary disease [Mistchenko et al. 1998]. Importantly, in a number of preclinical studies where adenoviral vectors were delivered to the respiratory tract, a rapid MIP-2-chemokine-dependent accumulation of neutrophils in lung parenchyma was observed. Adenoviral vectors delivered intravenously induce acute dose-dependent hepatotoxicity. Studies by Muruve and co-workers demonstrated that liver damage in response to adenovirus infection was due primarily to neutrophil recruitment and accumulation in the liver [Muruve et al. 1999; Zaiss et al. 2002]. Indeed, animal preinjection with anti-MIP-2 antibodies prior to virus administration alleviated liver pathology, thus confirming that tissue injury occurred largely due to chemokine production and neutrophil recruitment [Muruve et al. 1999]. Due to the critical role that CXC chemokines play in the induction of tissue injury following adenovirus infection, significant efforts were made to understand the molecular mechanisms of their gene induction. An early study, Amin et al. [1995] showed that human epithelial A549 cells infected with an adenoviral vector express significantly higher levels of IL-8 than those of mock-infected cells. A further study by Bruder and Kovesdi [1997] revealed that the Raf/MAPK signaling pathway is involved in activation of IL-8 gene transcription following adenovirus infection. Activation of Raf-1 and phosphorylation of p42 MAPK occurred as early as 20 minutes after cell infection with adenovirus, suggesting that activation of this pathway and IL-8 induction may play critical roles in adenovirus-induced inflammation in vivo. Induction of CXC chemokines in vitro was also observed following cell infection with different adenovirus serotypes. Metcalf and colleagues have analyzed the induction on IL-8 in A549 cells following infection with both Ad5 and Ad7 virus serotypes. They found that following infection of these cells with Ad7, IL-8 gene transcription was rapidly up-regulated [Booth and Metcalf 1999]. Again, the Ras/Raf/MEK/Erk pathway was found to be involved in activation of IL-8 gene transcription in response to adenovirus infection [Alcorn et al. 2001; Booth et al. 2004]. Infection of human corneal stromal fibroblasts with Ad19 resulted in rapid up-regulation of IL-8 mRNA by 300- and 1000-fold over mock-infected control cells 4 and 24 hours post-infection, respectively [Chodosh et al. 2000]. Analysis of signaling pathways mediating activation of IL-8 mRNA transcription in response to Ad19 infection showed a critical role of Src and Erk1/2 kinases, since specific inhibitors of these kinases completely blocked IL-8 transcriptional activation [Natarajan et al. 2003]. Although any of the early steps of adenovirus infection, including virus binding to CAR [Tamanini et al. 2006], cellular integrins [Liu et al. 2003], or virus internalization [Wu et al. 2006], were apparently sufficient to trigger signaling cascades activating IL-8 gene transcription, a study by Schwarz et al. [1999] demonstrated that IL-8 activation may, in fact, be downstream of and directly dependent on other early cytokine activation such as IL-1 of TNF-α. In our study on antiadenoviral inflammatory responses in mice following intravenous virus delivery, we found that the levels of MIP-2 mRNA observed in liver 30 minutes post-virus injection were markedly reduced in either TNF-receptor I –or IL-1-receptor I–knockout animals. Moreover, preinjection of mice with anti-IL-1 antibodies prior to adenovirus delivery reduced the levels of MIP-2 gene transcription significantly compared to animals preinjected with control antibody [Shayakhmetov et al. 2005]. Taken together, these data suggest that while a critical role of CXC chemokines in pathogenesis of adenovirus-induced inflammation and tissue injury is clear, the molecular mechanisms responsible for their activation require further investigation.

4.3.6 MCP-1 and IP-10 Chemokines and IL-12: Linking Innate and Adaptive Antiadenoviral Responses

The regulation of leukocyte migration and their activation by chemokines are recognized as potentially important functions in the induction of acute and chronic inflammatory reactions. In response to adenovirus infection, numerous chemokines are produced by cells to attract PMN cells, lymphocytes, and monocytes to the infection site to limit the virus spread, initiate tissue repair, and facilitate priming of cells of the adaptive immune system. In different model systems of adenovirus infection, CCL2 (monocyte chemotactic protein-1, MCP-1) and CXCL10 (IP-10) were the most activated chemokines present in infected tissues and secreted into blood following adenovirus delivery. In a study by Muruve et al., 6 hours after intravenous adenovirus administration, the levels of hepatic MCP-1 and IP-10 mRNA were elevated 25- and 100-fold, respectively, compared to mock-injected animals [Muruve et al. 1999; Zaiss et al. 2002]. Zhang et al. [2003] have found further that adenovirus infection of murine beta cells and pancreatic islets increased expression of multiple chemokines and their receptors, including MCP-1, CCR2, and RANTES. Chintakuntlawar et al. [2007] reported that Ad37 infection of mouse corneas resulted in rapid up-regulation of MCP-1 mRNA expression both 4 and 16 hours following virus delivery. MCP-1 and IP-10 are important chemokines that attract mononuclear cells to the sites of inflammation to facilitate priming of the adaptive immune system and resolve the inflammation. Indeed, upon administration of dexamethasone in mice prior to adenovirus infection, the histopathology scores of the lung were improved significantly, concomitant with reduced levels of MCP-1 and MIP−1α chemokines [Otake et al. 1998]. Overexpression of IP-10 from adenoviral vector in the lungs following intranasal delivery revealed the important roles of this chemokine in the attraction of mononuclear cells and the exacerbation of inflammation [Palmer et al. 1999]. Harvey et al. [2005] reported that IL-10 and related I-TAC chemokines secreted by primary human conjunctival epithelial cells can inactivate Ad5 and Ad3 virus particles directly, suggesting that secretion of these chemokines may have a dual effect: the attraction of leukocytes to the site of infection and the direct inactivation of the virus. Direct adenovirus particle interaction with cellular receptors appears to be sufficient to induce expression of IP-10, since ultraviolet–psoralen-inactivated adenoviral vectors induced identical levels of IP-10 gene expression in mouse renal epithelial cells, as an infectious control virus, expressing a transgene [Borgland et al. 2000]. Further studies revealed that NF-κB activation and ERK1/2 and p38 MAPK kinase signaling are necessary for adenovirus-induced IL-10 gene transcription to occur [Borgland et al. 2000; Tibbles et al. 2002; Liu et al. 2005]. In vitro studies of chemokine gene induction by capsid-modified adenoviral vectors demonstrated that vectors that are unable to bind integrins, due to an RGD motif deletion within the penton base, are deficient at up-regulating chemokine gene expression, suggesting that integrins are likely to trigger the signaling events leading to NF-κB activation and chemokine production following adenovirus infection [Liu et al. 2003]. Similarly, infection of human corneal fibroblasts with Ad19 led to the rapid phosphorylation of mitogen-activated protein kinases MKK7 and JNK, and activation of the transcription factor c-Jun. Specific inhibition of this signaling cascade abolished the transcriptional activation of the MCP-1 chemokine following adenovirus infection [Xiao and Chodosh 2005]. Although both MCP-1 and IP-10 play an important role in the activation of acute inflammatory host responses, they may also affect the type and magnitude of adaptive responses. Specifically, IP-10 was found to play an important role in modulating the generation and trafficking of effector T cells [Dufour et al. 2002], while MCP-1 can differentially alter the development of Th1- and Th2-type responses in vivo [Matsukawa et al. 2000].

IL-12 is a heterodimeric pro-inflammatory cytokine that induces the production of interferon-γ (IFN-γ), which promotes the differentiation of Th1 cells and activation of NK cells [Trinchieri 2003]. Therefore, IL-12 forms a link between innate and adaptive immunity. IL-12 is produced by macrophages and dendritic cells during natural adenovirus infection [Coutelier et al. 1995] as well as in response adenoviral vector delivery in vivo [Peng et al. 2001; Zhang et al. 2001; Shifrin et al. 2005]. Despite elevated levels of IL-12 observed in mouse plasma as early as 6 hours post-adenoviral vector delivery [Zhang et al. 2001], our data suggest that IL-12 is unlikely to be involved in the initiation of antiadenovirus innate host responses [Shayakhmetov et al. 2004, 2005]. Indeed, analysis of chemokine and cytokine gene activation in both liver and spleen revealed that IL-12 p40 mRNA is induced at later time points then are IL-1, TNF-α, MIP-2, and KC. Moreover, IL-12 involvement in modulating adaptive immune responses to intravenously injected adenovirus is likely to be redundant. Specifically, the characteristic IgG2a response to adenovirus infection was unimpaired in IL-12-knockout mice compared to wild-type animals [Xing et al. 2000]. Also, upon adenovirus infection in vitro, lymphocytes from draining lymph nodes and spleens of IL-12-knockout mice secreted levels of IFN-γ comparable to those produced by lymphocytes recovered from wild-type mice. It is noteworthy that in IL-12-knockout animals, the Th1 responses following adenovirus delivery via the respiratory tract were also unaffected, suggesting that other cytokines or chemokines may compensate for the lack of IL-12 in promoting Th1-type lymphocyte differentiation [Xing et al. 2000].

4.4 CLINICAL MANIFESTATIONS OF SEVERE TOXICITY FOLLOWING HIGH-DOSE ADENOVIRAL VECTOR DELIVERY VIA AN INTRAVASCULAR ROUTE

Intravascular delivery of high doses of adenoviral vectors induces acute, systemic, dose-limiting toxicity that can be fatal for the host [Schnell et al. 2001; Morral et al. 2002; Raper et al. 2003; Brunetti-Pierri et al. 2004]. Although the clinical manifestations, time of onset, and pathological changes in studied organs are rather stereotypical, the magnitude of response and severity of damage differ dramatically between species, depending on the applied vector doses. While the adenovirus dose of 1×10^{13} virus particles per kilogram is well tolerated upon intravascular delivery in mice, this dose can cause lethal toxicity in baboons [Morral et al. 2002; Brunetti-Pierri et al. 2004]. Moreover, in a clinical study of adenoviral vector delivery in humans, one patient suffered lethal toxicity upon administration of the much lower dose of 6×10^{11} virus particles per kilogram [Raper et al. 2003]. Importantly, studies in nonhuman primates revealed that the host responses intensify abruptly, and administration of only two-fold lower doses (5×10^{12} virus particles per kilogram) induces responses without major clinical sequelae [Brunetti-Pierri et al. 2004]. One of the earliest biochemical markers indicating a host response to a high-dose adenovirus injection is an elevated level of lactate dehydrogenase (LDH). In baboons given both high and low doses of adenoviral vectors, LDH levels were elevated more that fourfold over baseline within 1 hour of virus delivery [Brunetti-Pierri et al. 2004]. It is worth noting that Manickan et al. [2006] described Kupffer cell death within 10 minutes of a high-dose intravenous injection of adenoviral vector in mice. Thus, it is conceivable that the LDH released from dead Kupffer cells may contribute, at least in part, to the elevated LDH levels observed in baboons. Another hallmark of activation of host responses after intravenous adenovirus delivery is disseminated intravascular coagulation (DIC). Analysis of prothrombin time, activated partial thromboplastin time, and D-dimer levels all revealed a noticeable change between 1 and 2 hours after intravenous adenovirus delivery [Schnell et al. 2001; Brunetti-Pierri et al. 2004]. Importantly, thrombocytopenia was observed after adenovirus administration in all clinical trials and animal disease models when the number of circulating platelets declined significantly as early as 6 hours after adenovirus delivery. However, the most prominent marker of host response activation following adenovirus administration is the activation of pro-inflammatory cytokines and chemokines, which orchestrate the recruitment of circulating leukocytes to infected organs and exacerbate tissue damage. In the case of fatal systemic inflammatory response to intravascular adenovirus delivery during a clinical trial, the markedly elevated levels of IL-6 were found in serum by 4 hours after adenovirus administration [Raper et al. 2003]. Analysis of other cytokines and chemokines revealed that only IL-10 levels were elevated by 48 hours after adenovirus delivery, but levels of TNF-α and IL-8 were not changed significantly compared to a baseline control [Raper et al. 2003; Brunetti-Pierri et al. 2004]. Similar results were found in baboons, where levels of IL-6 were elevated by 1 hour and peaked by 3 hours after intravenous adenovirus delivery [Schnell et al. 2001; Brunetti-Pierri et al. 2004]. The levels of IL-12 were also elevated by 24 hours after adenovirus delivery. Upon necropsy evaluation of adenoviral DNA distribution to the organs, liver and spleen contained the highest amount of virus genomes. These data are consistent with the findings in mice and rats that liver and spleen were the tissues most efficiently transduced by adenoviral vectors after intravenous injection. Taken together, it is clear that after intravascular delivery, adenovirus induces acute and robust innate immune and inflammatory responses. However, it is unclear how specific markers of anti-adenoviral response depend upon each other. Specifically, elimination of Kupffer cells in mice appears to attenuate TNF-α activation and clearance of adenoviral DNA from the liver. However, it has no effect on the early induction and serum levels of IL-6 or IL-12 observed after adenovirus administration. Similarly, adenovirus administration into splenectomized or complement C3-knockout mice does not result in thrombocytopenia, but the molecular mechanisms underlying these findings remain unclear. Moreover, despite the well-documented activation of inflammatory cytokines and chemokines after intravenous adenovirus delivery, the initial events leading to adenovirus recognition by the host as well as temporal regulation and key mediators of inflammatory antiadenoviral cascade remain poorly defined. Indeed, experiments in knockout mice showed that adenovirus-induced inflammation is markedly reduced in all three strains of mice lacking either TNF-RI, IL-1-RI, or IFN-I-R. Clearly, future studies are needed to address these issues comprehensively, since better understanding of innate host responses will aid in developing safe and efficient adenoviral vectors for gene therapy applications.

4.5 ADAPTIVE RESPONSES TO ADENOVIRAL VECTORS

Adenovirus vector delivery in vivo induces strong humoral and cell-mediated immune responses to both the viral capsid proteins and the vector-encoded transgenes. Although the former poses significant limitations for the therapeutic use of adenovirus when repeated vector administration is required, the latter has proven to be beneficial for the induction of immunity to the adenovirus-encoded transgenes when adenovirus is used as a platform for vaccine development.

Following in vivo delivery, adenovirus particles are rapidly cleared by residential tissue macrophages and dendritic cells [Worgall et al. 1997a,b; Zhang et al. 2001]. These principal cells of the innate immune system are professional antigen-presenting cells and the key to activating adaptive immune responses. After adenovirus particle capture, macrophages secrete pro-inflammatory cytokines and chemokines (discussed above) that promote inflammatory host responses and limit systemic dissemination of the virus. Before encountering an antigen, dendritic cells reside in tissues in an "immature" form (iDCs). Adenovirus interaction with iDCs induces their maturation and migration into lymphoid organs, where they present adenovirus-associated antigens to CD4$^+$ T cells in a complex with MHC class II receptors. The direct interaction of mature DCs (mDCs) and CD4$^+$ T cells with simultaneous ligation of antigen-specific T-cell receptor and CD28 receptor provide stimulatory signals for T-cell activation and differentiation. Depending on the panel of cytokines released by mDC upon antigen presentation, CD4$^+$ T cells undergo differentiation into either Th1 or Th2 subtypes. When mDCs produce IL-12, upon presentation of an antigen, CD4$^+$ T cells differentiate into a pro-inflammatory Th1 subtype, which, through secretion of IL-2, IFN-γ, and TNF-α, promote macrophage activation and generation of cytotoxic CD8$^+$ T cells (CTL). CTLs are capable of recognizing adenovirus antigens complexed with MHC class I receptors on antigen-presenting cells or any cell where adenovirus gene expression occurs. Mature DCs and activated CD4$^+$ T cells further induce activation of adenovirus antigen-specific CD8$^+$ T cells, resulting in the generation of effector CTLs which kill cells transduced by adenoviral vectors or expressing the virus-encoded transgene.

To generate antiadenoviral humoral immunity (e.g., the secretion of neutralizing adenovirus-specific antibodies), direct interaction of naive B cells with virus antigens via the B-cell receptor is required. Following this initial interaction, adenovirus is internalized by B cells, processed and presented to Th2 CD4$^+$ T cells. Th2 T cells support virus-specific B-cell activation and differentiation into plasmocytes through secretion of IL-4, IL-5, IL-6, and IL-10 and direct stimulation via a co-stimulatory ligand–receptor interaction. After terminal differentiation, mature plasmocytes secrete adenovirus-specific antibodies, which inactivate adenovirus particles, promote adenovirus clearance, and prevent cell transduction following repeated vector application.

4.5.1 Humoral Immunity to Adenoviral Vectors

A stereotypic set of interactions, described above, leads to activation of adaptive immunity against adenoviral vectors, and the natural host exposure to adenovirus results in a remarkably strong early response and long-lasting immunity. Analysis of antibody prevalence for different adenovirus serotypes in humans populations revealed that from 60 to 90% of adults have neutralizing antibodies to human serotype 5 (Ad5) [Schmitz et al. 1983; Chirmule et al. 1999]. Importantly, Ad5 is the best studied adenovirus serotype, and the vast majority of adenoviral vectors developed and analyzed in preclinical and clinical studies to date are based on this serotype. Clearly, the high prevalence of neutralizing antibodies against Ad5 precludes efficient application of Ad5-based vectors in gene therapy settings which require virus exposure to blood. It is worth noting that the presence of neutralizing antibodies apparently has little effect on adenoviral transduction of localized tumors (upon direct intratumoral injection) or upon vector delivery to "immuno-privileged" sites such as eyes or brain [Bennett et al. 1996; Thomas et al. 2000, 2001; Suber et al. 2001; Bennett 2003]. However, when Ad2 vectors were applied through intrabronchial instillations in rhesus monkeys, all animals developed a significant humoral immune response [Kaplan et al. 1996]. Virus-neutralizing antibodies were detected in the serum and bronchoalveolar lavage of all vector-treated monkeys and included both IgG and secretory IgA, suggesting that host cell exposure to adenovirus activates a wide profile of cytokines, supporting Ig isotype switching. Indeed, Zhu et al. [2007b] have demonstrated that type I IFNs play a critical role in stimulating humoral immune responses to adenoviral vectors in vivo. Specifically, type I IFNs were required for early B-cell activation, germinal center formation, Ig isotype switching, and plasma cell differentiation. Of interest, the signaling of type I IFNs on DCs was required for the production of adenovirus-specific IgM, whereas Ig isotype switching and the formation of neutralizing antibodies required type I IFN signaling on both $CD4^+$ T and B cells.

In vitro analyses of immunological targets for adenovirus-specific neutralizing antibodies revealed that capsid surface proteins (i.e., the hexon, the penton base, and the fiber) are the principal targets of the immune system that enable antibody-mediated virus neutralization. Cryo-electron microscopy analysis of structural aspects of antibody-mediated adenovirus neutralization revealed that 240 molecules of hexon-specific IgG (or one antibody molecule per hexon trimer) were necessary to completely neutralize infectivity of one adenovirus particle in vitro [Varghese et al. 2004]. Those data imply that complete virion coverage with antibody is required for blocking the virus disassembly after internalization into the cell. Similar approaches also revealed that penton-base-specific neutralizing antibodies interact with penton-base proteins within the exposed RGD-containing loop, which is involved in virus binding to cellular integrins [Stewart et al. 1997; Nemerow and Stewart 2001] However, anti-penton-base antibody neutralization is incomplete due to steric hindrance preventing the binding of five Ab molecules to a single adenovirus penton. Adenovirus-neutralizing antibodies against fiber epitopes probably prevent efficient virus interaction with cellular attachment receptors. Importantly, in vivo studies suggest that the neutralizing antibodies against hexon epitopes are largely responsible for virus neutralization, creating a barrier for repeated virus administration in gene therapy settings [Gall et al. 1996; Mastrangeli et al. 1996; Sumida et al. 2004; Schoggins et al. 2005]. Indeed, administration of hexon-modified adenoviral vectors into rhesus monkeys preimmunizied with adenovirus possessing an identical penton base and fiber allows for efficient gene delivery and, thus, escape from adenovirus neutralization in vivo [Roberts et al. 2006].

Although neutralizing antibodies represent clear obstacle for efficient adenovirus transduction, not all adenovirus-specific antibodies found in serum are capable of neutralizing virus infectivity in vitro. Using Western blotting, surface plasmon resonance, and enzyme-linked immunosorbent assays, Perreau and Kremer [2006] have found high levels of nonneutralizing antibodies against canine adenovirus CAV-2 in human plasmas, which possess no neutralizing antibodies against this canine adenovirus. These data provide strong evidence that non-neutralizing antiadenoviral antibodies are likely to be present in human plasma independent of host preexposure to adenovirus. The importance of these nonneutralizing (also called *opsonizing*) antibodies is clearly underappreciated, likely due to low virus neutralizing activity. However, the opsonizing antibodies they may form a bridge between adenovirus particles and cells of the innate immune system, expressing Fc receptors (such as monocytes, neutrophils, etc. [Cotter et al. 2005]), or directly activate components of the complement system and stimulate pro-inflammatory responses [Jiang et al. 2004a,b].

4.5.2 Cellular Immunity to Adenoviral Vectors

Natural adenoviral infections, as well as adenoviral vector administration, induce potent cellular immune responses. The clearance of a natural adenoviral infection is critically dependent on the host's ability to generate $CD8^+$ CTLs, and when this function is impaired, the adenoviral infection may lead to a fatal outcome in humans [Feuchtinger et al. 2006, 2007]. An important consequence of exposure to adenovirus is the generation of memory T cells (T_M), which are maintained at various levels through a person's lifetime. Flomenberg and co-workers found that the C-terminal region of the adenovirus hexon H910-924 represents a dominant epitope that activates $CD4^+$ T-cell responses [Olive et al. 2002]. This epitope is highly conserved among different adenovirus serotypes and is restricted by HLA DP4, the most common class II allele in human populations [Tang et al. 2004]. Accordingly, memory adenovirus-specific $CD4^+$ T cells are detected in peripheral blood mononuclear cells from the majority of healthy adults [Flomenberg et al. 1995]. Leen et al. [2004] have identified five HLA class I–restricted epitopes from other conserved regions of the adenovirus hexon. Three of these epitopes were localized within the N-terminal part of the hexon. Importantly, Tang et al. [2006] have found that $CD8^+$ CTL responses to the penton base and fiber are markedly weaker than the responses to the hexon protein, suggesting that the hexon is a major immunodominant adenovirus capsid protein target for CTLs in healthy adults. The presence of both memory adenovirus-specific $CD4^+$ T cells and $CD8^+$ CTLs is a major obstacle to the use of adenoviral vectors for gene therapy applications when prolonged transgene expression or repeated vector administration is required [Yang et al. 1994a,b]. This is due primarily to the elimination of adenoviral vector-transduced cells that present fragments of both the virus capsid proteins and transgene on the MHC-class I molecules.

Due to the marked conservation of hexon immunodominant epitopes between different human and even animal adenovirus serotypes, the memory $CD4^+$ and $CD8^+$ T cells represent important barriers limiting the utility of adenoviral vectors. Although early studies showed that the sequential administration of adenoviral vectors based on different human adenoviral serotypes can escape preexisting humoral immunity [Vogels et al. 2003], the memory T-cell responses are not easy to overcome. Currently, a number of approaches are being tested to modulate both humoral and cellular antiadenoviral immune responses (reviewed comprehensively by Zhou and Ertl [2006]). Among the most promising are the development of adenoviral vectors based on animal serotypes (chimpanzee or canine adenovirus-based vectors) and transient immunosuppression of the host.

4.6 CONCLUSIONS

Adenoviruses are promising vectors for gene therapy. They are some of the best studied viruses and the most common vectors used in clinical studies worldwide. The principal advantage of adenoviral vectors over other virus-based gene delivery systems is their remarkable capacity to transduce human cells. Virtually all human cell types can be transduced at high efficiency with various serotypes of adenoviral vectors. The major drawback for this vector system, however, is high immunogenicity. During millions of years of coevolution with their hosts, adenoviruses developed an extensive set of immunomodulatory genes that interfere with virus detection by cells of the immune system, thus ensuring their evolutionary survival. However, in gene therapy settings, when large doses (compared to virus doses initiating natural infection) of purified virus particles are delivered via various routes, the host mounts potent innate and adaptive immune responses. These responses are the major obstacle for efficient application of adenoviral vector systems in gene therapy. Despite dramatic progress in understanding the molecular mechanisms responsible for the induction of antiadenoviral inflammatory responses, many questions still need to be answered. Further work is required to better define the sensors of adenovirus in human cells. Moreover, the design and analysis of novel, practical approaches to reducing the activation of inflammation following in vivo adenovirus delivery remain a high-priority task for many gene therapy groups. Although it is clear that there might not be a simple solution to escape antiadenoviral adaptive immunity, novel approaches are currently being tested to evaluate transient immunomodulation or the use of vectors based on nonhuman serotypes for the improvement of the vector performance in vivo. Although adenovirus will undoubtedly remain the vector of choice for many potential gene therapy applications, the realization of its true therapeutic potential and its successful clinical use will continue to be critically dependent on our ability to modulate both adenovirus-induced innate responses and adaptive antiadenoviral immunity.

REFERENCES

Akira S and Takeda K. 2004. Toll-like receptor signalling. *Nat Rev Immunol* 4:499–511.

Alcorn MJ, Booth JL, et al. 2001. Adenovirus type 7 induces interleukin-8 production via activation of extracellular regulated kinase 1/2. *J Virol* 75:6450–6459.

Alexopoulou L, Holt AC, et al. 2001. Recognition of double-stranded RNA and activation of NF-kappa B by Toll-like receptor 3. *Nature* 413:732–738.

Amin R, Wilmott R, et al. 1995. Replication-deficient adenovirus induces expression of interleukin-8 by airway epithelial-cells in-vitro. *Hum Gene Ther* 6:145–153.

Barton GM and Medzhitov R. 2002. Toll-like receptors and their ligands. *Curr Top Microbiol Immunol* 270:81–92.

Basner-Tschakarjan E, Gaffal E, et al. 2006. Adenovirus efficiently transduces plasmacytoid dendritic cells resulting in TLR9-dependent maturation and IFN-alpha production. *J Gene Med* 8:1300–1306.

Ben-Gary H, McKinney RL, et al. 2002. Systemic interleukin-6 responses following administration of adenovirus gene transfer vectors to humans by different routes. *Mol Ther* 6:287–297.

Benihoud K, Saggio I, et al. 1998. Efficient, repeated adenovirus-mediated gene transfer in mice lacking both tumor necrosis factor alpha and lymphotoxin alpha. *J Virol* 72:9514–9525.

Benihoud K, Salone B, et al. 2000. The role of IL-6 in the inflammatory and humoral response to adenoviral vectors. *J Gene Med* 2:194–203.

Benihoud K, Esselin S, et al. 2007. Respective roles of TNF-alpha and IL-6 in the immune response-elicited by adenovirus-mediated gene transfer in mice. *Gene Ther* 14:533–551.

Bennett J. 2003. Immune response following intraocular delivery of recombinant viral vectors. *Gene Ther* 10:977–982.

Bennett J, Pakola S, et al. 1996. Humoral response after administration of E1-deleted adenoviruses: immune privilege of the subretinal space. *Hum Gene Ther* 7:1763–1769.

Bergelson JM. 1999. Receptors mediating adenovirus attachment and internalization. *Biochem Pharmacol* 57:975–959.

Bergelson JM, Cunningham JA, et al. 1997. Isolation of a common receptor for coxsackie B viruses and adenoviruses 2 and 5. *Science* 275:1320–1323.

Bhat NR and Fan F. 2002. Adenovirus infection induces microglial activation: involvement of mitogen-activated protein kinase pathways. *Brain Res* 948:93–101.

Booth JL and Metcalf JP. 1999. Type-specific induction of interleukin-8 by adenovirus. *Am J Respir Cell Mol Biol* 21:521–527.

Booth JL, Coggeshall KM, et al. 2004. Adenovirus type 7 induces interleukin-8 in a lung slice model and requires activation of Erk. *J Virol* 78:4156–4164.

Borgland SL, Bowen GP, et al. 2000. Adenovirus vector-induced expression of the C-X-C chemokine IP-10 is mediated through capsid-dependent activation of NF-kappaB. *J Virol* 74:3941–3947.

Bowen GP, Borgland SL, et al. 2002. Adenovirus vector-induced inflammation: capsid-dependent induction of the C-C chemokine RANTES requires NF-kappa B. *Hum Gene Ther* 13:367–379.

Brakebusch C and Fassler R. 2003. The integrin–actin connection, an eternal love affair. *EMBO J* 22:2324–2333.

Bruder JT and Kovesdi I. 1997. Adenovirus infection stimulates the Raf/MAPK signaling pathway and induces interleukin-8 expression. *J Virol* 71:398–404.

Brunetti-Pierri N, Palmer DJ, et al. 2004. Acute toxicity after high-dose systemic injection of helper-dependent adenoviral vectors into nonhuman primates. *Hum Gene Ther* 15:35–46.

Cartmell T, Southgate T, et al. 1999. Interleukin-1 mediates a rapid inflammatory response after injection of adenoviral vectors into the brain. *J Neurosci* 19:1517–1523.

Cerullo V, Seiler MP, et al. 2007. Toll-like receptor 9 triggers an innate immune response to helper-dependent adenoviral vectors. *Mol Ther* 15:378–385.

Chang CH, Huang Y, et al. 2002. Interleukin-1 alpha released from epithelial cells after adenovirus type 37 infection activates intercellular adhesion molecule 1 expression on human vascular endothelial cells. *J Virol* 76:427–431.

Chintakuntlawar AV, Astley R, et al. 2007. Adenovirus type 37 keratitis in the C57BL/6J mouse. *Invest Ophthalmol Vis Sci* 48:781–788.

Chirmule N, Propert KJ, et al. 1999. Immune responses to adenovirus and adeno-associated virus in humans. *Gene Ther* 6:1574–1583.

Chodosh J, Astley RA, et al. 2000. Adenovirus keratitis: a role for interleukin-8. *Invest Ophthalmol Vis Sci* 41:783–789.

Cotter MJ, Zaiss AK, et al. 2005. Neutrophils interact with adenovirus vectors via Fc receptors and complement receptor 1. *J Virol* 79:14622–14631.

Coutelier JP, Vanbroeck J, et al. 1995. Interleukin-12 gene-expression after viral-infection in the mouse. *J Virol* 69:1955–1958.

Crystal RG, McElvaney NG, et al. 1994. Administration of an adenovirus containing the human CFTR cDNA to the respiratory tract of individuals with cystic fibrosis [see comments]. *Nat Genet* 8:42–51.

Davison E, Diaz RM, et al. 1997. Integrin alpha5beta1-mediated adenovirus infection is enhanced by the integrin-activating antibody TS2/16. *J Virol* 71:6204–6207.

Davison E, Kirby I, et al. 2001. Adenovirus type 5 uptake by lung adenocarcinoma cells in culture correlates with Ad5 fibre binding is mediated by alpha(v)beta1 integrin and can be modulated by changes in beta1 integrin function. *J Gene Med* 3:550–559.

Driesse MJ, Esandi MC, et al. 2000. Intra-CSF administered recombinant adenovirus causes an immune response-mediated toxicity. *Gene Ther* 7:1401–1409.

Dufour JH, Dziejman M, et al. 2002. IFN-gamma-inducible protein 10 (IP-10; CXCL10)-deficient mice reveal a role for IP-10 in effector T cell generation and trafficking. *J Immunol* 168:3195–3204.

Elkon KB, Liu CC, et al. 1997. Tumor necrosis factor alpha plays a central role in immune-mediated clearance of adenoviral vectors. *Proc Nat Acad Sci U S A* 94:9814–9819.

Feuchtinger T, Richard C, et al. 2006. Hexon specific T-cells for adoptive T-cell transfer as a treatment of adenovirus infection after allogeneic stem cell transplantation. *Blood* 108:2853 (ASH Annual Meeting Abstracts).

Feuchtinger T, Lang P, et al. 2007. Adenovirus infection after allogeneic stem cell transplantation. *Leuk Lymphoma* 48:244–255.

Fitzgerald KA, Rowe DC, et al. 2003. LPS-TLR4 signaling to IRF-3/7 and NF-kappa B involves the toll adapters TRAM and TRIF. *J Exp Med* 198:1043–1055.

Flomenberg P, Piaskowski V, et al. 1995. Characterization of human proliferative T-cell responses to adenovirus. *J Infect Dis* 171:1090–1096.

Gaggar A, Shayakhmetov D, et al. 2003. CD46 is a cellular receptor for group B adenoviruses. *Nat Med* 9:1408–1412.

Gall J, KassEisler A, et al. 1996. Adenovirus type 5 and 7 capsid chimera: Fiber replacement alters receptor tropism without affecting primary immune neutralization epitopes. *J Virol* 70:2116–2123.

Ginsberg HS, Moldawer LL, et al. 1991. A mouse model for investigating the molecular pathogenesis of adenovirus pneumonia. *Proc Natl Acad Sci U S A* 88:1651–1655.

Hartman ZC, Black EP, et al. 2007a. Adenoviral infection induces a multi-faceted innate cellular immune response that is mediated by the Toll-like receptor pathway in A549 cells. *Virology* 358:357–372.

Hartman ZC, Kiang A, et al. 2007b. Adenovirus infection triggers a rapid, MyD88-regulated transcriptome response critical to acute-phase and adaptive immune responses in vivo. *J Virol* 81:1796–1812.

Harvey SAK, Romanowski EG, et al. 2005. Adenovirus-directed ocular innate immunity: the role of conjunctival defensin-like chemokines (IP-10, I-TAC) and phagocytic human defensin-alpha. *Invest Ophthalmol Vis Sci* 46:3657–3665.

Hemmi H, Takeuchi O, et al. 2000. A Toll-like receptor recognizes bacterial DNA. *Nature* 408:740–745.

Holden NS, Catley MC, et al. 2004. ICAM-1 expression is highly NF-kappa B–dependent in A549 cells: no role for ERK and p38 MAPK. *Eur J Biochem* 271:785–791.

Huang S, Kamata T, et al. 1996. Adenovirus interaction with distinct integrins mediates separate events in cell entry and gene delivery to hematopoietic cells. *J Virol* 70:4502–4508.

Iacobelli-Martinez M and Nemerow GR. 2007. Preferential activation of Toll-like receptor nine by CD46-utilizing adenoviruses. *J Virol* 81:1305–1312.

Iacobelli-Martinez M, Nepomuceno RR, et al. 2005. CD46-utilizing adenoviruses inhibit C/EBP beta-dependent expression of proinflammatory cytokines. *J Virol* 79:11259–11268.

Isaacs A and Lindenmann J. 1957. Virus interference: 1. The interferon. *Proc R Soc London Ser B Biol Sci* 147:258–267.

Jiang HX, Wang Z, et al. 2004a. Recombinant adenovirus vectors activate the alternative complement pathway, leading to the binding of human complement protein C3 independent of anti-Ad antibodies. *Mol Ther* 10:1140–1142.

Jiang HX, Everett R, et al. 2004b. Ad interactions with the complement systems of humans and mice. *Mol Ther* 9:S387–S388.

Kajon AE, Gigliotti AP, et al. 2003. Acute inflammatory response and remodeling of airway epithelium after subspecies B1 human adenovirus infection of the mouse lower respiratory tract. *J Med Virol* 71:233–244.

Kaplan JM, St George JA, et al. 1996. Humoral and cellular immune responses of non-human primates to long-term repeated lung exposure to Ad2/CFTR-2. *Gene Ther* 3:117–127.

Kojaoghlanian T, Flomenberg P, et al. 2003. The impact of adenovirus infection on the immunocompromised host. *Rev Med Virol* 13:155–171.

Krug A, French AR, et al. 2004. TL-139-dependent recognition of MCMV by IPC and DC generates coordinated cytokine responses that activate antiviral NK cell function. *Immunity* 21:107–119.

Leen AM, Sili U, et al. 2004. Conserved CTL epitopes on the adenovirus hexon protein expand subgroup cross-reactive and subgroup-specific CD8(+) T cells. *Blood* 104:2432–2440.

Li E, Stupack D, et al. 1998a. Adenovirus endocytosis requires actin cytoskeleton reorganization mediated by Rho family GTPases. *J Virol* 72:8806–8812.

Li E, Stupack DG, et al. 1998b. Adenovirus cell entry requires the Rho family of small GTPases. *Mol Biol Cell* 9:344A–344A.

Li E, Stupack DG, et al. 2000. Association of p130CAS with phosphatidylinositol-3-OH kinase mediates adenovirus cell entry. *J Biol Chem* 275:14729–14735.

Li E, Brown SL, et al. 2001. Integrin alpha(v)beta1 is an adenovirus coreceptor. *J Virol* 75:5405–5409.

Lieber A, He CY, et al. 1997. The role of Kupffer cell activation and viral gene expression in early liver toxicity after infusion of recombinant adenovirus vectors. *J Virol* 71:8798–8807.

Lieber A, He CY, et al. 1998. Inhibition of NF-kappaB activation in combination with bcl-2 expression allows for persistence of first-generation adenovirus vectors in the mouse liver. *J Virol* 72:9267–9277.

Liu Q and Muruve DA. 2003. Molecular basis of the inflammatory response to adenovirus vectors. *Gene Ther* 10:935–940.

Liu Q, Zaiss AK, et al. 2003. The role of capsid–endothelial interactions in the innate immune response to adenovirus vectors. *Hum Gene Ther* 14:627–643.

Liu Q, White LR, et al. 2005. Akt/protein kinase B activation by adenovirus vectors contributes to NF kappa B-dependent CXCL10 expression. *J Virol* 79:14507–14515.

Lozier JN, Csako G, et al. 2002. Toxicity of a first-generation adenoviral vector in rhesus macaques. *Hum Gene Ther* 13:113–124.

Manickan E, Smith JS, et al. 2006. Rapid Kupffer cell death after intravenous injection of adenovirus vectors. *Mol Ther* 13:108–117.

Mastrangeli A, Harvey BG, et al. 1996. "Sero-switch" adenovirus-mediated in vivo gene transfer: circumvention of anti-adenovirus humoral immune defenses against repeat adenovirus vector administration by changing the adenovirus serotype. *Hum Gene Ther* 7:79–87.

Matsukawa A, Lukacs NW, et al. 2000. Adenoviral-mediated overexpression of monocyte chemoattractant protein-1 differentially alters the development of Th1 and Th2 type responses in vivo. *J Immunol* 164:1699–1704.

McElvaney NG and Crystal RG. 1995. IL-6 release and airway administration of human Cftr Cdna adenovirus vector. *Nat Med* 1:182–184.

Meier O and Greber UF. 2003. Adenovirus endocytosis. *J Gene Med* 5:451–462.

Metcalf JP. 1996. Adenovirus E1A 13S gene product upregulates tumor necrosis factor gene. *Am J Physiol Lung Cell Mol Physiol* 14:L535–L540.

Miggin SM and O'Neill LAJ. 2006. New insights into the regulation of TLR signaling. *J Leukocyte Biol* 80:220–226.

Mistchenko AS, Diez RA, et al. 1994. Cytokines in adenoviral disease in children: association of interleukin-6, interleukin-8, and tumor necrosis factor alpha levels with clinical outcome. *J Pediatr* 124:714–720.

Mistchenko AS, Robaldo JF, et al. 1998. Fatal adenovirus infection associated with new genome type. *J Med Virol* 54:233–236.

Morral N, O'Neal WK, et al. 2002. Lethal toxicity, severe endothelial injury, and a threshold effect with high doses of an adenoviral vector in baboons. *Hum Gene Ther* 13:143–154.

Muruve DA, Barnes MJ, et al. 1999. Adenoviral gene therapy leads to rapid induction of multiple chemokines and acute neutrophil-dependent hepatic injury in vivo. *Hum Gene Ther* 10:965–976.

Natarajan K, Rajala MS, et al. 2003. Corneal IL-8 expression following adenovirus infection is mediated by c-Src activation in human corneal fibroblasts. *J Immunol* 170:6234–6243.

Nemerow GR. 2000. Cell receptors involved in adenovirus entry. *Virology* 274:1–4.

Nemerow GR and Stewart PL. 1999. Role of alpha(v) integrins in adenovirus cell entry and gene delivery. *Microbiol Mol Biol Rev* 63:725–734.

Nemerow GR and Stewart PL. 2001. Antibody neutralization epitopes and integrin binding sites on nonenveloped viruses. *Virology* 288:189–191.

Nemunaitis J, Cunningham C, et al. 2001. Intravenous infusion of a replication-selective adenovirus (ONYX-015) in cancer patients: safety, feasibility and biological activity. *Gene Ther* 8:746–759.

Nociari M, Ocheretina O, et al. 2007. Sensing infection by adenovirus: Toll-like receptor-independent viral DNA recognition signals activation of the interferon regulatory factor 3 master regulator. *J Virol* 81:4145–4157.

Olive M, Eisenlohr L, et al. 2002. The adenovirus capsid protein hexon contains a highly conserved human CD4(+) T-cell epitope. *Hum Gene Ther* 13:1167–1178.

Otake K, Ennist DL, et al. 1998. Nonspecific inflammation inhibits adenovirus-mediated pulmonary gene transfer and expression independent of specific acquired immune responses. *Hum Gene Ther* 9:2207–2222.

Palmer K, Emtage PCR, et al. 1999. Transient gene transfer of non-ELR chemokines to rodent lung induces mononuclear cell accumulation and activation. *J Interferon Cytokine Res* 19:1381–1390.

Pasare C and Medzhitov R. 2004. Toll-like receptors: linking innate and adaptive immunity. *Microbes Infect* 6:1382–1387.

Peng YF, Falck-Pedersen E, et al. 2001. Variation in adenovirus transgene expression between BALB/c and C57BL/6 mice is associated with differences in interleukin-12 and gamma interferon production and NK cell activation. *J Virol* 75:4540–4550.

Perreau M and Kremer EJ. 2006. The conundrum between immunological memory to adenovirus and their use as vectors in clinical gene therapy. *Mol Biotechnol* 34:247–256.

Perreau M, Mennechet F, et al. 2007. Contrasting effects of human, canine, and hybrid adenovirus vectors on the phenotypical and functional maturation of human dendritic cells: implications for clinical efficacy. *J Virol* 81:3272–3284.

Pitkaranta A and Hovi T. 1993. Induction of interferon in human-leukocyte cultures by natural pathogenic respiratory viruses. *J Interferon Res* 13:423–426.

Raper SE, Chirmule N, et al. 2003. Fatal systemic inflammatory response syndrome in a ornithine transcarbamylase deficient patient following adenoviral gene transfer. *Mol Genet Metab* 80:148–158.

Rea D, Havenga MJ, et al. 2001. Highly efficient transduction of human monocyte-derived dendritic cells with subgroup B fiber-modified adenovirus vectors enhances transgene-encoded antigen presentation to cytotoxic T cells. *J Immunol* 166:5236–5244.

Ritzenthaler JD and Roman J. 2001. Interleukin-1beta gene transcription in U937 cells is modulated by type I collagen and cytoskeletal integrity via distinct signaling pathways. *J Interferon Cytokine Res* 21:105–116.

Roberts DM, Nanda A, et al. 2006. Hexon-chimaeric adenovirus serotype 5 vectors circumvent pre-existing anti-vector immunity. *Nature* 441:239–243.

Roelvink PW, Lizonova A, et al. 1998. The coxsackievirus–adenovirus receptor protein can function as a cellular attachment protein for adenovirus serotypes from subgroups A, C, D, E, and F. *J Virol* 72:7909–7915.

Roelvink PW, Mi Lee G, et al. 1999. Identification of a conserved receptor-binding site on the fiber proteins of CAR-recognizing adenoviridae. *Science* 286:1568–1571.

Roman J, Ritzenthaler JD, et al. 1999. Differential modes of regulation of interleukin-1beta expression by extracellular matrices. *Immunology* 98:228–237.

Roman J, Ritzenthaler JD, et al. 2000. Transcriptional regulation of the human interleukin 1beta gene by fibronectin: role of protein kinase C and activator protein 1 (AP-1). *Cytokine* 12:1581–1596.

Ruuskanen O MO and Akusjarvi G. 2002. Adenoviruses. In *Clinical Virology*, 2nd ed., Richman DD, et al. eds. ASM Press, Washington, DC, pp. 515–534.

Sakurai F, Akitomo K, et al. 2007. Downregulation of human CD46 by adenovirus serotype 35 vectors. *Gene Ther* 14:912–919.

Schmitz H, Wigand R, et al. 1983. Worldwide epidemiology of human adenovirus infections. *Am J Epidemiol* 117:455–466.

Schnell MA, Zhang Y, et al. 2001. Activation of innate immunity in nonhuman primates following intraportal administration of adenoviral vectors. *Mol Ther* 3:708–722.

Schoggins JW and Falck-Pedersen E. 2006. Fiber and penton base capsid modifications yield diminished adenovirus type 5 transduction and proinflammatory gene expression with retention of antigen-specific humoral immunity. *J Virol* 80:10634–10644.

Schoggins JW, Nociari M, et al. 2005. Influence of fiber detargeting on adenovirus-mediated innate and adaptive immune activation. *J Virol* 79:11627–11637.

Schwarz YA, Amin RS, et al. 1999. Interleukin-1 receptor antagonist inhibits interleukin-8 expression in A549 respiratory epithelial cells infected in vitro with a replication-deficient recombinant adenovirus vector. *Am J Resp Cell Mol Biol* 21:388–394.

Segerman A, Atkinson JP, et al. 2003. Adenovirus type 11 uses CD46 as a cellular receptor. *J Virol* 77:9183–9191.

Shayakhmetov DM, Li ZY, et al. 2003. The interaction between the fiber knob domain and the cellular attachment receptor determines the intracellular trafficking route of adenoviruses. *J Virol* 77:3712–723.

Shayakhmetov DM, Li ZY, et al. 2004. Analysis of adenovirus sequestration in the liver, transduction of hepatic cells, and innate toxicity after injection of fiber-modified vectors. *J Virol* 78:5368–7381.

Shayakhmetov DM, Li ZY, et al. 2005. Interference with the IL-1-signaling pathway improves the toxicity profile of systemically applied adenovirus vectors. *J Immunol* 174:7310–7319.

Shifrin AL, Chirmule N, et al. 2005. Innate immune responses to adenoviral vector-mediated acute pancreatitis. *Pancreas* 30:122–129.

Stewart PL, Chiu CY, et al. 1997. Cryo-EM visualization of an exposed RGD epitope on adenovirus that escapes antibody neutralization. *EMBO J* 16:1189–1198.

Suber ML, Hurwitz MY, et al. 2001. Immune consequences of intraocular administration of modified adenoviral vectors. *Hum Gene Ther* 12:833–838.

Sumida SM, Truitt DM, et al. 2004. Neutralizing antibodies and $CD8^+$ T lymphocytes both contribute to immunity to adenovirus serotype 5 vaccine vectors. *J Virol* 78:2666–2673.

Suomalainen M, Nakano MY, et al. 2001. Adenovirus-activated PKA and p38/MAPK pathways boost microtubule-mediated nuclear targeting of virus. *EMBO J* 20:1310–1319.

Takaoka A, Wang Z, et al. 2007. DAI (DLM-1/ZBP1) is a cytosolic DNA sensor and an activator of innate immune response. *Nature* 448:501–514.

Tamanini A, Rolfini R, et al. 2003. MAP kinases and NF-kappaB collaborate to induce ICAM-1 gene expression in the early phase of adenovirus infection. *Virology* 307:228–242.

Tamanini A, Nicolis E, et al. 2006. Interaction of adenovirus type 5 fiber with the coxsackievirus and adenovirus receptor activates inflammatory response in human respiratory cells. *J Virol* 80:11241–11254.

Tang J, Olive M, et al. 2004. Adenovirus hexon T-cell epitope is recognized by most adults and is restricted by HLA DP4, the most common class II allele. *Gene Ther* 11:1408–1415.

Tang J, Olive M, et al. 2006. Human $CD8^+$ cytotoxic T cell responses to adenovirus capsid proteins. *Virology* 350:312–322.

Thomas CE, Schiedner G, et al. 2000. Peripheral infection with adenovirus causes unexpected long-term brain inflammation in animals injected intracranially with first-generation, but not with high-capacity, adenovirus vectors: toward realistic long-term neurological gene therapy for chronic diseases. *Proc Nat Acad Sci U S A* 97:7482–7487.

Thomas CE, Schiedner G, et al. 2001. Preexisting antiadenoviral immunity is not a barrier to efficient and stable transduction of the brain, mediated by novel high-capacity adenovirus vectors. *Hum Gene Ther* 12:839–846.

Tibbles LA, Spurrell JC, et al. 2002. Activation of p38 and ERK signaling during adenovirus vector cell entry lead to expression of the C-X-C chemokine IP-10. *J Virol* 76:1559–1568.

Tomko RP, Xu R, et al. 1997. HCAR and MCAR: the human and mouse cellular receptors for subgroup C adenoviruses and group B coxsackieviruses. *Proc Natl Acad Sci U S A* 94:3352–3356.

Trinchieri G. 2003. Interleukin-12 and the regulation of innate resistance and adaptive immunity. *Nat Rev Immunol* 3:133–146.

Varghese R, Mikyas Y, et al. 2004. Postentry neutralization of adenovirus type 5 by an antihexon antibody. *J Virol* 78:12320–12332.

Varnavski AN, Zhang Y, et al. 2002. Preexisting immunity to adenovirus in rhesus monkeys fails to prevent vector-induced toxicity. *J Virol* 76:5711–5719.

Vogels R, Zuijdgeest D, et al. 2003. Replication-deficient human adenovirus type 35 vectors for gene transfer and vaccination: efficient human cell infection and bypass of preexisting adenovirus immunity. *J Virol* 77:8263–8271.

Wang X and Bergelson JM. 1999. Coxsackievirus and adenovirus receptor cytoplasmic and transmembrane domains are not essential for coxsackievirus and adenovirus infection. *J Virol* 73:2559–2562.

Wickham TJ, Mathias P, et al. 1993. Integrins alpha v beta 3 and alpha v beta 5 promote adenovirus internalization but not virus attachment. *Cell* 73:309–319.

Worgall S, Leopold PL, et al. 1997a. Role of alveolar macrophages in rapid elimination of adenovirus vectors administered to the epithelial surface of the respiratory tract. *Hum Gene Ther* 8:1675–1684.

Worgall S, Wolff G, et al. 1997b. Innate immune mechanisms dominate elimination of adenoviral vectors following in vivo administration. *Hum Gene Ther* 8:37–44.

Wu WX, Booth JL, et al. 2006. Calcium-dependent viral internalization is required for adenovirus type 7 induction of IL-8 protein. *Virology* 355:18–29.

Xiao JN and Chodosh J. 2005. JNK regulates MCP-1 expression in adenovirus type 19-infected human corneal fibroblasts. *Invest Ophthalmol Vis Sci* 46:3777–3782.

Xing Z, Braciak T, et al. 1994. Adenovirus-mediated cytokine gene-transfer at tissue sites: overexpression of IL-6 induces lymphocytic hyperplasia in the lung. *J Immunol* 153:4059–4069.

Xing Z, Zganiacz A, et al. 2000. IL-12-independent Th1-type immune responses to respiratory viral infection: requirement of IL-18 for IFN-gamma release in the lung but not for the differentiation of viral-reactive Th1-type lymphocytes. *J Immunol* 164:2575–2584.

Yang YP, Ertl HCJ, et al. 1994a. Mhc class I-restricted cytotoxic T-lymphocytes to viral-antigens destroy hepatocytes in mice infected with E1-deleted recombinant adenoviruses. *Immunity* 1:433–442.

Yang YP, Nunes FA, et al. 1994b. Cellular-immunity to viral-antigens limits E1-deleted adenoviruses for gene-therapy. *Proc Nat Acad Sci U S A* 91:4407–4411.

Yurochko AD, Liu DY, et al. 1992. Integrins as a primary signal transduction molecule regulating monocyte immediate-early gene induction. *Proc Natl Acad Sci U S A* 89:9034–9038.

Zaiss AK, Liu Q, et al. 2002. Differential activation of innate immune responses by adenovirus and adeno-associated virus vectors. *J Virol* 76:4580–4590.

Zhang HG, Zhou T, et al. 1998. Inhibition of tumor necrosis factor alpha decreases inflammation and prolongs adenovirus gene expression in lung and liver. *Hum Gene Ther* 9:1875–1884.

Zhang N, Schroppel B, et al. 2003. Adenovirus transduction induces expression of multiple chemokines and chemokine receptors in murine beta cells and pancreatic islets. *Am J Transplantation* 3:1230–1241.

Zhang Y, Chirmule N, et al. 2001. Acute cytokine response to systemic adenoviral vectors in mice is mediated by dendritic cells and macrophages. *Mol Ther* 3:697–707.

Zhou DM and Ertl HCJ. 2006. Therapeutic potential of adenovirus as a vaccine vector for chronic virus infections. *Expert Opin Biol Ther* 6:63–72.

Zhu JG, Huang XP, et al. 2007a. Innate immune response to adenoviral vectors is mediated by both Toll-like receptor-dependent and -independent pathways. *J Virol* 81:3170–3180.

Zhu JG, Huang XP, et al. 2007b. Type IIFN signaling on both B and CD4T cells is required for protective antibody response to adenovirus. *J Immunol* 178:3505–3510.

Zsengeller Z, Otake K, et al. 2000. Internalization of adenovirus by alveolar macrophages initiates early proinflammatory signaling during acute respiratory tract infection. *J Virol* 74:9655–9667.

5

IMMUNE RESPONSE TO LENTIVIRAL VECTORS

LUNG-JI CHANG, PH.D.

Department of Molecular Genetics and Microbiology, University of Florida, Gainesville, Florida

5.1 INTRODUCTION: LENTIVIRAL VECTORS FOR GENE DELIVERY

Traditional retroviral vectors derived from oncogenic murine leukemia virus have been used in multiple clinical trials treating genetic disorders and cancer [Klatzmann et al. 1998; Gaspar and Thrasher 2005; Parney et al. 2006; Schwarzwaelder et al. 2007]. Onco-retroviral vectors have known limitations, however, including lack of nuclear entry in nondividing (quiescent) cells and preferred integration into a promoter region, resulting in uncontrolled cellular gene activation. In a clinical trial for X-linked severe combined immunodeficiency (SCID-X1), ex vivo transduction of $CD34^+$ hematopoietic stem cells with onco-retroviral vectors expressing gamma chain (γc) gene has successfully corrected the deficiency in more than 10 pediatric patients [Hacein-Bey-Abina et al. 2002]. However, several patients unexpectedly developed T-cell clonal expansion leading to leukemia. Further investigation indicates that the onco-retroviral vectors specifically integrated into chromosomal locations adjacent to the LMO2

Gene Therapy Immunology, Edited by Roland Herzog

proto-oncogene promoter, which led to aberrant transcription and expression of LMO2 [Hacein-Bey-Abina et al. 2003; Berns 2004]. This high leukemic frequency after onco-retroviral gene transfer into hematopoietic cells highlights the importance of understanding safety profiles of gene transfer vectors prior to clinical applications.

Lentiviral vectors (LVs), on the other hand, are becoming more popular than onco-retroviral vectors because LVs can efficiently target slowly dividing and nondividing cells [Verma and Somia 1997; Buchschacher and Wong-Staal 2000; Chang and Gay 2001] and display increased transgene expression with longer-term stability [Zaiss et al. 2002].

The most studied LVs are derived from proviral DNA of human immunodeficiency virus type 1 (HIV-1). Unlike onco-retroviruses, HIV-1 has not been linked directly to cancer, although in AIDS patients, all of the infected cells contain randomly integrated provirus(es). Even when AIDS patients develop oncogenic malignancies after reactivation of dormant transforming viruses, such as human papilloma virus, Epstein–Barr virus, or human herpes virus, integration by HIV-1 has not been associated with cellular abnormality. In a rare incidence, HIV-1 provirus was found in non-Hodgkin's lymphoma cells of an AIDS patient without a diagnosis of alternative viral etiology; however, no evidence could connect the cancer malignancy to HIV-1 integration [Herndier et al. 1992].

Gene transfer into developing fetuses may present a different picture. Themis et al. report that LVs derived from equine infectious anemia virus, but not HIV-1, are associated with a high incidence of hepatoma in mice after neonatal gene transfer [Themis et al. 2005]. The molecular mechanism behind equine infectious anemia virus vector-associated liver oncogenesis has not been resolved.

Accumulated evidence now supports the idea that integration of HIV-1-derived LVs does not lead to cancer, and LVs apparently have safer integration profiles than those of onco-retroviral vectors [Bushman 2007; Cattoglio et al. 2007].

5.2 IMMUNE RESPONSE TO LENTIVIRAL VECTORS

Host immune response may affect the efficacy and safety of gene transfer vectors. Genes and viral proteins in the vectors can both contribute to host immune reactivity. For LV preparation, the replication-defective viral RNA genomes are assembled within viral Gag and Pol proteins and pseudotyped with vesicular stomatitis virus G envelope proteins, and these virion-associated proteins are therefore part of the delivery vehicles. Earlier generations of LVs carry some of the viral genes, which are expressed after transduction and can potentially induce a cellular immune response. In later improved LV systems, all of the lentiviral genes and some regulatory sequences, including a viral promoter in the long terminal repeat (LTR), are deleted from the vector backbone [Zufferey et al. 1998; Cui et al. 1999; Iwakuma et al. 1999]. These advanced LVs do not encode any viral proteins, and all viral components required for vector function are encoded by helper constructs provided in trans [Naldini and Verma 2000;

Chang and Gay 2001]. Ex vivo application of LV-transduced cells or transgene products is unlikely to trigger an antiviral response due to the absence of viral proteins (Fig. 5-1, ex vivo applications). However, direct in vivo injection of LVs may trigger a T-helper response via class II major histocompatibility complex (MHC class II) and a humoral immune response to the viral proteins. The strength of the host immune response is in direct correlation with the amount of the vector injected and the location of injection. Cross-presentation of exogenous antigens through the MHC class I pathway can induce a CD8 cytotoxic T-cell response, and ready access of professional antigen presentation cells may further promote a strong antivector immunity (Fig. 5-1, in vivo applications).

Although viral proteins, such as Gag, Pol, Tat, and Rev, are present in only minute amounts in vector particles, professional antigen-presenting cells such as dendritic cells (DCs) may efficiently process and present the viral antigens through the MHC class II pathway or cross-presented via the MHC class I pathway (Fig. 5-1) [Yewdell et al. 1999; Buseyne et al. 2001]. In fact, defective HIV-1 particles are able to prime DCs to induce an MHC class I–restricted, HIV-specific CD8 cytotoxic T-cell response [Buseyne et al. 2001]. Moreover, transduction of DCs with an improved version of self-inactivating LVs can induce a primary immune response against viral antigens, apparently by processing the minute amount of viral proteins in the vector particles. The latter has been demonstrated by co-culturing LV-transduced DCs with autologous T cells, and detecting primary CD4 and CD8 T cell response specific to HIV-1 Gag and Pol proteins [Chen et al. 2006]. Therefore, in vivo injection of LVs may prime antigen presentation cells and induce a primary CD4 and CD8 T-cell response, in addition to the activation of an innate immune response (Fig. 5-1).

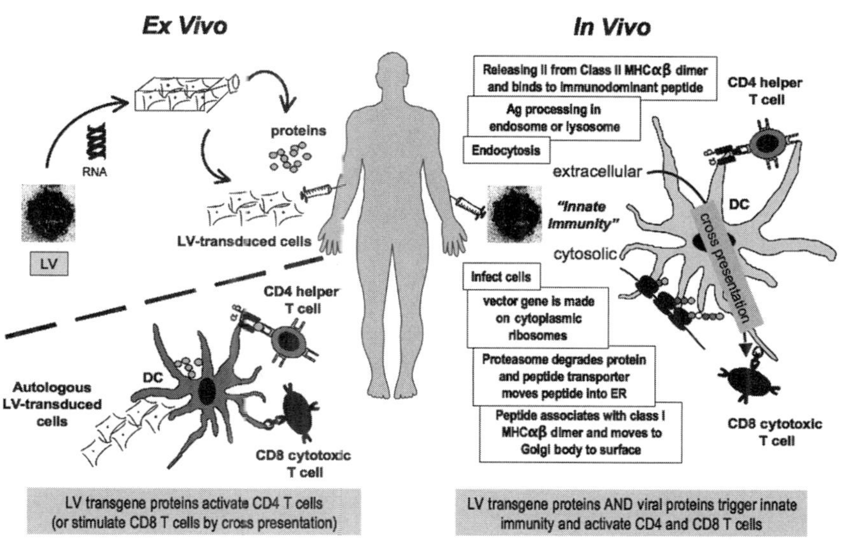

Figure 5-1 In vivo and ex vivo lentiviral vector–mediated host immunity.

TABLE 5-1 In Vivo Analysis of Lentiviral Vector Immunity

Tissue Target	Delivery Method	Immune Response	Reference
Monkey brain	Local injection	Negative	Kordower et al. [2000]
Cat eye	Local injection	Negative	Khare et al. [2007]
Rat Brain	Local injection	Negative	Naldini et al. [1996]
Rat liver and muscle	Local injection	Negative	Kafri et al. [1997]
Mouse in utero	Yolk sac vessel	Negative	Han et al. [2007]
Mouse eye	Local injection	Negative	Bemelmans et al. [2006]
Mouse thymus	Intrathymic	Negative	Marodon et al. [2006]
Mouse neonatal	Intravenous injection	Negative	Carbonaro et al. [2006]

While transduction of DCs with LVs can induce a primary immune response to vector-associated proteins, there has been limited evidence of host anti-LV immunity in vivo (see examples in Table 5-1). In a Parkinson's disease model, LV delivery of glial cell–derived neurotrophic factor (GDNF) into the brains of rhesus monkeys has prevented nigrostriatal degeneration for several months with little to no immune response found against the vectors [Kordower et al. 2000]. The absence of antivector immunity in monkey brains could be due to reduced cellular immunity in this immune-privileged organ.

In contrast, lentiviral gene transfer into mouse livers lacks long-term gene transfer efficacy, which is due to activation of cellular immunity and clearance of the transgene-modified cells [Brown et al. 2007b]. It appears that an adverse immunity is induced by off-target lentiviral transduction of hematopoietic cells (antigen-presenting cells) in the liver; specific suppression of vector RNA in hematopoietic lineage of cells by inserting a hematopoietic-specific micro-RNA target sequence in the vector genome effectively abrogates this host antitransgene effect [Brown et al. 2007a]. Alternatively, LVs can be engineered with increased target specificity by pseudotyping with tissue-specific envelope proteins and/or carrying a tissue-specific promoter to diminish possible off-target gene delivery [Han et al. 2007; Pariente et al. 2007].

5.3 MODULATION OF DENDRITIC CELL IMMUNITY WITH LENTIVIRAL VECTORS

DCs are key antigen-presenting cells in the development of an immune response [Steinman 1991; Banchereau and Steinman 1998; Mellman and Steinman 2001]. Several thousands of patients have entered clinical trials employing DC therapies, yet only limited success has been attained [Ridgway 2003]. The reason is that most patients have experienced a high load of pathogenic antigens: for example, high viral load in HIV patients and high cancer burden in late-stage cancer patients. These patients' immune systems would have been highly tolerized toward the disease antigens and may also display defective DC functions. Modification of DC or its precursors may overcome this problem [Girolomoni and Ricciardi-Castagnoli 1997; van Schooten et al. 1997; Toes et al. 1998; Lanzavecchia and Sallusto 2001].

Various approaches that have been used to modify DC functions include applications with biological molecules such as inactivated bacteria, cytokines, chemokines, Toll-like receptor ligands, and ligands of signaling pathways known to mediate immune interactions [Miller et al. 1998; Pulendran et al. 2001]. These exogenous factors may not effectively correct a defective DC's function, however. Intracellular modification of DC or its precursors with genetic tools, on the other hand, may overcome such an intrinsic defect of DCs [Wan et al. 2000; Chen et al. 2004; Gabrilovich 2004; Breckpot et al. 2007].

Many studies have reported efficient lentiviral transduction of immature DCs and bone marrow $CD34^+$ cells without altering their functions [Chinnasamy et al. 2000; Gruber et al. 2000; Schroers et al. 2000; Chang and Gay 2001; Dyall et al. 2001]. However, careful analysis of phenotypes and T-cell activation functions of DCs after lentiviral transduction indicates that lentiviral transduction can down-regulate DC immunity [Chen et al. 2004; Tan et al. 2005]. The immediate effect of lentiviral transduction of DCs includes down-regulation of surface expression of CD1a, CD80, CD86, ICAM-1, and DC-SIGN, or intracellular up-regulation of indoleamine 2,3-dioxygenase enzyme which suppresses T-cell activities. Some of these surface markers are co-stimulatory molecules essential to activation of T cells. As a result, DC-mediated Th1 effector functions are down-regulated after lentiviral gene transfer. This immunological downturn, however, may be reversed through lentiviral delivery of Th1 regulators into DCs such as interleukin-12, interferon-γ, indoleamine 2,3-dioxygenase enzyme, or small interfering RNAs suppressing interleukin-10. Immune modification of DCs with LVs encoding these immune modulatory molecules effectively up-regulates Th1 effector functions [Chen et al. 2004; Tan et al. 2005].

Lentiviral integration into DC endows prolonged antigen presentation with extended antigenic memory and increased activation potential, which results in enhanced effector functions and memory differentiation of T cells. Sustained antigen signaling from activated DCs to T cells is essential to the development of a long-lasting immunity, which is assisted in part by the expansion of a MHC class II–restricted memory T-cell response. Obst et al. [2007] have demonstrated increased CD4 T-cell priming and expansion in vivo by enforcing persistent antigen presentation on DCs. The potential of lentiviral modification of DC functions is unlimited. For examples, over-expression of anti-apoptotic genes or chaperone genes in DCs with LVs can prolong DC survival with increased antigen processing efficiency and MHC-peptide stability [Shi et al. 2006] (see also Han et al. 2008, and Wang and Chang, unpublished observations). In vivo applications of such modified DCs may improve significantly the therapeutic potential of DC vaccines.

5.4 MODULATION OF T-CELL IMMUNITY WITH LENTIVIRAL VECTORS

Adaptive immunity is established through immune cell receptor–mediated antigen-specific responses. Functional modifications of different lineages of hematopoietic cells, including cytotoxic, helper, and regulatory T cells, may help control autoimmune disease, infectious disease, and cancer. A direct approach to up-regulate antigen-specific T-cell immunity is to ectopically endow desired T-cell receptor (TCR) functions to peripheral blood T cells through high-efficiency gene transfer, followed by infusion of modified T cells [Willemsen et al. 2003; Rossig and Brenner 2004; Miles et al. 2006; Morgan et al. 2006; Stauss et al. 2007]. Antigen-specific immune effector cells can be engineered with naturally occurring MHC-restricted, ligand-specific TCR-α and β genes, or alternatively, with genetically reconstructed TCR signaling fusion proteins independent of MHC requirements [Heemskerk et al. 2007; Murphy et al. 2007; Spaapen et al. 2007].

Immunotherapy by TCR gene transfer requires that target cells express MHC-restricted epitopes. If the target cells down-regulate or completely lose expression of MHC molecules, the effort will be futile. In virus-infected cells or cancer cells, down-regulation of MHC class I or II molecules is a known mechanism of escape of immune surveillance. The limitation of MHC presentation may be overcome by engineering a chimeric fusion TCR gene to target specific surface molecules in the absence of MHC restriction. For example, a fusion gene encoding a combination of three domains—specific antibody single-chain Fv (scFv), CD28 transmembrane domain, and TCR/CD3ζ signaling domain—could deliver a T-cell activation signal through binding to any target cells that express antigens specific to the scFv (T-body) [Zhang et al. 2004; Landmeier et al. 2007]. This T-body approach requires surface expression of specific target molecules but not MHC molecules. LVs are highly favorable in engineered T-cell therapy, due to their high efficiency and stable long-term gene transfer capability [Yang and Baltimore 2005]. Many of these innovative immunotherapeutic strategies are entering clinical trials worldwide.

5.5 METHODS OF LENTIVIRAL GENE TRANSFER INTO IMMUNE CELLS

The efficiency of lentiviral transduction is controlled by both entry and postentry mechanisms in the target cells. Expanded tropism of LV entry is based on pseudotyping with vesicular stomatitis virus G envelope protein, which targets a broad spectrum of host cells. Lentiviral targeting hematopoietic cells is dependent on the metabolic state and differentiation stage of the immune cells. In general, LVs transduce proliferating hematopoietic cells with high efficiency but not cells in a terminally differentiated or resting state. LVs transduce resting T cells at low efficiency, yet the transduction efficiency can be improved upon G1-phase cell cycle progression by treating the resting cells with growth-promoting factors such as interleukin-7 [Unutmaz et al. 1999]. Similarly, efficient lentiviral gene transfer into DCs is dependent on the maturation state of the target cells; mature DCs are difficult to transduce, but monocytic precursors or immature DCs are efficiently transduced with LVs [Chinnasamy et al. 2000; Chen et al. 2004].

Although compared with onco-retroviral vectors, LVs transduce unstimulated hematopoietic stem and presursor cells at higher efficiency, preincubation of hematopoietic stem and precursor cells with growth factors can further improve gene delivery efficiency [Douglas et al. 1999; Haas et al. 2000; Zielske and Gerson 2003; Hanawa et al. 2004]. Besides the metabolic state of the target cells, the titer of LV is also a determining factor for high-efficiency hematopoietic cell gene transfer [Haas et al. 2000]. Concentrated vector preparation improves lentiviral transgene delivery in a fashion exceeding linear correlations. In addition, low-speed centrifugation during lentiviral transduction has also been shown to increase LV gene delivery efficiency to certain cell types: for example, mouse hematopoietic stem cells and human embryonic stem cells [Xiong et al. 2005]. Therefore, it is necessary to evaluate various cell-handling procedures to achieve optimal efficiency of lentiviral gene transfer.

5.6 CONCLUSIONS

Clinical application of LVs requires extensive knowledge of host immune response to the vector to ensure safety. Direct in vivo injections of LVs may elicit antivector immunity toward viral proteins or transgene-encoded products. For in vivo lentiviral gene delivery, local application is favored over systemic injection because of the low vector stability and tissue permeability. Although successes of systemic delivery with LVs have been demonstrated in mice, the difference in size between mouse and human presents an almost insurmountable barrier to systemic lentiviral application in the clinics. As LVs establish prolonged and stable transgene expression, in vivo lentiviral gene transfer must also emphasize targeting specificity to avoid nonspecific damages. Clearly, the concerns over LV immunity are diminished in ex vivo applications, as the therapeutic materials can be delivered as purified transgenic proteins or LV-modified cells. Ex vivo modification of therapeutic cells with LVs is preferred to in vivo vector injection, as the former approach avoids vector immunity and allows extensive safety and efficacy assessment of the genetic materials prior to their clinical delivery. Extensive studies of the integration profile of HIV-1-derived LVs strongly suggest that such LVs are safe in targeting human cells. Future emphasis should be given to resolving potential issues with host immune reactivity to lentiviral transgenes—specifically, when immune modulatory genes are involved—to ensure clinical safety and the absence of nonspecific adverse effects.

REFERENCES

Banchereau J and Steinman RM. 1998. Dendritic cells and the control of immunity. *Nature* 392:245–252.

Bemelmans AP, Kostic C , et al. 2006. Lentiviral gene transfer of RPE65 rescues survival and function of cones in a mouse model of Leber congenital amaurosis. *PLoS Med* 3: e347.

Berns A. 2004. Good news for gene therapy. *N Engl J Med* 350:1679–1680.

Breckpot K, Aerts JL, et al. 2007. Lentiviral vectors for cancer immunotherapy: transforming infectious particles into therapeutics. *Gene Ther* 14:847–862.

Brown BD, Cantore A, et al. 2007a. A microRNA-regulated lentiviral vector mediates stable correction of hemophilia B mice. *Blood* 110:4144–4152.

Brown BD, Sitia G, et al. 2007b. In vivo administration of lentiviral vectors triggers a type I interferon response that restricts hepatocyte gene transfer and promotes vector clearance. *Blood* 109:2797–2805.

Buchschacher GL Jr and Wong-Staal F. 2000. Development of lentiviral vectors for gene therapy for human diseases. *Blood* 95:2499–2504.

Buseyne F, Le Gall S, et al. 2001. MHC-I-restricted presentation of HIV-1 virion antigens without viral replication. *Nat Med* 7:344–349.

Bushman FD. 2007. Retroviral integration and human gene therapy. *J Clin Invest* 117:2083–2086.

Carbonaro DA, Jin X , et al. 2006. In vivo transduction by intravenous injection of a lentiviral vector expressing human ADA into neonatal ADA gene knockout mice: a novel form of enzyme replacement therapy for ADA deficiency. *Mol Ther* 13: 110–1120.

Cattoglio C, Facchini G, et al. 2007. Hot spots of retroviral integration in human $CD34^+$ hematopoietic cells. *Blood* 110:1770–1778.

Chang L-J and Gay EE. 2001. The molecular genetics of lentiviral vectors: current and future perspectives. *Curr Gene Ther* 1:237–251.

Chen X, He J, et al. 2004. Alteration of T cell immunity by lentiviral transduction of human monocyte-derived dendritic cells. *Retrovirology* 1:37.

Chen X, Wang B, et al. 2006. Induction of primary anti-HIV CD4 and CD8T cell responses by dendritic cells transduced with self-inactivating lentiviral vectors. *Cell Immunol* 243:10–18.

Chinnasamy N, Chinnasamy D, et al. 2000. Efficient gene transfer to human peripheral blood monocyte–derived dendritic cells using human immunodeficiency virus type 1–based lentiviral vectors. *Hum Gene Ther* 11:1901–1909.

Cui Y, Iwakuma T, et al. 1999. Contributions of viral splice sites and cis-regulatory elements to lentivirus vector function. *J Virol* 73:6171–6176.

Douglas J, Kelly P, et al. 1999. Efficient transduction of human lymphocytes and $CD34^+$ cells via human immunodeficiency virus–based gene transfer vectors. *Hum Gene Ther* 10:935–945.

Dyall J, Latouche JB, et al. 2001. Lentivirus-transduced human monocyte-derived dendritic cells efficiently stimulate antigen-specific cytotoxic T lymphocytes. *Blood* 97:114–121.

Gabrilovich D. 2004. Mechanisms and functional significance of tumour-induced dendritic-cell defects. *Nat Rev Immunol* 4:941–952.

Gaspar HB and Thrasher AJ. 2005. Gene therapy for severe combined immunodeficiencies. *Expert Opin Biol Ther* 5:1175–1182.

Girolomoni G and Ricciardi-Castagnoli P. 1997. Dendritic cells hold promise for immunotherapy. *Immunol Today* 18:102–104.

Gruber A, Kan-Mitchell J, et al. 2000. Dendritic cells transduced by multiply deleted HIV-1 vectors exhibit normal phenotypes and functions and elicit an HIV-specific cytotoxic T-lymphocyte response in vitro. *Blood* 96:1327–1333.

Haas DL, Case SS, et al. 2000. Critical factors influencing stable transduction of human CD34(+) cells with HIV-1-derived lentiviral vectors. *Mol Ther* 2:71–80.

Hacein-Bey-Abina S, Le Deist F, et al. 2002. Sustained correction of X-linked severe combined immunodeficiency by ex vivo gene therapy. *N Engl J Med* 346:1185–1193.

Hacein-Bey-Abina S, Von Kalle C, et al. 2003. LMO2-associated clonal T cell proliferation in two patients after gene therapy for SCID-X1. *Science* 302:415–419.

Han S, Wang B, et al. 2008. Overcoming immune tolerance against multiple myeloma with lentiviral calnexin-engineered dendritic cells. *Mol Ther* 16: 269–279.

Han XD, Lin C, et al. 2007. Fetal gene therapy of alpha-thalassemia in a mouse model. *Proc Natl Acad Sci U S A* 104:9007–9011.

Hanawa H, Hematti P, et al. 2004. Efficient gene transfer into rhesus repopulating hematopoietic stem cells using a simian immunodeficiency virus-based lentiviral vector system. *Blood* 103:4062–4069.

Heemskerk MH, Hagedoorn RS, et al. 2007. Efficiency of T-cell receptor expression in dual-specific T cells is controlled by the intrinsic qualities of the TCR chains within the TCR–CD3 complex. *Blood* 109:235–243.

Herndier BG, Shiramizu BT, et al. 1992. Acquired immunodeficiency syndrome-associated T-cell lymphoma: evidence for human immunodeficiency virus type 1–associated T-cell transformation. *Blood* 79:1768–1774.

Iwakuma T, Cui Y, et al. 1999. Self-inactivating lentiviral vectors with U3 and U5 modifications. *Virology* 261:120–132.

Kafri T, Blomer U, et al. 1997. Sustained expression of genes delivered into liver and muscle by lentiviral vectors. *Nat Genet* 17: 314–317.

Khare PD, Loewen N, et al. 2007. Durable, safe, multigene lentiviral vector expression in feline trabecular meshwork. *Mol Ther* 16: 97–106.

Klatzmann D, Valery CA, et al. 1998. A phase I/II study of herpes simplex virus type 1 thymidine kinase "suicide" gene therapy for recurrent glioblastoma. Study Group on Gene Therapy for Glioblastoma. *Hum Gene Ther* 9:2595–2604.

Kordower JH, Emborg ME, et al. 2000. Neurodegeneration prevented by lentiviral vector delivery of GDNF in primate models of Parkinson's disease. *Science* 290:767–773.

Landmeier S, Altvater B, et al. 2007. Gene-engineered varicella-zoster virus reactive $CD4^+$ cytotoxic T cells exert tumor-specific effector function. *Cancer Res* 67:8335–8343.

Lanzavecchia A and Sallusto F. 2001. Regulation of T cell immunity by dendritic cells. *Cell* 106:263–266.

Marodon G, Fisson S, et al. 2006. Induction of antigen-specific tolerance by intrathymic injection of lentiviral vetors. *Blood* 108: 2972–2978.

Mellman I and Steinman RM. 2001. Dendritic cells: specialized and regulated antigen processing machines. *Cell* 106:255–258.

Miles JJ, Silins SL, et al. 2006. Engineered T cell receptors and their potential in molecular medicine. *Curr Med Chem* 13:2725–2736.

Miller PW, Sharma S, et al. 1998. Dendritic cells augment granulocyte–macrophage colony-stimulating factor (GM-CSF)/herpes simplex virus thymidine kinase–mediated gene therapy of lung cancer. *Cancer Gene Ther* 5:380–389.

Morgan RA, Dudley ME, et al. 2006. Cancer regression in patients after transfer of genetically engineered lymphocytes. *Science* 314:126–129.

Murphy A, Westwood JA, et al. 2007. Antitumor activity of dual-specific T cells and influenza virus. *Cancer Gene Ther* 14:499–508.

Naldini L, Blomer U, et al. 1996. In vivo gene delivery and stable transduction of non-dividing cells by a lentiviral vector. *Science* 272:263–267.

Naldini L and Verma IM. 2000. Lentiviral vectors. *Adv Virus Res* 55: 599–609.

Obst R, van Santen HM, et al. 2007. Sustained antigen presentation can promote an immunogenic T cell response, like dendritic cell activation. *Proc Natl Acad Sci U S A* 104:15460–15465.

Pariente N, Morizono K, et al. 2007. A novel dual-targeted lentiviral vector leads to specific transduction of prostate cancer bone metastases in vivo after systemic administration. *Mol Ther* 15:1973–1981.

Parney IF, Chang LJ, et al. 2006. Technical hurdles in a pilot clinical trial of combined B7–2 and GM-CSF immunogene therapy for glioblastomas and melanomas. *J Neurooncol* 78:71–80.

Pulendran B, Banchereau J, et al. 2001. Modulating the immune response with dendritic cells and their growth factors. *Trends Immunol* 22:41–47.

Ridgway D. 2003. The first 1000 dendritic cell vaccinees. Cancer Invest 21:873–886.

Rossig C and Brenner MK. 2004. Genetic modification of T lymphocytes for adoptive immunotherapy. *Mol Ther* 10:5–18.

Schroers R, Sinha I, et al. 2000. Transduction of human PBMC-derived dendritic cells and macrophages by an HIV-1-based lentiviral vector system. *Mol Ther* 1:171–179.

Schwarzwaelder K, Howe SJ, et al. 2007. Gammaretrovirus-mediated correction of SCID-X1 is associated with skewed vector integration site distribution in vivo. *J Clin Invest* 117:2241–2249.

Shi H, Cao T, et al. 2006. Hyperthermia enhances CTL cross-priming. *J Immunol* 176:2134–2141.

Spaapen R, van den Oudenalder K, et al. 2007. Rebuilding human leukocyte antigen class II–restricted minor histocompatibility antigen specificity in recall antigen-specific T cells by adoptive T cell receptor transfer: implications for adoptive immunotherapy. *Clin Cancer Res* 13:4009–4015.

Stauss HJ, Cesco-Gaspere M, et al. 2007. Monoclonal T-cell receptors: new reagents for cancer therapy. *Mol Ther* 15:1744–1750.

Steinman RM. 1991. The dendritic cell system and its role in immunogenicity. *Annu Rev Immunol* 9:271–296.

Tan PH, Beutelspacher SC, et al. 2005. Modulation of human dendritic-cell function following transduction with viral vectors: implications for gene therapy. *Blood* 105:3824–3832.

Themis M, Waddington SN, et al. 2005. Oncogenesis following delivery of a nonprimate lentiviral gene therapy vector to fetal and neonatal mice. *Mol Ther* 12:763–771.

Toes RE, van der Voort EI, et al. 1998. Enhancement of tumor outgrowth through CTL tolerization after peptide vaccination is avoided by peptide presentation on dendritic cells. *J Immunol* 160:4449–4456.

Unutmaz D, KewalRamani VN, et al. 1999. Cytokine signals are sufficient for HIV-1 infection of resting human T lymphocytes. *J Exp Med* 189:1735–1746.

van Schooten WC, Strang G, et al. 1997. Biological properties of dendritic cells: implications to their use in the treatment of cancer. *Mol Med Today* 3:254–260

Verma IM and Somia N. 1997. Gene therapy: promises, problems and prospects. *Nature* 389:239–242.

Wan Y, Bramson J, et al. 2000. Genetically modified dendritic cells prime autoreactive T cells through a pathway independent of CD40L and interleukin 12: implications for cancer vaccines. *Cancer Res* 60:3247–3253.

Willemsen RA, Debets R, et al. 2003. Genetic engineering of T cell specificity for immunotherapy of cancer. *Hum Immunol* 64:56–68.

Xiong C, Tang D-Q, et al. 2005. Genetic engineering of human embryonic stem cells with lentiviral vectors. *Stem Cell Dev* 14:367–377.

Yang L and Baltimore D. 2005. Long-term in vivo provision of antigen-specific T cell immunity by programming hematopoietic stem cells. *Proc Natl Acad Sci U S A* 102:4518–4523.

Yewdell JW, Norbury CC, et al. 1999. Mechanisms of exogenous antigen presentation by MHC class I molecules in vitro and in vivo: implications for generating $CD8^+$ T cell responses to infectious agents, tumors, transplants, and vaccines. *Adv Immunol* 73:1–77.

Zaiss A-K, Son S, et al. 2002. RNA 3′-readthrough of oncoretrovirus and lentivirus: implications in vector safety and efficacy. *J Virol* 76:7209–7219.

Zhang T, He X, et al. 2004. Transgenic TCR expression: comparison of single chain with full-length receptor constructs for T-cell function. *Cancer Gene Ther* 11:487–496.

Zielske SP and Gerson SL. 2003. Cytokines, including stem cell factor alone, enhance lentiviral transduction in nondividing human LTCIC and NOD/SCID repopulating cells. *Mol Ther* 7:325–333.

Zufferey R, Dull T, et al 1998. Self-inactivating lentivirus vector for safe and efficient in vivo gene delivery. *J Virol* 72:9873–9880.

6

IMMUNE RESPONSES TO ADENO-ASSOCIATED VIRUS VECTORS

Shih-Wen Lin, Ph.D., and Hildegund Ertl, M.D.
The Wistar Institute, University of Pennsylvania, Philadelphia, Pennsylvania

6.1 INTRODUCTION

The immune system protects against foreign agents such as viruses or bacteria. Gene delivery vehicles that are commonly used for gene replacement therapy, as well as some of the therapeutic proteins, are foreign to the host and thus treated by the immune system like an invading pathogen [Bessis et al. 2004]. For successful gene replacement therapy, induction of innate and adaptive immune responses against the gene replacement carrier and the therapeutic protein have to be avoided, which has meant that commonly used viral gene transfer vehicles have encountered difficulties, as was demonstrated initially with replication-defective adenoviral vectors [Raper et al. 2003]. Vectors based on adenoviruses of the common human serotype 5 have been used extensively for gene

Gene Therapy Immunology, Edited by Roland Herzog

replacement therapy [Barnett et al. 2002]. Early trials with E1-deleted adenoviral vectors conducted in immunocompromised rodents yielded promising results by achieving long-term production of the transgene product at high levels [Brown et al. 1997]. Nevertheless, similar experiments conducted in immunocompetent animals showed only transient transgene product expression [Tripathy et al. 1996] that could not be rescued by reapplication of the adenoviral gene replacement vectors. In immunocompetent animals, the E1-deleted vectors induced a potent $CD8^+$ T-cell response directed against antigens of adenovirus as well as to the transgene product, which rapidly eliminated the transduced cells within 10 to 14 days. A concomitant activation of B cells led to production of adenovirus-neutralizing antibodies, which impaired transduction of cells upon reapplication of the same vector [Fitzgerald et al. 2003]. As could have been predicted, the immune system thus responded to E1-deleted adenoviral vectors as it would have responded to a dangerous replication-competent virus. The exceptionally potent $CD8^+$ T- and B-cell responses to the transgene product of E1-deleted adenoviral vectors, which are now being utilized as vaccine carriers [Tatsis and Ertl 2004], relate to some of the features of adenovirus. The vectors induce a strong inflammatory response. They directly transduce immature dendritic cells, which then mature into antigen-presenting cells. The noncytopathic nature of E1-deleted adenovirus allows for prolonged antigen presentation, which further augments the adaptive immune response to epitopes of adenovirus and the transgene product. Even completely gutted adenoviral vectors may induce $CD8^+$ T cells [Kafri et al. 1998], which should eventually result in removal of the transduced cells.

Vectors based on adeno-associated viruses (AAVs) have yielded very promising results in gene replacement therapy of immunocompetent experimental animals [Fisher et al. 1997; High 2002]. In recombinant AAV (rAAV) gene transfer vehicles, the viral coding sequences have been removed so that only the transgene product can be expressed. rAAV vectors have achieved long-term transgene expression in vivo, indicating that they are comparatively nonimmunogenic [Wang et al. 2004; Zaiss and Muruve 2005], which may in part relate to their inability to induce activation of the innate immune system. Nevertheless, other studies have shown that immune responses can be induced to rAAV vectors as well as to rAAV vector-encoded proteins [Manning et al. 1997; Xin et al. 2001], and this is currently being exploited for the development of vaccines.

6.2 CHARACTERISTICS OF ADENO-ASSOCIATED VIRUSES

Adeno-associated viruses (AAVs) are single-stranded DNA viruses of the parvovirinae subfamily that infect both dividing and nondividing cells. They are dependoviruses that infect concomitantly with a helper virus such as adenovirus or herpes virus in nature [Carter 1974]. Helper viruses are needed to allow for transcription from the dependovirus genome and thus for replication of the virus. AAVs' single-stranded DNA genome of about 5 kb is flanked by 145-base palindromic inverted terminal repeat (ITR) elements [Smith-Arica and Bartlett 2001; Goncalves 2005]. ITRs initiate DNA replication and are required for encapsidation of the genome; they are minimally needed *in cis* to generate recombinant AAV (rAAV) vectors, in which all other viral sequences are supplied *in trans* [X. Liu et al. 2000; Gao et al. 2002b]. The genome contains two open reading frames (ORFs). One encodes proteins needed for DNA replication and for integration. The other encodes the three capsid proteins, which are generated from a single ORF by alternative splicing and distinct translation initiation sites. Of the three capsid proteins vp1 to 3, vp3 is the most abundant of the proteins and comprises 80% of the capsid; vp1 and vp2 are present at equal ratios of 10% [Timpe et al. 2005].

Humans are naturally exposed to AAVs, which they acquire together with a helper virus. AAV infections are not known to cause clinical sequelae [Blacklow 1988]. AAVs establish persistent infections and can be isolated from various tissues of primates. The virus can remain in an episomal form or it can integrate into the host cell genome [Weitzman et al. 1994; Young et al. 2000]. A unique aspect of the AAV2 virus (wild-type) is that it commonly, albeit not exclusively, integrates at a specific site on human chromosome 19 called AAVS1 [Wonderling and Owens 1997]. This site is located near a DNase I hypersensitive chromatin region, the core of which corresponds to a sequence displaying transcriptional enhancer-like properties, suggesting that AAVS1 constitutes a transcription-competent environment where AAV sequences may be transcribed, resulting in the production of AAV-derived proteins [Lamartina et al. 2000]. In mice, specific integration of AAV2 vectors into a specific region of chromosome 12 has been described [Donsante et al. 2007]. This region is rich for micro-RNA and small nucleolar RNA encoding sequences, which are overexpressed upon integration of the AAV vectors' genome. Integration into this region causes a marked increase in the hepatocellular carcinoma of infected animals [Donsante et al. 2007]. Natural infections with AAVs are not known to be associated with any particular type of cancer.

So far, six distinct serotypes have been identified in humans, AAV1 through AAV-6. Of those, AAV2-based vectors have been used most commonly for gene therapy. Recently, a number of additional serotypes have been isolated from nonhuman primates [Gao et al. 2005], which show divergence from serotypes derived from humans, especially in the hypervariable region of the capsid protein, the target for virus-neutralizing antibodies. AAVs can also infect other species, including reptiles. AAV serotypes are subdivided into different clades (A to F), with the commonly used AAV2 belonging to clade B, AAV1 to clade A, AAV7 to clade D, AAV8 to clade E, and AAV9 to clade F. The various AAV serotypes display different cell and tissue tropisms in vivo and in vitro, as was shown using AAV vectors in transfection studies. For example, AAV1 and AAV7 efficiently transduce skeletal muscle [Louboutin et al. 2005], while AAV2, AAV4, and AAV5 transduce cells of the central nervous system [Taymans et al. 2007]. The AAV7, 8, and 9, and Rh10 vectors transduce neurons [Cearley and Wolfe 2006], but not astrocytes or oligodendrocytes of the brain. AAV8 preferentially targets liver cells [Gao et al. 2002a], and AAV6 targets apical airway cells [Thorsen et al. 2006].

Although many serotypes have been isolated and vectored from primates and other animals, vectors based on AAV serotype 2 have been studied most extensively. AAV2 infects cells by attaching to the cell surface receptor heparin sulfate proteoglycan (HSPG). A co-receptor, alphaVbeta5 integrin, and activation of the small GTP-binding protein Rac1 allows internalization [Summerford et al. 1999]. Fibroblast growth factor receptor 1 has been identified as an additional co-receptor for AAV2 [Qing et al. 1999]. Transducing virions can enter through clathrin-coated pits or through other pathways. Once within the cell, AAV particles traffic to the late endosome, where pH-dependent penetration of the endosome can occur for the virus to traffic to the nucleus [Douar et al. 2001]. Intracellular movement of AAV2 to the nucleus via microfilaments and microtubules is dependent on activation of the phosphatidyliositol-3 (PI3) kinase pathway [Bartlett et al. 2000; Sanlioglu et al. 2000]. Other AAVs of clades A, C, D, E, and F do not bind the HSPG receptor, and it is not yet known how they attach and enter their target cells.

6.3 COMPONENTS OF rAAV VECTORS

In rAAVs used for gene transfer, the ORFs are removed and replaced with the gene of interest and regulatory elements flanked by the ITRs. The resulting vector can be grown in cells that provide the proteins encoded by the AAV in trans and which provide helper virus functions commonly through the E1, E2, E4, and virus-associated RNA of adenovirus [Geoffroy and Salvetti 2005; Wang and Lieber 2006]. Single-stranded (ss) AAV vectors most commonly used for gene delivery are able to package DNA inserts of up to 4.7 kb in size. The ss genome is inactive transcriptionally until it is converted into double-stranded (ds) DNA, a process that is time consuming and causes a delay in transgene product expression. rAAV vectors with self-complementary dsDNA packaged have been developed. These vectors circumvent the delay of transgene product expression associated with conversion of ss to ds DNA. They, furthermore, show superior transduction of certain cell types. An obvious disadvantage of dsAAV vectors is that their payload (i.e., the amount of foreign sequence that can be packaged) is only half that of traditional ssAAV vectors.

6.4 IMMUNE RESPONSES TO AAV

rAAV vectors have been used successfully in gene replacement therapy to treat diseases resulting from genetic deficiencies, such as hemophilia and muscular dystrophy [Kay et al. 2000; Cordier et al. 2001], and at least in experimental animals, have achieved long-term expression of the therapeutic proteins. Paradoxically, rAAV vectors have also been used as vaccine carriers and in these studies they were shown to induce transgene product-specific T- and B-cell responses. The aims of gene replacement therapy and vaccination are mutually exclusive, although the basic methodology (i.e., introduction of a foreign gene) can be identical. The overall focus of this chapter is to dissect the immune response in rAAV gene transfer as well as the advantages and limitations of rAAV in achieving these opposing goals.

6.4.1 Innate Immune Responses to rAAV Vectors

The innate immune system serves as a first line of defense against microbes. It consists of an army of soluble and cellular components, including complement, monocytes and macrophages, natural killer (NK) cells, dendritic cells (DCs), granulocytes, and polymorphonuclear leukocytes (PMNs), which can all produce cytokines and chemokines. The innate system is activated immediately after infection and usually operates locally at the site of infection. The main purpose of the innate immune system is to block or inhibit initial infection and to recruit other innate and adaptive immune cells. The innate response also directs the flavor of adaptive immune responses.

Innate immune responses are non-antigen-specific and are initiated by pathogen-associated molecular patterns (PAMPs) which are structurally conserved molecules expressed on or by microbes. PAMPs include lipopolysacharides and lipoproteins, peptidoglycans, single- and double-stranded RNA, unmethylated CpG motifs on DNA molecules, or viral glycoproteins, all of which are absent or rare in mammals. These PAMPs interact with pattern recognition receptors (PRRs) such as Toll-like receptors, located either on the cell surface or in endosomes or NOD-like receptors in the cytoplasm. Interactions between PAMPs and PRRs result in activation of NF-κB, which in turn leads to production of pro-inflammatory cytokines and chemokines, and to maturation of dendritic cells into professional antigen-presenting cells.

Some AAVs, such as AAV2, can transduce dendritic cells directly upon binding of HSPG, whereas others, such as AAV1, 7, or 8, fail to transduce dendritic cells directly. Both types of AAV appear to lack PAMPs, and intramuscular injection of rAAVs into mice fails to elicit a strong cellular infiltrate at the site of inoculation. One study showed that in DBA/2 mice, a rAAV vector expressing lacZ administered intravenously induced chemokines and cytokines in the liver, including TNF-α, RANTES, IP-10, MIP-1b, MIP-2, and MCP-1, followed by infiltration of neutrophils into the liver. The chemokine mRNA levels and infiltration returned to baseline within 6 hours [Zaiss et al. 2002] and depended on the presence of Kupffer cells. It remains to be seen if this finding can be reproduced with vectors derived from other serotypes of AAV or with rAAV2 vectors expressing other transgene products. In vitro, other rAAV vectors have been shown not to induce the expression of chemokines and cytokines from epithelium-derived cells, although additional in vitro studies with THP-1 cells (human promonocytic cells) showed them to produce various chemokine and inflammatory cytokine mRNAs upon transduction by rAAV vectors [Zaiss et al. 2002].

rAAV vectors do not appear to induce maturation of immature dendritic cells, although results remain controversial. Lack of dendritic cell maturation was shown in in vitro experiments in which AAV2-treated dendritic cells failed to up-regulate co-stimulatory molecules such as CD80, CD86, CD54, CD1a, CD40, and MHC classes I and II [Ponnazhagan et al. 2001]. Lack of up-regulation of CD54, CD80, CD86, and CD1a was also observed upon in vitro transfection of mouse or human myeloid and plasmacytoid dendritic cells with dsAAV1, 2, or 6 vectors [Aldrich et al. 2006; Veron et al. 2007], indicating lack of their maturation.

These results in part contradict another report, which showed that only AAVs of clade B (such as AAV2) [and not those of clade A (AAV1 and AAV6)] can transfect dendritic cells directly [Vandenberghe et al. 2006]. It should be pointed out, however, that maturation of dendritic cells does not require direct interaction with a pathogen but can also be achieved through cytokines produced by other cells, such as type I interferons. Furthermore, dendritic cells modulate a multitude of surface proteins during maturation, which either facilitate or dampen activation of cells of the adaptive immune system. Upon activation, dendritic cells can also produce a plethora of factors. Furthermore, dendritic cells are divided into different subsets, with divergent roles during a primary immune response, which can be distinguished by their morphology and expression of certain cell surface markers and PRRs. Myeloid dendritic cells, characterized as $CD11c^{high}$ and $CD11b^{high}$, are the main subsets that present antigen, and plasmacytoid dendritic cells, $CD11b^{low}$ and $CD123^{high}$, are a main source of type 1 interferons. Considering the complexity of dendritic cells and their activation pathways, and the contradictory results obtained by different laboratories, additional studies are warranted to ensure that, indeed, rAAV vectors fail to affect in vivo maturation of dendritic cells, which are believed pivotal for activation of primary immune responses. The role of the transgene and its regulatory elements especially, as well as the transgene product, all of which may carry immunostimulatory sequences, need to be tested more thoroughly for vector constructs designed for gene replacement therapy before generalized conclusions about interactions between rAAV vectors and the innate immune system can be drawn.

During natural infections, AAVs generally coinfect with a helper virus such as an adenovirus, which triggers robust innate immune responses. One would thus expect that the innate responses to the helper virus facilitate activation of adaptive immune responses to AAVs. rAAV vectors have been shown to induce B- and T-cell responses to both capsid components and the transgene product, which are described in more detail below. This suggests either that AAVs cause some maturation of dendritic cells, although this has not been supported by experimental evidence, or that direct activation of dendritic cells by AAV vectors is superfluous for the activation of naive B and T cells, which would be against the well-established immunological tenet that two signals, an antigen and a co-stimulator, are required to initiate a primary immune response, whereas antigen alone leads to anergy. In our studies with adenoviral vectors that drive maturation of dendritic cells through type 1 interferons, we observed that mice that were unable to respond to type 1 interferon due to a genetic inactivation of the type 1 interferon receptor failed to show maturation of dendritic cells treated with adenoviral vectors [Hensley et al. 2005, 2007]. Nevertheless, the mice mounted a robust T- and B-cell response to the transgene product encoded by the adenovirus. Again, these results appear to contradict the need for two signals. It should be pointed out, though, that we observed small subsets of mature dendritic cells in our naive mice (kept under pathogen-free but not germ-free conditions), which could have been transduced by the adenoviral vectors and which sufficed to initiate adaptive immune responses. A similar scenario, at least in theory, can be envisioned for initiation of T- and B-cell responses by rAAV vectors, although this seems unlikely, as we explain later in the chapter.

6.4.2 Adaptive Immune Responses to rAAV Vectors

While the innate immune system may slow down a viral infection, resolution of the infection usually requires the participation of adaptive immune responses. Most viral infections trigger B- and T-cell responses. Whereas B cells prevent infections through the secretion of neutralizing antibodies, T cells, especially $CD8^+$ T cells, are best suited to clear a viral infection through the release of antiviral cytokines such as interferons or through direct lysis of infected cells.

Humoral Immunity to AAV and rAAV Vectors B cells can be separated into B1 cells, which are found in the peritoneal cavity, and B2 cells, which are found in lymphoid tissues. B cells in the spleen can be subdivided into marginal zone B cells and follicular B cells. Marginal zone splenic B cells and B1 cells respond to antigen very early and independent of T helper cells by secretion of IgM antibodies, which, in general, have low affinity to the antigen. This response peaks after 3 to 4 days and is then followed by antibodies originating from B2 follicular B cells. Once B1 or marginal zone B cells become activated, they differentiate terminally into plasma cells. They do not contribute to the memory response but undergo programmed cell death. B2 cells produce antibodies of high quality, with a delay, and their differentiation into antibody-producing cells generally requires help from $CD4^+$ T cells. Several avenues can lead to T-helper-independent activation of B cells. Viruses with complex structures that carry repeats of a pattern may activate B cells directly by cross-linking of the Ig receptors. Other viruses may express antigens cross-reacting with common environmental antigens, triggering a memory rather than a primary B-cell response [Vos et al. 2000].

Immunoglobulin molecules serving as B-cell receptors (BCRs) on B-cell membranes can recognize viral particles. Once bound to a viral particle, the BCR is internalized, leading to a display of viral peptides on MHC class II molecules. These complexes, in turn, are recognized by $CD4^+$ T helper cells, which then provide co-stimulation through the secretion of cytokines and up-regulation of cell surface molecules such as CD40 ligand (CD40L), which interacts with CD40 on B cells. The activated B cells then expand clonally and differentiate into plasma cells that secrete antibodies, or they form germinal centers crucial for generating long-term antibody responses and B-cell memory. During clonal expansion the immunoglobulin genes hypermutate, and B cells that produce antibodies with high affinity are selected for preferentially. Furthermore, immunoglobulin genes rearrange to form different antibody isotypes, which have distinct functions. Antibody responses persist for long periods of time after removal of the bulk of the antigen, in part through constant reactivation via antibody–antigen complexes deposited on follicular dendritic cells within lymphatic tissues. Reencounter of the antigen causes rapid reactivation of memory B cells, and secondary antibody responses emerge far more rapidly than primary responses and result in higher antibody titers.

As a result of natural exposure, humans and nonhuman primates commonly carry neutralizing antibodies to AAVs. Epidemiological studies show that 30% of the human population has neutralizing antibodies to AAV2; other studies showed similar prevalence rates of neutralizing antibodies to AAV6 and slightly lower prevalence rates to AAV5 [Halbert et al. 2006]. The majority of humans (80%) have binding antibodies to AAVs [Moskalenko et al. 2000]. Prevalence depends on the age group and geographic location. We tested human sera from sub-Saharan Africa for neutralization of AAV1, 2, 5, 7, 8, and 9 and found that approximately 30% of sera carried neutralizing antibodies against these viruses, including those of nonhuman primate origin (Fig. 6-1). The latter indicates either cross-species transmission, or more likely, serological cross-reactivity between different AAV serotypes, as had been described previously [Gao et al. 2004b].

Even low titers of neutralizing antibodies to AAV can impair the efficacy of AAV-mediated gene transfer, as was shown in mice that received rAAV vectors into the liver [Scallan et al. 2006] or the central nervous system [Peden et al. 2004].

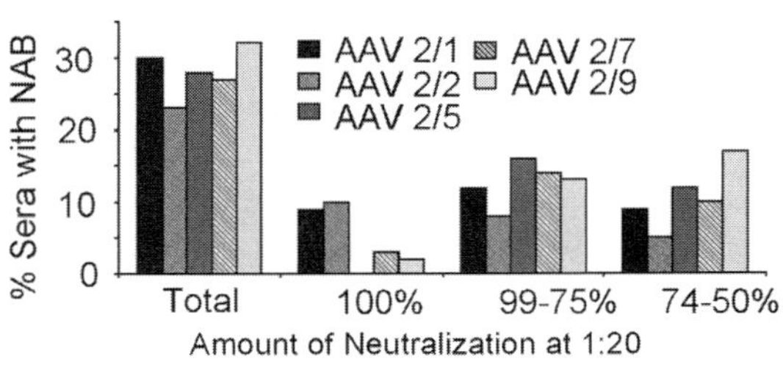

Figure 6-1 Neutralizing antibody formation to AAV. Cells from an HEK-293-derived cell line (8431 cells) were infected with AAV vectors expressing EGFP that were preincubated with a 1:20 dilution of human sera from Cameroon. Levels of neutralizing antibodies were estimated by counting the number of EGFP-expressing cells after infection with vectors that were incubated with the experimental serum or control serum. Data show the percent of sera that neutralized (first column). The graph also shows the percent of sera that caused a complete loss of infection (100%), a 75 to 99% reduction in infection, or a 50 to 74% reduction in infection. Positive sera were then tested at serial dilutions to determine their anti-AAV titers.

Neutralizing antibodies can in part be overcome by PEGylation of AAV particles [Lee et al. 2005]. In animal models, neutralizing antibodies to AAV2 could be circumvented by using vectors pseudotyped with AAV3 or AAV6 capsid in AAV2-immune mice [Halbert et al. 2000], with AAVrh10 capsid in AAV2- and AAV5-immune mice [De et al. 2006], or with AAV8 capsid in AAV2-immune dogs [Wang et al. 2005a]. Considering the prevalence of neutralizing antibodies to human and nonhuman primate isolates of AAV and the high degree of serological cross-reactivity among the various AAVs, it may become rather complex to overcome preexisting immunity through the use of different AAV serotypes for gene transfer.

rAAV vectors given to naive animals can induce both T-cell-independent and T-cell-dependent B cell responses. One study showed that depleting $CD4^+$ T cells completely inhibits induction of AAV capsid-specific antibodies upon AAV vector application [Chirmule et al. 2000]. Another study showed that AAV delivery through the portal vein yielded a B-cell response that was partially T-cell independent [Xiao et al. 2000]. The route of rAAV-mediated gene delivery may play a role in eliciting anti-AAV-capsid antibodies. In a study of rhesus macaques, all animals exposed to wild-type AAV (except through the intranasal route) developed a humoral immune response to AAV capsid proteins [Hernandez et al. 1999]. In patients, rAAV-mediated gene transfer was shown to result in an increase of AAV-neutralizing antibodies in patients with undetectable to moderate titers of preexisting antibodies to AAV, suggesting that the vector had caused an expansion of memory B cells present due to natural infections or induced a B-cell response in immunologically naive individuals [Manno et al. 2003]. In contrast, intracranial infusion of a rAAV vector into patients with Canavan disease failed to elicit an increase in circulating antibodies to AAV in about 70% of patients treated [McPhee et al. 2006], indicating that vector administration to the central nervous system, an immunologically privileged site, is less immunogenic than vector administration to muscle, liver, or lung.

rAAV vectors not only induce antibody responses against their capsid antigen but can also cause activation of B cells against the transgene product. This can be a major complication of gene therapy, as neutralizing antibodies against the transgene product may not only negate beneficial effects of the gene transfer, but in the case of hemophilia may rob patients of traditional treatment options. Induction of neutralizing antibodies (also termed inhibitors) against the transgene product has been studied most thoroughly in animal models of hemophilia B, which can be corrected by genetic transfer of factor IX. Studies in mice showed that intramuscular administration of a rAAV vector expressing human factor IX resulted in inhibitor formation, whereas intraportal vein application targeting the vector to the liver did not [Ge et al. 2001]. Inhibitor formation was also demonstrated in hemophilia B mice with a large deletion mutation upon intramuscular administration of mouse factor IX. In this model the development of inhibitors could be prevented by transient immunosuppression [Fields et al. 2001]. Inhibitor formation was seen in dogs with hemophilia that obtained large intramuscular doses per site of an rAAV2 vector expressing canine factor IX;

inhibitor formation was prevented by using lower vector doses per injection site or by transient immunosuppression [Herzog et al. 2002].

In one study, gene transfer of an rAAV vector resulted in antibody-mediated autoimmunity in primates. Intramuscular administration of rAAV vectors carrying the hormone erythropoietin (EPO) into cynomolgus macaques caused severe anemia in some animals, due to an antibody response to endogenous and transgene-derived EPO [Chenuaud et al. 2004; Gao et al. 2004a].

Lack of inhibitor formation upon hepatic transfer of rAAV vectors expressing factor IX was linked to the induction of $CD4^+$ $CD25^+$ $FoxP3^+$ regulatory T cells (Tregs), and depletion of such T cells caused formation of inhibitors in mice that received an rAAV2 factor IX vector through the portal vein [Cao et al. 2007]. Nonhuman primates that received rAAV2 factor IX gene transfer into the liver develop long-term expression of factor IX without inhibitor formation. In one study, rAAV gene transfer was coupled with an immunosuppressive regimen composed of mycophenolate mofetil, a DNA synthesis inhibitor, sirolimus (rapamycin), which inhibits the response to IL-2, and daclizumab, a humanized monoclonal antibody to the IL-2Rα receptor (CD25) of T cells. Unlike those that were not immunosuppressed, these animals developed inhibitors against factor IX, again indicating that lack of a transgene product–specific B-cell response depends on Tregs that were inactivated or depleted by the antibody to CD25 [Mingozzi et al. 2007a].

rAAV vectors have been used as vaccine carriers. Such vectors, unlike those used for gene replacement therapy, carry genes that express foreign proteins and may contribute to activation of innate immunity, which may then drive adaptive immune responses. rAAV2 vectors expressing the MSP4 antigen of *Plasmodium falciparum* or the MSP4/5 antigen of *P. yoelii* given intramuscularly induced long-lasting antibody responses, although they were not protective against challenge of mice with *P. yoelli*; attempts to boost the antibody response by prime boost regimens were unsuccessful [Logan et al. 2007]. The major capsid protein L1 of human papilloma virus (HPV) type 16, which elicits protective antibodies against the virus, expressed by a rAAV5 vector, induced a long-lasting antibody response both systemically and at mucosal surfaces upon intranasal application to mice [Kuck et al. 2006]. Whether or not the quality of these antibodies was comparable to those induced by L1-virus-like particles, which form the basis of commercially available preventive vaccine to HPVs, including HPV-16, was not assessed.

Overall, the data available show that infections with AAV readily induce capsid-specific neutralizing antibodies which impair rAAV-mediated gene transfer. Data also show that AAV gene transfer boosts preexisting AAV-specific B cells or induces a primary B-cell response against capsid components that will affect repeated use of AAV vectors. Depending on the route of immunization, AAV vectors can also induce transgene product-specific antibody responses, which is advantageous for their use as vaccine carriers but is potentially detrimental for gene replacement therapy.

Cellular Immune Responses to AAVs While humoral immune responses, especially neutralizing antibodies, prevent viral infections and thus reduce gene transfer by viral vectors, cell-mediated immune responses can eliminate vector-transduced cells. Induction of antigen-specific T-cell responses requires presentation of viral antigens by professional antigen-presenting cells, which are in general dendritic cells [Banchereau and Steinman 1998; Lanzavecchia and Sallusto 2001; Liu 2001; Mellman and Steinman 2001]. Dendritic cells, which are derived from bone marrow progenitors, are dispersed throughout an organism but are exceptionally common in tissues that form a boundary to the outside world, such as the skin and mucosal surfaces. Dendritic cells within these tissues are immature; they take up antigen but fail to present the antigen to naive T cells. They express only low levels of co-stimulatory signals and they lack CCR7 receptor expression, which promotes homing to lymphoid tissues, where activation of T cells takes place. They express other chemokine receptors, such as CCR1, CCR2, CCR5, and CXCR1, which lead to their recruitment to inflammatory sites where MIP-1α, MIP-1β, and RANTES are produced. Invasion of pathogens triggers maturation of dendritic cells through interactions between PAMPs on the microbes and PRRs on or in the dendritic cells. Alternatively, maturation of dendritic cells can be a consequence of pro-inflammatory cytokines or cell damage or death, causing the release of heat shock proteins that can interact with PRRs. Some viruses, including some serotypes of AAVs, can infect dendritic cells directly. Other serotypes of AAVs cannot infect dendritic cells directly. Their presentation relies on either phagocytosis of viral particles or pinocytosis of antigen released from infected cells. Once dendritic cells receive a maturation signal, they initially up-regulate and then down-regulate expression of CCR1, CCR5, and CXCR1, and thus at first they become more sensitive, and then resistant to recruitment by pro-inflammatory chemokines. While down-regulating CCR1, CCR5, and CXCR1, they increase expression of CCR7, which renders them responsive to SLC (secondary lymphoid tissue chemokine) and ELC (EB11-ligand chemokine), which are both produced in T-cell-rich areas of lymphoid tissues to which mature dendritic cells migrate [Sallusto et al. 1998, 2000; Sozzani et al. 1998, 2000]. Once mature, dendritic cells upregulate expression of MHC class II and co-stimulatory molecules on their cell surface.

$CD4^+$ T cells that provide help for activation of B cells and $CD8^+$ T cells are stimulated by peptides presented by MHC class II molecules [Castellino and Germain 1995; Castellino et al. 1997; Watts and Powis 1999; Pieters 2000]. After synthesis of the α and β subunits, MHC class II molecules assemble in the endoplasmic reticulum with a polypeptide called the invariant chain. The MHC class II invariant chain complexes are translocated to an endosomal–lysosomal storage area. Antigen taken up by cells progresses from early to late endosomes and then to lysosomes, where they are broken down into peptides which can bond with MHC class II dimers upon release of the invariant chains. MHC class II–peptide complexes are then moved to the cell surface, where they can be recognized by the receptor of $CD4^+$ T cells. MHC class II peptide complexes are long-lived, with an average half-life of more than 10 hours, as was shown in vitro.

$CD8^+$ T cells recognize antigenic peptides associated with MHC class I determinants that are expressed on the majority of cells. Unlike MHC class II molecules, MHC class I molecules associate primarily with peptides derived from proteins synthesized de novo. Newly synthesized MHC class I heavy chains associate in the endoplasmic reticulum with calnexin, which promotes appropriate folding of the protein. The folded heavy chain then binds β2 microglobulin. Correct folding of the MHC class I heavy chain is facilitated by calreticulin. The resulting complex binds to tapasin, providing a link to the transporter associated with antigen presentation (TAP), which connects the endoplasmic reticulum with the cytoplasma where viral proteins are being synthesized [Cresswell et al. 1999; Solheim 1999; Grandea and Van Kaer 2001]. Newly produced proteins that are faulty or incorrectly folded are degraded in the cytoplasm by a complex of proteolytic enzymes that assemble into a proteasome complex [York et al. 1999]. Peptides 8 to 13 amino acids in length, which are derived upon enzymatic cleavage of proteins, are transported into the endoplasmic reticulum though TAP [Elliott 1997; Abele and Tampe 1999; Reits et al. 2000]. Once peptides reach the endoplamic reticulum, they bind to the groove of MHC class I [Murray and McMichael 1992]. Upon binding of peptides, the MHC class I heavy chain–β2 microglobulin complex releases calreticulin and tapasin and is transported through the Golgi apparatus to the cell surface. During most viral infections, the response is commonly dominated by T cells that recognize only one or two peptides from many that could provide potential targets [Fairchild and Wraith 1996].

MHC class I binding epitopes of AAV2 capsid antigens (Table 6-1) have been defined [Sabatino et al. 2005] for several mouse ($H-2^b$, as in C57Bl/6 mice, and $H-2^d$, as in DBA/2, BALB/c, or B10.D2 mice) and human haplotypes through experimentation and the use of predictive algorithms. Most of the epitopes were shown to be located in vp3, the most abundant capsid protein. Furthermore, many of these epitopes are in conserved regions of the capsid protein, allowing for cross-reactive recognition of multiple serotypes by T cells.

Although due to their lack of coding AAV sequences, rAAV vectors would not be expected to induce $CD8^+$ T cells through the described pathway, dendritic cells can present exogenous antigen in the context of an MHC class I determinant

TABLE 6-1 Mouse AAV2 Capsid $CD8^+$ T-Cell Epitopes Mapped for C57Bl/6 and BALB/c Strains

Mouse Strain	Amino Acid Position	Peptide Sequence	MHC Restriction
C57Bl/6	702–710	SNYNKSVNV	K^b
C67Bl/6	511–525	NGRDSLVNPGPAMAS	D^b
BALB/c	372–380	VPQYGYLTL	L^d
BALB/c	306–320	FRPKRLNFKLFNIQV	L^d
BALB/c	426–440	HSQSLDRLMNPLIDQ	L^d

through the process of cross-priming [Brossart and Bevan 1997]. Presentation of exogenous antigen through cross-priming is proteasome- and TAP-dependent and takes place in the endoplasmic reticulum. Peptides that contain a signal sequence can cross from the cytoplasm into the endoplasmic reticulum independent of TAP. When they reach the endoplasmic reticulum, these peptides are degraded further by peptidases until they reach a size that allows for binding to the cleft of MHC class I molecules. rAAV vectors, which are known to escape endosomes, reach the cytoplasm, where some vector particles become ubiquitinated and targeted for degradation by proteasomes [Yan et al. 2002]. AAVs would thus be expected to activate capsid-specific $CD8^+$ T cells through this alternative processing pathway. Alternatively, it has been suggested that AAV vector preparations can be contaminated with AAV particles that package capsid-encoding genome sequences which are synthesized within transduced cells, thus allowing for presentation of peptides from de novo synthesized proteins [C. Li et al. 2007].

Dendritic cells that display antigenic peptides in association with MHC class I molecules activate $CD8^+$ T cells with the corresponding receptors. In general, activation of $CD8^+$ T cells requires help from $CD4^+$ T cells. Some viruses, such as Sendai virus, induce $CD8^+$ T-cell responses without T help. $CD8^+$ T cells induced without T help differentiate into functionally active effector cells, but their ability to mount a memory response is impaired [Sun and Bevan 2004].

Dendritic cells are crucial to activate naive T cells during a primary immune response. Antigen-experienced T cells can be reactivated by antigen displayed on a variety of cell types, including B cells [Matzinger 2002] or macrophages. A study by Vandenberghe et al. [2006] showed that nonhuman primates mount robust T-cell responses to the capsid antigens of AAV2 but only weak-to-undetectable T-cell responses to other serotypes, such as AAV8, due to lack of binding of HSPG and failure to transduce dendritic cells directly. The authors conclude that serotypes that do not bind to HSPG are less susceptible to immune-mediated elimination. This may not be justified, as recall responses in humans with preexisting immunity to AAVs due to natural infections do not require presentation of antigen by dendritic cells.

Effector and Memory T Cells After activation by antigen displayed on professional antigen-presenting cells, T cells proliferate extensively. $CD8^+$ T cells proliferate far more vigorously than do $CD4^+$ T cells, and at the height of the immune response, depending on the antigen and the amount of antigen, up to 20 to 40% of all central $CD8^+$ T cells comprise those with specificity to a single epitope of the pathogen.

$CD4^+$ T cells mature either into Th1- or Th2-type cells [Flavell 1999; Moser and Murphy 2000; Dong and Flavell 2001], depending on the type of innate immune response that is elicited by the infectious agent. IL-12 promotes activation of Th1 cells [Trinchieri 1998], whereas IL-4 sponsors differentiation into Th2 cells [Chatelain et al. 1992]. If both are present concomitantly, IL-4 overrides the functions of IL-12. IL-10 inhibits the activity of IL-12 and thus favors the generation of Th2 cells [O'Garra 1998]. Th1 cells release IFN-γ and lymphotoxin, aid activation of $CD8^+$ T cells, and promote generation of antibodies of the IgG2a isotype in mice. Th2 cells secrete IL-4, IL-5, and IL-10, promote B cells that secrete IgG1, IgE, or IgA, and activate mast cells and eosinophils. Most viruses trigger release of interferons and therefore generate a Th1 response or a mixed response that is Th1 dominated. Some early reports indicated that AAVs might trigger a Th2 response, although this would be counterintuitive. The type of response to natural infections with AAV is probably determined by the helper virus, which induces a robust innate immune response. As was shown with E1-deleted vectors in mice, adenoviruses, which most commonly serve as helper viruses to AAVs, induce a Th1-biased response if given systemically, or a mixed response upon mucosal application. A primary response to AAV would thus be expected to be Th1-dominated or mixed, as was indeed shown experimentally [Chirmule et al. 1999]. Regardless of the cytokine milieu at the time of reactivation, recall responses mimic the type of primary response. The type of recall response of AAV-specific $CD4^+$ T cells upon AAV-mediated gene transfer would probably be similar to that of a primary $CD4^+$ T cell response to natural infections with AAV.

$CD4^+$ T cells combat viral infections primarily through the release of antiviral cytokines such as IFN-γ and through the recruitment of other effector cells, such as macrophages, neutrophils, or NK cells. $CD8^+$ T cells are best suited to eliminate virus-infected cells through a number of mechanisms. They can kill them by the release of perforin or granzyme. Activated $CD8^+$ T cells express fas ligand (CD95) on their surface, and interactions of CD95 with fas expressed on virus-infected cells induce their death by apoptosis [Topham et al. 2001]. Upon engagement of their receptors, most $CD8^+$ T cells release IFN-γ, which not only reduces viral replication but also clears persistent infection with certain viruses, such as lymphocytic choriomeningitis virus [Saron et al. 1997] or hepatitis B virus [Guidotti and Chisari 2000]. Once the effector phase has been terminated by removal or elimination of the infectious agent, most of the virus-specific $CD8^+$ T cells undergo activation-induced cell death [Ju et al. 1999], and frequencies of antigen-specific $CD8^+$ and $CD4^+$ T cells decline sharply until they reach the steady-stage level during the immunological memory phase. T cells are maintained at remarkably stable frequencies during memory, even in the absence of antigen, through homeostatic proliferation promoted by IL-7 and IL-15.

Based on phenotypic markers, memory T cells can be divided into effector memory cells and central memory cells. Effector memory cells are $CD62L^{low}$, circulate in the blood, are present in tissues, and assume effector functions without further proliferation. Resting memory T cells are $CD62L^{high}$ and reside primarily in lymphatic tissues. Although they can assume effector function quite rapidly upon reencounter of antigen, they presumably proliferate in vivo upon reactivation before they egress the lymphatic tissues and migrate to the site of infection (Fig. 6-2 and Table 6-2). Although this is still open to debate, experimental evidence suggests that effector memory cells are present after infection only transiently and then are gradually replaced by central memory cells [Roberts et al. 2005].

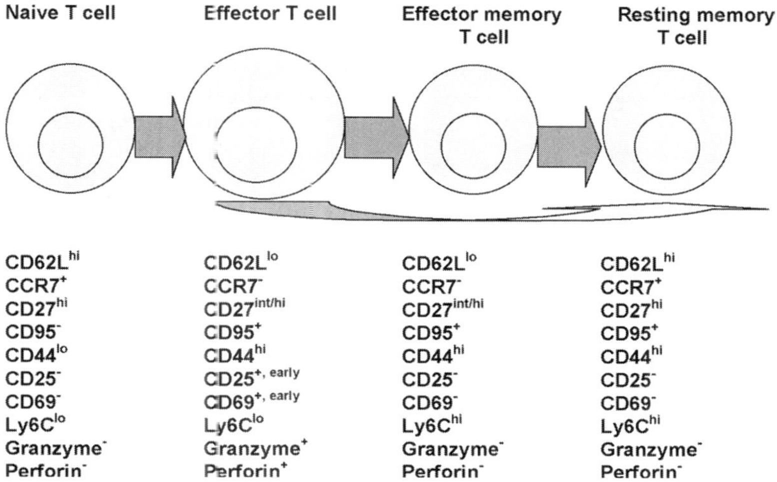

Figure 6-2 $CD8^+$ T-cell activation. $CD8^+$ T cells are classified as naive, effector, effector memory, or central memory cells, based on cell surface and intracellular markers. It should be pointed out that expression of these markers is partly tissue dependent and may vary between mice and humans.

Human peripheral blood mononuclear cells and human splenocytes have been tested for T cells to AAV capsid antigens using sensitive detection methods that at least in theory should detect one AAV-specific T cell in 10^6 mononuclear cells. AAV-specific $CD8^+$ T cells could be detected in the blood of some human subjects, and more frequently, in spleens. Frequencies were very low and in vitro expansion was needed for their detection. Also, a number of samples derived from humans with antibodies to AAV indicative for a previous infection were negative for AAV-specific T cells [Mingozzi et al. 2007b]. This contrasts with memory T-cell responses to other persistent infections, such as those with herpesviruses, to which most humans have robust and readily detectable numbers of circulating memory T cells. The latter are probably boosted periodically upon reactivation of the persisting virus. The lack of high frequencies of AAV-specific T cells could suggest that although AAVs persist, the viruses are not reactivated or are reactivated only very rarely. However, this is counterintuitive because evolution favors traits that enhance survival of a species, and viral persistence without occasional reactivation followed by replication would be pointless. Alternatively, persisting AAVs may occasionally be reactivated upon infection of the person with a helper virus but may have evolved to subvert expansion of memory responses. Viruses, especially the larger, more complex DNA viruses, have a number of strategies to evade a host immune system. In particular, herpesviruses and adenoviruses, both of which serve as helper viruses for AAVs, encode proteins that interfere with activation of innate and adaptive immune responses. It remains

TABLE 6-2 CD8$^+$ T-Cell Activation Markers[a]

Marker	Also Known as:	Function
CD62L	L-selectin, LECAM-1, LAM-1	Binds a series of glycoproteins, including CD34, GlyCAM-1, and MAdCAM-1; is important for homing of naive lymphocytes via endothelial venules to peripheral lymph nodes and Peyer's patches
CCR7	EBI-1, CD197	Receptor for 6Ckine/SLC (secondary lymphoid–tissue chemokine) and MIP–3β/ELC (EBI1–ligand chemokine); expressed predominantly on naive T cells
CD27	S152, T14, TNF-R	Binds to CD70, a member of the TNF ligand superfamily; found primarily on peripheral blood T cells and on a subpopulation of B cells and NK cells
CD95	APO-1, Fas, TNFRSF6, APT1	Expressed, typically at high levels, on activated T and B cells; mediates apoptosis-inducing signals
CD44	ECMR III, H-CAM, HUTCH-1, Hermes, Lu, In-related, Pgp-1, gp85	Involved in leukocyte attachment to and rolling on endothelial cells, homing to peripheral lymphoid organs and to sites of inflammation
CD25	IL2R, Tac antigen	Expressed, typically at high levels, on stimulated T cells and some subsets of regulatory T cells
CD69	AIM, activator inducer molecule	Transiently expressed on activated leukocytes, including T cells; cross-linking induces cytotoxic activity and co-stimulates cytokine production; controls egress of lymphocytes from lymph nodes
Ly6C	Ly-6C	Induces clustering of LFA-1; involved in subtype-specific adhesion of CD8$^+$ T cells
Granzyme		Exogenous serine proteases that are released by cytoplasmic granules within cytotoxic T cells and natural killer cells to induce apoptosis within virus-infected cells, thus destroying them
Perforin		Cytolytic mediator produced by killer lymphocytes; stored in and released by cytoplasmic granules

[a]These cellular surface and intracellular markers are used to phenotype CD8$^+$ T cells and determine their activation states.

to be investigated whether any of the AAV-encoded proteins interfere with the immune system or whether AAVs are in part shielded through the immunoevasive mechanisms employed by their helper viruses.

T-Cell Responses to the Capsid Antigen of AAV Vectors AAV vectors have been shown to cause long-term expression of the therapeutic protein in experimental animals, and it was initially assumed that due to lack of de novo synthesis of viral proteins, they failed to elicit $CD8^+$ T-cell responses to the vectors' capsid antigens. In a human gene therapy trial in which patients received a rAAV2 vector expressing factor IX under a hepatocyte-specific promoter into the portal artery, the first patient of the highest-dose group developed therapeutic levels of circulating factor IX by 2 weeks after gene transfer. Shortly afterward, the patient developed a subclinical transaminitis and factor IX levels declined to levels before gene transfer. The transaminitis resolved concomitantly. The next patient in the same trial received a lower dose of the rAAV2F.IX vector. This dose did not result in detectable levels of circulating factor IX. Nevertheless, this patient also developed a mild transaminitis with the same kinetics as those of the high-dose patient. In the second patient, blood mononuclear cells were tested before and after gene transfer for T cells to AAV capsid and factor IX. Before gene transfer, T cells to peptide libraries from AAV capsid or factor IX could not be detected in blood. After gene transfer, T cells specific to AAV capsid became detectable in blood; their frequency initially increased in blood and then returned to baseline. T cells specific to factor IX could not be detected at any time. The patient's AAV-specific T cells were at first detected by ELISpot assays for IFN-γ, which do not allow distinction between $CD4^+$ or $CD8^+$ T cells. Upon their in vitro expansion, T cells were analyzed further by intracellular cytokine staining, a T-cell detection method that is less sensitive than the ELISpot assay but allows for the phenotyping of cells. This assay showed clearly that the T cells belonged to the $CD8^+$ subset. It was concluded that the loss of factor IX-producing hepatocytes was probably mediated by the AAV-specific $CD8^+$ T cells that had been present at low frequencies in patients due to natural infections and that had become reactivated by the gene transfer [Mingozzi et al. 2007b].

$CD8^+$ T cell–mediated rejection of AAV vector–transduced cells had thus far not been observed in experimental animals, and the argument was that unlike humans, animals are not naturally infected by AAVs and therefore lack AAV capsid–specific memory T cells. Several groups tried to develop a mouse model to recapitulate the findings of the hemophilia trial. Our group induced $CD8^+$ T cells to AAVs by either immunizing mice with AAV2 or AAV8 vectors that expressed an immunogenic protein, or with E1-deleted adenoviral vectors expressing AAV2 or AAV8 capsid antigens. High frequencies of AAV capsid–specific $CD8^+$ T cells could readily be induced by AAV2 vectors or by the adenoviral vectors, whereas AAV8 vectors induced only marginal frequencies of capsid-specific $CD8^+$ T cells, which others had observed. T cells cross-reacted between AAV2 and AAV8, again confirming previous results. Nevertheless, if immunized mice carrying high frequencies of AAV capsid–specific $CD8^+$ T cells were injected after a short interval with an AAV vector expressing human factor IX, which was serologically distinct from the AAV capsid used for immunization but shared $CD8^+$ T-cell epitopes, AAV capsid–specific $CD8^+$ T cells failed to expand, mice did not show an increase in transaminases, and sustained expression of factor IX was observed [H. Li et al. 2007]. These findings were reproduced rapidly by two other groups, suggesting that effector $CD8^+$ T cells to AAV capsid do not eliminate rAAV-transduced hepatocytes. It should be pointed out, however, that the mouse experiments differed in several crucial aspects from the human clinical trial. Humans are exposed to AAVs during childhood and thus carry memory T cells to AAV capsid; mice were immunized and treated with the rAAV vector at the height of the effector phase following immunization to AAV capsid. Humans in the gene transfer trial received the rAAV vector through the portal artery, whereas the mice were injected intravenously, so one could argue that the surgical procedures of portal artery administration resulted in an inflammatory reaction that was missing in intravenously injected mice. Humans had low titers of neutralizing antibodies to AAV2, which again were missing in experimental animals. These antibodies may redirect uptake of rAAVs to different cell types and thereby affect induction or reactivation of adaptive immune responses.

This finding in hemophilia patients may have been recapitulated in a recent trial in which baboons were injected in the myocardium with a rAAV2 construct encoding a human TNF receptor II IgG-Fc fusion protein or as a control with empty AAV2 capsid. Animals that received the transgene-carrying vector developed a myocarditis, with a pronounced $CD8^+$ T-cell infiltrate, which was also seen in animals that received empty capsid. Unfortunately, animals were not tested for a T-cell response to AAV capsid or the transgene product, and therefore the target antigen of the infiltrating $CD8^+$ T cells remains elusive [McTiernan et al. 2007].

Cellular Immune Response to the Transgene Product of AAV Vectors Gene transfer by rAAV vectors can result in the induction of transgene product–specific T cells. Delivery of ovalbumin (OVA) to skeletal muscle by an rAAV2 vector stimulated $CD4^+$ and $CD8^+$ T cells. Surprisingly, OVA-specific $CD4^+$ T-cell activation could be detected as early as 5 days after gene transfer by ssAAV2 vectors, which would not be expected to produce significant amounts of transgene product within this short time [Wang et al. 2005b, 2007]. rAAV vectors expressing the highly immunogenic influenza A virus hemagglutinin also induced a $CD4^+$ T-cell response, albeit with a delay compared to an adenoviral vector expressing the same transgene product [Sarukhan et al. 2001]. The response to hemagglutinin as expressed by rAAV vectors depended on cross-priming and could be abrogated by blockade of the CD40–CD40L pathway. Induction of transgene product–specific $CD8^+$ T cells was also observed upon intramuscular injection of mice with a rAAV2 vector expressing β-galactosidase. In this model, activation of $CD8^+$ T cells was also CD40L dependent and was not observed in CD40L-knockout mice [Zhang et al. 2000].

Because transfer of rAAV vectors to skeletal muscle can result in specific T- and B-cell responses to an immunogenic transgene product, rAAV vectors were tested as vaccine carriers. rAAV2 vectors expressing gag of human immunodeficiency virus 1 [Xin et al. 2002], the herpes simplex virus glycoprotein B [Manning et al. 1997], or the E7 protein of human papillomavirus (HPV) type 16 fused to a heat shock protein D. [Liu et al. 2000] elicited a $CD8^+$ T-cell response in mice that was found to be $CD4^+$ T-cell dependent, at least in the HPV-16 E7 model. Delivery of antigens from simian immunodeficiency virus (SIV) induced SIV-specific B- and T-cell responses in nonhuman primates and provided partial protection against challenge [Johnson et al. 2005]. Notwithstanding, in a subsequent phase I clinical trial, rAAV2 vectors expressing antigens of HIV-1 were found to be weakly immunogenic and at the highest dose elicited only low levels of HIV-specific T-cell responses in about 30% of the volunteers. rAAV1 vectors expressing antigens of HIV-1 have been reported to induce more robust HIV-specific $CD8^+$ T-cell responses than rAAV2 vectors, which may reflect their higher tropism to skeletal muscle cells, and additional HIV-1 vaccine trials with rAAV1 vectors are being planned [Pastor 2007].

Investigators have induced $CD8^+$ T-cell responses by dendritic cells that were transduced in vitro with rAAV vectors expressing prostate-specific antigen [Mahadevan et al. 2007], the core protein of hepatitis B or C virus [Liu et al. 2006; You et al. 2006], the breast cancer antigen BA46 [Liu et al. 2005], and the E7 [Chiriva-Internati et al. 2002] and E6 [Liu, Y. et al. 2001] antigens of HPV-16. Surprisingly, they also repeatedly reported that transduction of immature dendritic cells by rAAV2 vectors caused their maturation, as they showed by up-regulation of co-stimulatory molecules and secretion of cytokines. This finding is in stark contrast to that of other groups, which reported that AAV vectors do not drive maturation of dendritic cells.

We tested rAAV vectors of different serotypes expressing gag of HIV-1 for the induction of transgene product–specific $CD8^+$ T cells in mice. Mice immunized intramuscularly developed detectable frequencies of gag-specific $CD8^+$ T cells, especially after immunizations with rAAV serotypes with high tropism for muscle cells, such as vectors based on rAAV1 or rAA7, whereas rAAV2 vectors performed poorly. Nevertheless, the gag-specific $CD8^+$ T-cell response was impaired in exhibiting reduced capacity for cytokine release, lysis, or proliferation upon antigen reexposure. These results were recapitulated with rAAV8 vectors [Lin et al. 2007]. Our results indicate that $CD8^+$ T cells induced to the transgene product of an rAAV vector are partially exhausted, probably as a result of continued production of transgene product by persisting rAAV vectors. Needless to say, a vaccine that induces a $CD8^+$ T-cell response that is incapable of expanding upon reencounter of the antigen, such as that upon a natural infection, may increase rather than decrease the susceptibility of the person vaccinated.

6.4.3 Induction of Regulatory T Cells by AAV Vectors

The immune system is designed to respond to infections by microbes while maintaining tolerance to self-antigens. Self-tolerance is maintained by several mechanisms, such as elimination of autoreactive T cells during development in the thymus and by stringent control of T-cell activation, which requires not only ligation of antigen receptors but also second signals from cells of the innate immune system, which in turn are induced by PAMPs. A further safeguard against autoimmunity is provided by regulatory T cells. Different types of regulatory T cells (Tregs) have been described. Sakaguchi and his colleagues first identified $CD4^+CD25^+$ regulatory T cells [Sakaguchi et al. 1995; Takahashi et al. 1998], which comprise about 5 to 10% of peripheral $CD4^+$ T cells in mice and humans. These cells are commonly termed *naturally occurring Tregs*, as opposed to *induced Tregs*. $CD4^+$ $CD25^+$ Tregs can be distinguished from activated $CD4^+$ T cells, which also up-regulate CD25 on their cell surface, by expression of the forkhead transcription factor (Fox)p3, which is crucial for the development of Tregs. Elegant studies from several groups showed that transfer of $CD4^+$ $CD25^+$ Tregs can prevent autoimmune disease in animals [Fowell et al. 1991]. Others showed that $CD25^+$ $CD4^+$ Tregs also modulate T-cell responses to foreign antigens and that their functional inactivation increases responses to vaccination. The mode of action of Tregs remains under investigation. Tregs have been described to secrete immunoinhibitory cytokines such as IL-10, and they have been shown to inhibit T-cell functions such as in vitro proliferation.

Other populations of T cells can exert regulatory functions upon other cell subsets. These include some subsets of $CD8^+$ T cells and NK T cells as well as $CD25^-$ $CD4^+$ Treg cells. Unlike $CD25^+$ Tregs induced by antigen, the latter subset dampens immune responses through secretion of immunosuppressive cytokines such as IL-10 and TGF-β.

Several groups reported that gene transfer of rAAV vectors results in the induction of regulatory T cells that cause tolerance to the transgene product. One group showed that a single muscle injection of an rAAV vector carrying the autoantigen glutamic acid decarboxylase (GAD) suppressed autoimmune diabetes in NOD mice. NOD mice develop diabetes spontaneously, which in many aspects resembles type I diabetes of humans. AAV-mediated gene transfer of GAD led to inactivation of GAD-specific T cells, an enhanced GAD-specific Th2 response, including an increase of T-cell-producing IL-4, IL-10, and TGF-β, a decrease of those producing IFN-γ, and an increase of $CD4^+$ $CD25^+$ Tregs cells [Han et al. 2005].

A recent series of elegant studies showed that rAAV vectors induce transgene product-specific tolerance through the induction of $CD4^+$ $CD25^+$ Tregs. rAAV-induced Tregs not only prevented immune responses to the transgene product delivered by the rAAV vector, but also blocked induction of responses to a highly immunogenic adenovirus vector expressing the same transgene product. Tregs were most efficiently induced by hepatic rAAV-mediated gene transfer. They were shown to express FoxP3, GITR, and CTLA4, and suppressed the activation of $CD4^+$ T helper cells, and in consequence, they suppressed antibody formation to the transgene product [Dobrzynski et al. 2006; Cao et al. 2007].

6.5 CONCLUSIONS

More than 20 clinical phase I or II trials are under way or at their final stages of planning to test ssAAV or dsAAV vectors expressing therapeutic proteins or vaccine antigens in human volunteers. Most reports on rAAV vectors explicitly state them to be exceptionally safe, although in the only rAAV gene therapy trial to date that objectively achieved expression of therapeutic levels of the transgene product, one patient, within weeks after vector infusion into the liver, developed a subclinical hepatitis and then lost the therapeutic benefit of the gene transfer, presumably caused by an immune response to the vector's capsid antigens. In other serious adverse reactions following AAV gene transfer, a death due to status epilepticus shortly after intracerebral application of rAAV vectors for treatment of Batten disease was reported by the Recombinant DNA Advisory Committee [2005], and more recently a death upon intraarticular injection of a rAAV vector expressing a TNF-α antagonist for treatment of rheumatoid arthritis [Weiss 2007]. Whether or not AAV gene transfer contributed to the death of these two patients remains unresolved. Clinical trials using rAAV2 vectors as vaccine carriers did not report any serious adverse reactions, but unfortunately, neither reported induction of potent immune responses.

Overall, we know remarkably little about the biology of natural AAV infections or immunological memory responses that humans harbor to antigens of AAV. Although we know more by far about rAAV vectors, the literature contains contradictory findings about how rAAV vectors interact with various cells of the immune system. Although rAAV vectors have performed exceptionally well in preclinical trials and have yielded promising results in clinical trials that targeted immunoprivileged sites such as the brain or the eye, additional basic studies on natural infections with AAVs as well as on the basic biological behavior of rAAV vectors are still warranted to improve their efficacy for as gene replacement vectors. The use of rAAV vectors as vaccine vehicles clearly needs additional preclinical studies to further understand the effects of rAAV vaccines on T-cell functionality.

REFERENCES

Abele R and Tampe R. 1999. Function of the transport complex TAP in cellular immune recognition. *Biochim Biophys Acta* 1461:405–419.

Aldrich WA, Ren C, et al. 2006. Enhanced transduction of mouse bone marrow–derived dendritic cells by repetitive infection with self-complementary adeno-associated virus 6 combined with immunostimulatory ligands. *Gene Ther* 13:29–39.

Banchereau J and Steinman RM. 1998. Dendritic cells and the control of immunity. *Nature* 392:245–252.

Barnett BG, Crews CJ, et al. 2002. Targeted adenoviral vectors. *Biochim Biophys Acta* 1575:1–14.

Bartlett JS, Wilcher R, et al. 2000. Infectious entry pathway of adeno-associated virus and adeno-associated virus vectors. *J Virol* 74:2777–2785.

Bessis N, GarciaCozar FJ, et al. 2004. Immune responses to gene therapy vectors: influence on vector function and effector mechanisms. *Gene Ther* 11 (Suppl 1):S10–S17.

Blacklow NR. 1988. In *Parvoviruses and Human Disease*, JR Pattison, Ed. CRC Press, Boca Raton, FL, pp. 117–132.

Brossart P and Bevan MJ. 1997. Presentation of exogenous protein antigens on major histocompatibility complex class I molecules by dendritic cells: pathway of presentation and regulation by cytokines. *Blood* 90:1594–1599.

Brown GR, Thiele DL, et al. 1997. Adenoviral vectors given intravenously to immunocompromised mice yield stable transduction of the colonic epithelium. *Gastroenterology* 112:1586–1594.

Cao O, Dobrzynski E, et al. 2007. Induction and role of regulatory $CD4^{+}CD25^{+}$ T cells in tolerance to the transgene product following hepatic in vivo gene transfer. *Blood* 110:1132–1140.

Carter BJ. 1974. Analysis of parvovirus mRNA by sedimentation and electrophoresis in aqueous and nonaqueous solution. *J Virol* 14:834–839.

Castellino F and Germain RN. 1995. Extensive trafficking of MHC class II-invariant chain complexes in the endocytic pathway and appearance of peptide-loaded class II in multiple compartments. *Immunity* 2:73–88.

Castellino F, Zhong G, et al. 1997. Antigen presentation by MHC class II molecules: invariant chain function, protein trafficking, and the molecular basis of diverse determinant capture. *Hum Immunol* 54:159–169.

Cearley CN and Wolfe JH. 2006. Transduction characteristics of adeno-associated virus vectors expressing cap serotypes 7, 8, 9, and Rh10 in the mouse brain. *Mol Ther* 13:528–537.

Chatelain R, Varkila K, et al. 1992. IL-4 induces a Th2 response in *Leishmania major*–infected mice. *J Immunol* 148:1182–1187.

Chenuaud P, Larcher T, et al. 2004. Autoimmune anemia in macaques following erythropoietin gene therapy. *Blood* 103:3303–3304.

Chiriva-Internati M, Liu Y, et al. 2002. Efficient generation of cytotoxic T lymphocytes against cervical cancer cells by adeno-associated virus/human papillomavirus type 16 E7 antigen gene transduction into dendritic cells. *Eur J Immunol* 32:30–38.

Chirmule N, Propert K, et al. 1999. Immune responses to adenovirus and adeno-associated virus in humans. *Gene Ther* 6:1574–1583.

Chirmule N, Xiao W, et al. 2000. Humoral immunity to adeno-associated virus type 2 vectors following administration to murine and nonhuman primate muscle. *J Virol* 74:2420–2425.

Cordier L, Gao GP, et al. 2001. Muscle-specific promoters may be necessary for adeno-associated virus-mediated gene transfer in the treatment of muscular dystrophies. *Hum Gene Ther* 12:205–215.

Cresswell P, Bangia N, et al. 1999. The nature of the MHC class I peptide loading complex. *Immunol Rev* 172:21–28.

De BP, Heguy A, et al. 2006. High levels of persistent expression of alpha1-antitrypsin mediated by the nonhuman primate serotype rh.10 adeno-associated virus despite pre-existing immunity to common human adeno-associated viruses. *Mol Ther* 13:67–76.

Dobrzynski E, Fitzgerald JC, et al. 2006. Prevention of cytotoxic T lymphocyte responses to factor IX–expressing hepatocytes by gene transfer–induced regulatory T cells. *Proc Natl Acad Sci U S A* 103:4592–4597.

Dong C and Flavell RA. 2001. Th1 and Th2 cells. *Curr Opin Hematol* 8:47–51.

Donsante A, Miller DG, et al. 2007. AAV vector integration sites in mouse hepatocellular carcinoma. *Science* 317:477.

Douar AM, Poulard K, et al. 2001. Intracellular trafficking of adeno-associated virus vectors: routing to the late endosomal compartment and proteasome degradation. *J Virol* 75:1824–1833.

Elliott T. 1997. How does TAP associate with MHC class I molecules? *Immunol Today* 18:375–379.

Fairchild PJ and Wraith DC. 1996. Lowering the tone: mechanisms of immunodominance among epitopes with low affinity for MHC. *Immunol Today* 17:80–85.

Fields PA, Arruda VR, et al. 2001. Risk and prevention of anti-factor IX formation in AAV-mediated gene transfer in the context of a large deletion of F9. *Mol Ther* 4:201–210.

Fisher KJ, Jooss K, et al. 1997. Recombinant adeno-associated virus for muscle directed gene therapy. *Nat Med* 3:306–312.

Fitzgerald JC, Gao GP, et al. 2003. A simian replication-defective adenoviral recombinant vaccine to HIV-1 gag. *J Immunol* 170:1416–1422.

Flavell RA. 1999. The molecular basis of T cell differentiation. *Immunol Res* 19:159–168.

Fowell D, McKnight AJ, et al. 1991. Subsets of CD4$^+$ T cells and their roles in the induction and prevention of autoimmunity. *Immunol Rev* 123:37–64.

Gao G, Lebherz C, et al. 2004a. Erythropoietin gene therapy leads to autoimmune anemia in macaques. *Blood* 103:3300–3302.

Gao G, Vandenberghe LH, et al. 2004b. Clades of adeno-associated viruses are widely disseminated in human tissues. *J Virol* 78:6381–6388.

Gao G, Vandenberghe LH, et al. 2005. New recombinant serotypes of AAV vectors. *Curr Gene Ther* 5:285–297.

Gao GP, Alvira MR, et al. 2002a. Novel adeno-associated viruses from rhesus monkeys as vectors for human gene therapy. *Proc Natl Acad Sci U S A* 99:11854–11859.

Gao GP, Lu F, et al. 2002b. Rep/Cap gene amplification and high-yield production of AAV in an A549 cell line expressing Rep/Cap. *Mol Ther* 5:644–649.

Ge Y, Powell S, et al. 2001. Factors influencing the development of an anti-factor IX (FIX) immune response following administration of adeno-associated virus-FIX. *Blood* 97:3733–3737.

Geoffroy MC and Salvetti A. 2005. Helper functions required for wild type and recombinant adeno-associated virus growth. *Curr Gene Ther* 5:265–271.

Goncalves MA. 2005. Adeno-associated virus: from defective virus to effective vector. *Virol J* 2:43.

Grandea AG, 3rd and Van Kaer L. 2001. Tapasin: an ER chaperone that controls MHC class I assembly with peptide. *Trends Immunol* 22:194–199.

Guidotti LG and Chisari FV. 2000. Cytokine-mediated control of viral infections. *Virology* 273:221–227.

Halbert CL, Rutledge EA, et al. 2000. Repeat transduction in the mouse lung by using adeno-associated virus vectors with different serotypes. *J Virol* 74:1524–1532.

Halbert CL, Miller AD, et al. 2006. Prevalence of neutralizing antibodies against adeno-associated virus (AAV) types 2, 5, and 6 in cystic fibrosis and normal populations: implications for gene therapy using AAV vectors. *Hum Gene Ther* 17:440–447.

Han G, Li Y, et al. 2005. Active tolerance induction and prevention of autoimmune diabetes by immunogene therapy using recombinant adenoassociated virus expressing glutamic acid decarboxylase 65 peptide GAD(500–585). *J Immunol* 174:4516–4524.

Hensley SE, Giles-Davis W, et al. 2005. Dendritic cell maturation, but not $CD8^+$ T cell induction, is dependent on type I IFN signaling during vaccination with adenovirus vectors. *J Immunol* 175:6032–6041.

Hensley SE, Cun AS, et al. 2007. Type I interferon inhibits antibody responses induced by a chimpanzee adenovirus vector. *Mol Ther* 15:393–403.

Hernandez YJ, Wang J, et al. 1999. Latent adeno-associated virus infection elicits humoral but not cell-mediated immune responses in a nonhuman primate model. *J Virol* 73:8549–8558.

Herzog RW, Fields PA, et al. 2002. Influence of vector dose on factor IX–specific T and B cell responses in muscle-directed gene therapy. *Hum Gene Ther* 13:1281–1291.

High K. 2002. AAV-mediated gene transfer for hemophilia. *Genet Med* 4:56S–61S.

Johnson PR, Schnepp BC, et al. 2005. Novel adeno-associated virus vector vaccine restricts replication of simian immunodeficiency virus in macaques. *J Virol* 79:955–965.

Ju ST, Matsui K, et al. 1999. Molecular and cellular mechanisms regulating T and B cell apoptosis through Fas/FasL interaction. *Int Rev Immunol* 18:485–513.

Kafri T, Morgan D, et al. 1998. Cellular immune response to adenoviral vector infected cells does not require de novo viral gene expression: implications for gene therapy. *Proc Natl Acad Sci U S A* 95:11377–11382.

Kay MA, Manno CS, et al. 2000. Evidence for gene transfer and expression of factor IX in haemophilia B patients treated with an AAV vector. *Nat Genet* 24:257–261.

Kuck D, Lau T, et al. 2006. Intranasal vaccination with recombinant adeno-associated virus type 5 against human papillomavirus type 16 L1. *J Virol* 80:2621–2630.

Lamartina S, Sporeno E, et al. 2000. Characteristics of the adeno-associated virus preintegration site in human chromosome 19: open chromatin conformation and transcription-competent environment. *J Virol* 74:7671–7677.

Lanzavecchia A and Sallusto F. 2001. Regulation of T cell immunity by dendritic cells. *Cell* 106:263–266.

Lee GK, Maheshri N, et al. 2005. PEG conjugation moderately protects adeno-associated viral vectors against antibody neutralization. *Biotechnol Bioeng* 92:24–34.

Li C, Hirsch M, et al. 2007. Adeno-associated virus type 2 (AAV2) capsid-specific cytotoxic T lymphocytes eliminate only vector-transduced cells coexpressing the AAV2 capsid in vivo. *J Virol* 81:7540–7547.

Li H, Murphy SL, et al. 2007. Pre-existing AAV capsid-specific $CD8^+$ T cells are unable to eliminate AAV-transduced hepatocytes. *Mol Ther* 15:792–800.

Lin J, Zhi Y, et al. 2007. Vaccines based on novel adeno-associated virus vectors elicit aberrant $CD8^+$ T cell responses in mice. *J Virol* 81:11840–11849.

Liu DW, Tsao YP, et al. 2000. Recombinant adeno-associated virus expressing human papillomavirus type 16 E7 peptide DNA fused with heat shock protein DNA as a potential vaccine for cervical cancer. *J Virol* 74:2888–2894.

Liu X, Voulgaropoulou F, et al. 2000. Selective Rep–Cap gene amplification as a mechanism for high-titer recombinant AAV production from stable cell lines. *Mol Ther* 2:394–403.

Liu YJ. 2001. Dendritic cell subsets and lineages, and their functions in innate and adaptive immunity. *Cell* 106:259–262.

Liu Y, Chiriva-Internati M, et al. 2001. Rapid induction of cytotoxic T-cell response against cervical cancer cells by human papillomavirus type 16 E6 antigen gene delivery into human dendritic cells by an adeno-associated virus vector. *Cancer Gene Ther* 8:948–957.

Liu Y, Chiriva-Internati M, et al. 2005. Use and specificity of breast cancer antigen/milk protein BA46 for generating anti-self-cytotoxic T lymphocytes by recombinant adeno-associated virus-based gene loading of dendritic cells. *Cancer Gene Ther* 12:304–312.

Liu Y, Zhou W, et al. 2006. An autoimmune domain-reduced HCV core gene remains effective in stimulating anti-core cytotoxic T lymphocyte activity. *Vaccine* 24:1615–1624.

Logan GJ, Wang L, et al. 2007. AAV vectors encoding malarial antigens stimulate antigen-specific immunity but do not protect from parasite infection. *Vaccine* 25:1014–1022.

Louboutin JP, Wang L, et al. 2005. Gene transfer into skeletal muscle using novel AAV serotypes. *J Gene Med* 7:442–451.

Mahadevan M, Liu Y, et al. 2007. Generation of robust cytotoxic T lymphocytes against prostate specific antigen by transduction of dendritic cells using protein and recombinant adeno-associated virus. *Cancer Immunol Immunother* 56:1615–1624.

Manning WC, Paliard X, et al. 1997. Genetic immunization with adeno-associated virus vectors expressing herpes simplex virus type 2 glycoproteins B and D. *J Virol* 71:7960–7962.

Manno CS, Chew AJ, et al. 2003. AAV-mediated factor IX gene transfer to skeletal muscle in patients with severe hemophilia B. *Blood* 101:2963–2972.

Matzinger P. 2002. The danger model: a renewed sense of self. *Science* 296:301–305.

McPhee SW, Janson CG, et al. 2006. Immune responses to AAV in a phase I study for Canavan disease. *J Gene Med* 8:577–588.

McTiernan CF, Mathier MA, et al. 2007. Myocarditis following adeno-associated viral gene expression of human soluble TNF receptor (TNFRII-Fc) in baboon hearts. *Gene Ther* 14:1613–1622.

Mellman I and Steinman RM. 2001. Dendritic cells: specialized and regulated antigen processing machines. *Cell* 106:255–258.

Mingozzi F, Hasbrouck NC, et al. 2007a. Modulation of tolerance to the transgene product in a non-human primate model of AAV-mediated gene transfer to liver. *Blood* 110:2334–2341.

Mingozzi F, Maus MV, et al. 2007b. CD8(+) T-cell responses to adeno-associated virus capsid in humans. *Nat Med* 13:419–422.

Moser M and Murphy KM. 2000. Dendritic cell regulation of Th1–Th2 development. *Nat Immunol* 1:199–205.

Moskalenko M, Chen L, et al. 2000. Epitope mapping of human anti-adeno-associated virus type 2 neutralizing antibodies: implications for gene therapy and virus structure. *J Virol* 74:1761–1766.

Murray N and McMichael A. 1992. Antigen presentation in virus infection. *Curr Opin Immunol* 4:401–407.

O'Garra A. 1998. Cytokines induce the development of functionally heterogeneous T helper cell subsets. *Immunity* 8:275–283.

Pastor EJ, Debelak DJ, et al. 2007. *Development and characterization of a relative potency assay for rAAV1 vectors for use as vaccines*. Presented at the 10th Annual Meeting of the American Society of Gene Therapy, Seattle, WA.

Peden CS, Burger C, et al. 2004. Circulating anti-wild-type adeno-associated virus type 2 (AAV2) antibodies inhibit recombinant AAV2 (rAAV2)-mediated, but not rAAV5-mediated, gene transfer in the brain. *J Virol* 78:6344–6359.

Pieters J. 2000. MHC class II–restricted antigen processing and presentation. *Adv Immunol* 75:159–208.

Ponnazhagan S, Mahendra G, et al. 2001. Adeno-associated virus type 2–mediated transduction of human monocyte-derived dendritic cells: implications for ex vivo immunotherapy. *J Virol* 75:9493–9501.

Qing K, Mah C, et al. 1999. Human fibroblast growth factor receptor 1 is a co-receptor for infection by adeno-associated virus 2. *Nat Med* 5:71–77.

Raper SE, Chirmule N, et al. 2003. Fatal systemic inflammatory response syndrome in a ornithine transcarbamylase deficient patient following adenoviral gene transfer. *Mol Genet Metab* 80:148–158.

Recombinant DNA Advisory Committee. 2005. National Institutes of Health, Bethesda, MD.

Reits EA, Vos JC, et al. 2000. The major substrates for TAP in vivo are derived from newly synthesized proteins. *Nature* 404:774–778.

Roberts AD, Ely KH, et al. 2005. Differential contributions of central and effector memory T cells to recall responses. *J Exp Med* 202:123–133.

Sabatino DE, Mingozzi F, et al. 2005. Identification of mouse AAV capsid-specific $CD8^+$ T cell epitopes. *Mol Ther* 12:1023–1033.

Sakaguchi S, Sakaguchi N, et al. 1995. Immunologic self-tolerance maintained by activated T cells expressing IL-2 receptor alpha-chains (CD25): breakdown of a single mechanism of self-tolerance causes various autoimmune diseases. *J Immunol* 155:1151–1164.

Sallusto F, Schaerli P, et al. 1998. Rapid and coordinated switch in chemokine receptor expression during dendritic cell maturation. *Eur J Immunol* 28:2760–2769.

Sallusto F, Langenkamp A, et al. 2000. Functional subsets of memory T cells identified by CCR7 expression. *Curr Top Microbiol Immunol* 251:167–171.

Sanlioglu S, Benson PK, et al. 2000. Endocytosis and nuclear trafficking of adeno-associated virus type 2 are controlled by rac1 and phosphatidylinositol-3 kinase activation. *J Virol* 74:9184–9196.

Saron MF, Fayolle C, et al. 1997. Anti-viral protection conferred by recombinant adenylate cyclase toxins from *Bordetella pertussis* carrying a $CD8^+$ T cell epitope from lymphocytic choriomeningitis virus. *Proc Natl Acad Sci U S A* 94:3314–3319.

Sarukhan A, Camugli S, et al. 2001. Successful interference with cellular immune responses to immunogenic proteins encoded by recombinant viral vectors. *J Virol* 75:269–277.

Scallan CD, Jiang H, et al. 2006. Human immunoglobulin inhibits liver transduction by AAV vectors at low AAV2 neutralizing titers in SCID mice. *Blood* 107:1810–1817.

Smith-Arica JR and Bartlett JS. 2001. Gene therapy: recombinant adeno-associated virus vectors. *Curr Cardiol Rep* 3:43–49.

Solheim JC. 1999. Class I MHC molecules: assembly and antigen presentation. *Immunol Rev* 172:11–19.

Sozzani S, Allavena P, et al. 1998. Differential regulation of chemokine receptors during dendritic cell maturation: a model for their trafficking properties. *J Immunol* 161:1083–1086.

Sozzani S, Allavena P, et al. 2000. Chemokines and dendritic cell traffic. *J Clin Immunol* 20:151–160.

Summerford C, Bartlett JS, et al. 1999. AlphaVbeta5 integrin: a co-receptor for adeno-associated virus type 2 infection. *Nat Med* 5:78–82.

Sun JC and Bevan MJ. 2004. Cutting edge: long-lived CD8 memory and protective immunity in the absence of CD40 expression on CD8T cells. *J Immunol* 172:3385–3389.

Takahashi T, Kuniyasu Y, et al. 1998. Immunologic self-tolerance maintained by $CD25^{+}CD4^{+}$ naturally anergic and suppressive T cells: induction of autoimmune disease by breaking their anergic/suppressive state. *Int Immunol* 10:1969–1980.

Tatsis N and Ertl HC. 2004. Adenoviruses as vaccine vectors. *Mol Ther* 10:616–629.

Taymans JM, Vandenberghe LH, et al. 2007. Comparative analysis of adeno-associated viral vector serotypes 1, 2, 5, 7, and 8 in mouse brain. *Hum Gene Ther* 18:195–206.

Thorsen F, Afione S, et al. 2006. Adeno-associated virus (AAV) serotypes 2, 4 and 5 display similar transduction profiles and penetrate solid tumor tissue in models of human glioma. *J Gene Med* 8:1131–1140.

Timpe J, Bevington J, et al. 2005. Mechanisms of adeno-associated virus genome encapsidation. *Curr Gene Ther* 5:273–284.

Topham DJ, Cardin RC, et al. 2001. Perforin and Fas in murine gammaherpesvirus-specific CD8(+) T cell control and morbidity. *J Gen Virol* 82:1971–1981.

Trinchieri G. 1998. Proinflammatory and immunoregulatory functions of interleukin-12. *Int Rev Immunol* 16:365–396.

Tripathy SK, Black HB, et al. 1996. Immune responses to transgene-encoded proteins limit the stability of gene expression after injection of replication-defective adenovirus vectors. *Nat Med* 2:545–550.

Vandenberghe LH, Wang L, et al. 2006. Heparin binding directs activation of T cells against adeno-associated virus serotype 2 capsid. *Nat Med* 12:967–971.

Veron P, Allo V, et al. 2007. Major subsets of human dendritic cells are efficiently transduced by self-complementary adeno-associated virus vectors 1 and 2. *J Virol* 81:5385–5394.

Vos Q, Lees A, et al. 2000. B-cell activation by T-cell-independent type 2 antigens as an integral part of the humoral immune response to pathogenic microorganisms. *Immunol Rev* 176:154–170.

Wang CH, Liu DW, et al. 2004. Can genes transduced by adeno-associated virus vectors elicit or evade an immune response? *Arch Virol* 149:1–15.

Wang H and Lieber A. 2006. A helper-dependent capsid-modified adenovirus vector expressing adeno-associated virus rep78 mediates site-specific integration of a 27-kilobase transgene cassette. *J Virol* 80:11699–11709.

Wang L, Calcedo R, et al. 2005a. Sustained correction of disease in naive and AAV2-pretreated hemophilia B dogs: AAV2/8-mediated, liver-directed gene therapy. *Blood* 105:3079–3086.

Wang L, Dobrzynski E, et al. 2005b. Systemic protein delivery by muscle-gene transfer is limited by a local immune response. *Blood* 105:4226–4234.

Wang L, Figueredo J, et al. 2007. Cross-presentation of adeno-associated virus serotype 2 capsids activates cytotoxic T cells but does not render hepatocytes effective cytolytic targets. *Hum Gene Ther* 18:185–194.

Watts C and Powis S. 1999. Pathways of antigen processing and presentation. *Rev Immunogenet* 1:60–74.

Weiss R. 2007. Suspended gene therapy test had drawn early questions. *Washington Post*, July 28, p. A09.

Weitzman MD, Kyostio SR, et al. 1994. Adeno-associated virus (AAV) Rep proteins mediate complex formation between AAV DNA and its integration site in human DNA. *Proc Natl Acad Sci U S A* 91:5808–5812.

Wonderling RS and Owens RA. 1997. Binding sites for adeno-associated virus Rep proteins within the human genome. *J Virol* 71:2528–2534.

Xiao W, Chirmule N, et al. 2000. Route of administration determines induction of T-cell-independent humoral responses to adeno-associated virus vectors. *Mol Ther* 1:323–329.

Xin KQ, Urabe M, et al. 2001. A novel recombinant adeno-associated virus vaccine induces a long-term humoral immune response to human immunodeficiency virus. *Hum Gene Ther* 12:1047–1061.

Xin KQ, Ooki T, et al. 2002. Oral administration of recombinant adeno-associated virus elicits human immunodeficiency virus-specific immune responses. *Hum Gene Ther* 13:1571–1581.

Yan Z, Zak R, et al. 2002. Ubiquitination of both adeno-associated virus type 2 and 5 capsid proteins affects the transduction efficiency of recombinant vectors. *J Virol* 76:2043–2053.

York IA, Goldberg AL, et al. 1999. Proteolysis and class I major histocompatibility complex antigen presentation. *Immunol Rev* 172:49–66.

You H, Liu Y, et al. 2006. HBV genes induce cytotoxic T-lymphocyte response upon adeno-associated virus (AAV) vector delivery into dendritic cells. *J Viral Hepat* 13:605–612.

Young SM Jr, McCarty DM, et al. 2000. Roles of adeno-associated virus Rep protein and human chromosome 19 in site-specific recombination. *J Virol* 74:3953–3966.

Zaiss AK and Muruve DA. 2005. Immune responses to adeno-associated virus vectors. *Curr Gene Ther* 5:323–331.

Zaiss AK, Liu Q, et al. 2002. Differential activation of innate immune responses by adenovirus and adeno-associated virus vectors. *J Virol* 76:4580–4590.

Zhang Y, Chirmule N, et al. 2000. CD40 ligand-dependent activation of cytotoxic T lymphocytes by adeno-associated virus vectors in vivo: role of immature dendritic cells. *J Virol* 74:8003–8010.

7

IMMUNE RESPONSES AFTER IN UTERO AND NEONATAL GENE TRANSFER

SIMON N. WADDINGTON, PH.D., AND
SUZANNE M. K. BUCKLEY, PH.D.

Department of Haematology, Haemophilia Centre and Haemostasis Unit, Royal Free and University College Medical School, London, UK

MEGHA S. NIVSARKAR, PH.D., AND CHARLES COUTELLE, M.D., PH.D.

Faculty of Medicine, Imperial College London, London, UK

7.1 INTRODUCTION

In utero or neonatal gene transfer has been proposed as a strategy for treatment of early-onset monogenetic diseases. There are several putative advantages of this approach: Early gene transfer may prevent the onset of terminal pathological changes, take advantage of a high vector/cell ratio, and provide unique access

Gene Therapy Immunology, Edited by Roland Herzog

to stem cell and progenitor cell compartments. In addition, and the subject of this chapter, is the fact that early gene transfer may predispose a mammal to immunological tolerance to the xenoantigen.

In 1953, Peter Medawar demonstrated that immunological tolerance to foreign homologous cells was acquired after inoculation in fetal life. Over the past few years, numerous studies have shown long-term expression of a transgenic protein after fetal or neonatal gene transfer. Nevertheless, several studies have demonstrated that the fetus is capable of mounting an immune response against pathogens, and there is evidence of immune response even in some gene transfer studies. In the early sections of this chapter we provide insight into why early gene transfer so often results in tolerization to transgenic protein. In the later sections we provide an extensive list of studies describing fetal and neonatal gene transfer. In the final section we highlight studies which are important in that they describe *failure* to achieve immune tolerance after early gene transfer.

7.2 HOW GENE TRANSFER MAY DIFFER BETWEEN IMMATURE AND MATURE MAMMALS

A summary of some of the mechanisms that both facilitate and obstruct gene transfer in the fetus and neonate compared with the adult is shown in Fig. 7-1.

7.2.1 Mechanisms Associated with Adaptive Immunity

There are numerous differences in both cell-mediated and humoral immunity between the adult and the fetus/neonate in both humans and mice. Generally, fetuses and neonates show lower and more transient antibody responses to T-cell-dependent protein antigens. Similarly, cell-mediated immune responses are of lower potency than those generated in adults. As part of the widely accepted principle that the fetal and neonatal immune system is generally immature, one possible explanation for poor potency of the immune response is that interaction between the immature dendritic cell and the antigen may be less effective.

The state of pregnancy is associated with a number of unique changes in the maternal immune system. Many of these immune events, which are critical to prevent rejection of the fetus and placenta by the mother, also affect the developing fetus and to some degree extend into neonatal life. Indeed, the fetoplacental unit is often referred to as an immunologically tolerated allograft. Furthermore, parturition shares many similar events with inflammation, including involvement of numerous Th1-associated cytokines. During pregnancy, mechanisms exist to prevent abortion by inhibiting Th1-associated events that enhance Th2-associated activity. Substances that effect this shift in immune function are secreted by the ovaries and placenta and other intrauterine structures. These substances include members of the TGF family [Ayatollahi et al. 2007], IL-10 [Murphy et al. 2005], progesterone [Arck et al. 2007], and progesterone-induced blocking factor (PIBF)

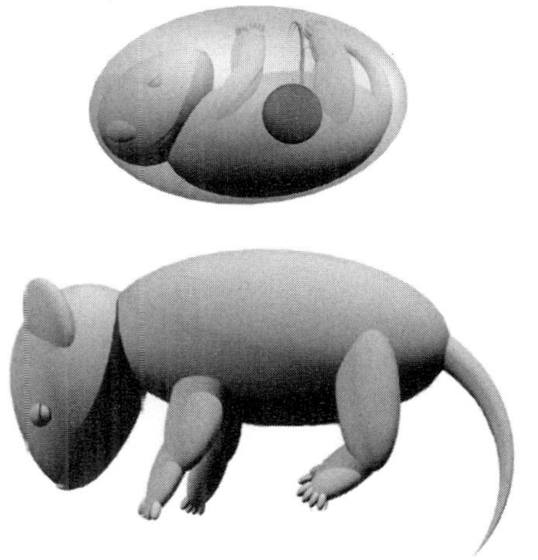

Figure 7-1 Selected summary of mechanisms that influence fetal or neonatal gene transfer.

[Szekeres-Bartho et al. 1997]. This immune milieu is an ideal environment for gene transfer but poses a problem for those aiming to vaccinate the young mammal by direct means. To overcome this, maternal vaccination to provide passive immunization of the fetus has been employed in the animal health industry for decades [Pravieux et al. 2007]. Apart from the fact that fetal and neonatal immunity is skewed toward a Th2 phenotype, other factors probably cause reduced immune response to delivered transgenes and vectors. These include the fact that there are reduced overall numbers of immune cells in early life, that cells participating in the immune response appear to be developmentally immature, and that memory cells are absent due to the naivety of the immune system [Adkins et al. 2003].

As iterated by Ponder et al., newborn humans and/or mice have a reduced secretion of cytokines by lymphocytes. The adult ratio of dendritic cells to thymocytes is only reached at 1 week of age, and the full complement of dendritic cells and plasmacytoid pre-dendritic cells is only acquired at 5 weeks of age. Also, neonatal dendritic cells were inefficient in producing IL-12p70 and IFN-γ and in antigen presentation [Dakic et al. 2004].

Selected studies illustrating such mechanisms are cited below. Newborn mice have a delayed CD4-mediated inflammatory response to pulmonary *Pneumocystis carinii* infection, probably as a consequence of several factors, including blunted TNF-α production, the reduced migration ability of T cells [Qureshi et al. 2003], inefficient phagocytosis and migration of lung antigen-presenting cells to the lymph nodes, as well as delayed chemokine and TNF-α mRNA production [Garvy and Qureshi 2000]. There is evidence that although B cells from human cord blood proliferate and up-regulate CD86 and MHC class II in response to unmethylated cytosine–phosphate–guanosine (CpG)–containing oligonucleotides, they also exhibit homing defects which would prevent them from entering peripheral lymphoid organs efficiently [Tasker and Marshall-Clarke 2003]. Plasmacytoid dendritic cells from human cord blood produced much less IFN-α in response to CpG oligonucleotides than did cells from adult blood [De Wit et al. 2004]. Although spontaneous in vitro proliferation of fetal and neonatal T lymphocytes has been observed to be greater than that of adults, fetal cells responded poorly when simulated with phytohaemagglutinin or allogeneic stimulator cells; IL-2, IL-4, and IFN-γ secretion was entirely absent in fetal T cells and only modest in those from neonates [Zhao et al. 2002].

Despite the wealth of data demonstrating early immune hyporesponsiveness, there is also evidence for a degree of early immune competency which might, in theory, curtail efficacy of fetal and neonatal gene therapy regimes and which, conversely, should provide encouragement for those endeavoring to develop genetic vaccines for early application. For example, human neonatal T cells were found to be capable of developing an adultlike immune CD8 response to *Trypanosoma cruzi*. Following intrauterine antigen exposure, increased concentrations of TNF-α, IL-1β, IL-6, IL-10, and $CD45RO^+$ cells were detected in preterm infants [Duggan et al. 2001].

Additionally, although infants show a limited IFN-γ response to hepatitis B surface antigen vaccination, they also show a greater immunological memory response. This might be specific to the particulate structure of the hepatitis B surface antigen since young infants produce relatively lower antibody responses than those of adults after vaccination against diphtheria, pertussis, tetanus, *Haemophilus influenzae* type B, and measles vaccines [Ota et al. 2004]. Human fetal B cells have reduced antibody repertoires, due to reduced junctional diversity; however, this a not a limiting determinant of the quality of antibody response to viruses of infants beyond the neonatal period [Weitkamp et al. 2003]. It has also been observed that white blood cells from preterm and term neonates show blunted IL-10 and TGF-β production after lipopolysaccharide (LPS) and phorbol myristoyl aceate/ionomycin stimulation, respectively. Furthermore, IL-10 was less effective in inhibiting IL-1α, IL-6, IL-8, and TNF-α produced in response to LPS [Schultz et al. 2004]. The controversy surrounding the capacity for immune sensitization stems not only from the unique phenotype of the fetal immune system, but also from a past inability to detect and immunophenotype antigen-specific $CD4^+$ and $CD8^+$ T cells. However, the advent of MHC classes I and II multimer reagents has now enabled such analysis. From pregnant mothers vaccinated against influenza, it was found that the fetus produced antivaccine antibodies; *H. influenza*–specific $CD4^+$ T cells were detected in cord blood [Rastogi et al. 2007].

In conclusion, although the early adaptive immune system appears to be predisposed to tolerance to transgenic protein, it remains highly complex and poorly understood compared with the adult immune system. Moreover, the relative maturity of immune systems of different animal models is often highly divergent from that of the human system, both throughout gestation and at birth.

7.2.2 Innate Immune Mechanisms

Innate and acquired immunity interact closely in a multitude of ways, forming a defensive continuum. The innate antiviral activity of human leucocytes was shown to be lower in umbilical cord blood than in blood from adults [Rybka et al. 2003]. However, it has been suggested that in most other ways, innate immunity is enhanced perinatally to compensate for the shortcomings of the acquired immune system. Innate immunity exists in the form of many barriers, including immune cells, cell layers, extracellular matrices, and antimicrobial compounds. For the fetus, the enclosing membranes are the first line of defense. When lacZ adenovirus was injected into the exocoelomic cavity between the amniotic and chorionic membranes, no transduction of fetal tissues was observed, probably because of the physical barrier of the membrane [Laurema et al. 2004]. Similarly, in our experience of intraamniotic injections into fetal mice, it is important to ensure penetration of the needle into the amniotic cavity, since virus inadvertently injected into the extraembryonic coelom would produce excellent transduction of the membranes but none in the fetus [Buckley et al. 2005]. The skin of the human fetus begins to stratify at week 9 and completes keratinization by week 14 [Bullard et al. 2003]. The barrier function of the skin has been described as the *raison d'être* of the epidermis [Madison 2003]. In mice, early intraamniotic injection of lacZ adenovirus resulted in skin expression, which decreased the later in gestation the injection was performed [Schneider et al. 1999; Buckley et al. 2005]. Similarly, neonatal but not adult muscle was found to strongly express β-galactosidase after delivery by herpex simplex virus vector. Evidence was provided to suggest that the immaturity of the basal lamina of the neonatal muscle was the reason for this disparity [Huard et al. 1996]. There is also evidence that the blood–brain barrier permeability decreases from the third trimester through to adulthood in sheep [Stonestreet et al. 1996] and rats [Kniesel et al. 1996].

Respiratory mucus protects the airways from dehydration but also from pathogens. Secretion begins in the fetal respiratory mucosae at 13 weeks of gestation, but the mucins expressed are quite different from those found in the adult and are thought to be involved in lung differentiation and maturation [Buisine et al. 1999]. Therefore, one might suppose that in utero the lung could be more vulnerable to infection by pathogens—or vectors. The fetus is bathed in amniotic fluid, which not only provides physical support but also possesses antibacterial and antifungal properties [Yoshio et al. 2003]. Lysozyme, which was identified in fractions of the amniotic fluid showing antimicrobial activity and is also found in human placenta and fetal membranes, shows antiviral activity against HIV and ectromelia virus [Lee-Huang et al. 1999]. Amniotic fluid was also found to inhibit in vitro infection of 3T3 cells by retroviral vectors [Douar et al. 1996]. This and other antimicrobial compounds have also been found in the cervical mucus plugs and the vernix caseosa (Latin for "cheesy varnish"), a lipid-rich deposit covering the skin of the baby at birth [Yoshio et al. 2003]. Other compounds include the recently discovered antimicrobial peptides of which humans possess two major classes, defensins and cathelicidins. The defensin cryptidin was found in fetal mice as early as 17.5 days gestation (term at approximately 20 days), expressed in the suprabasal keratinocytes of fetal and neonatal but not adult mice [Shirafuji et al. 1999]. In vitro, defensins have been shown to inhibit replication of HIV-1 [Zhang et al. 2002] and infection of 293 cells with adenovirus vector [Bastian and Schafer 2001]. Specifically the theta-defensin retrocyclin was found to inhibit early HIV infection, probably by preventing viral fusion or entry [Cole et al. 2002; Munk et al. 2003]. Cathelicidins, which have been shown to be greatly up-regulated in neonatal skin [Dorschner et al. 2003], have been shown to prevent infection of Vero76 cells by herpes simplex virus in vitro [Benincasa et al. 2003]. Human intestinal defensin expression was found to be much lower in the 24-week fetus than in the adult and was posited as a contributory factor in the high incidence of necrotizing enterocolitis in preterm infants [Mallow et al. 1996]. Other substances found in the vernix caseosa, in human colostrums, and in milk include fatty acids, which have been found to kill enveloped viruses in vitro. In fact, the stomach contents of infants show strong antiviral properties, due to release of fatty acids from the milk triglycerides. Indeed, it has been suggested that regurgitation of partially digested milk into the nasal passages may afford microbicidal protection (reviewed by Thormar and Hilmarsson [2007]).

7.2.3 Vector Receptors

To gain entry to the cell, viruses utilize a wide range of cell surface receptors, which generally serve critical purposes at some point or throughout life. However, as viruses and their hosts have coevolved over millennia, it is much easier to discuss the consequences than the reasons for differential receptor development throughout early ontogeny in the context of viral and, *ergo*, vector delivery. It was demonstrated that marker gene expression after adenoviral vector delivery was much greater in the neonate than the adult in almost all tissues, and similar differential expression of the αv integrin receptor, known to mediate vector endocytosis, was observed [Huard et al. 1995]. Similarly, it was found that skeletal muscle fibers were infected efficiently by adenoviral vectors in neonatal but less so in adult mice, and that this was probably due to the relatively high neonatal expression of the coxsackie and adenovirus receptor [Nalbantoglu et al. 1999].

7.2.4 Maternal Influence

Transplacental transport of maternal immunoglobulins to the developing fetus is important in protection of the newborn from infection, since neonatal antibody production is delayed. Fcγ receptors, which are believed to facilitate this transport, are expressed predominantly on fetal endothelial cells in the third trimester. This is thought to explain why preterm neonates have reduced levels of maternal immunoglobulin [Okoko et al. 2001]. In mice, transplacental passage of antibodies against herpes simplex virus was shown to protect the neonate against viral-induced mortality. After birth, mammals receive protective antibody from maternal milk; humans receive primarily IgA and mice primarily IgG [Yorty et al. 2004]. Therefore, preexisting maternal immunity to viral vector components might impede fetal or neonatal gene transfer by vector neutralization or antibody-dependent cellular cytotoxicity. Also, in addition to antibodies (and fatty acids, discussed above), maternal milk supplies the neonate with other antimicrobial and antiviral compounds, including lysozyme and lactoferrin, which shows antiviral activity against herpes simplex virus [Marchetti et al. 2004], HIV [Berkhout et al. 2002], and adenovirus [Di Biase et al. 2003]. At birth, the sterility of the fetal gut is lost rapidly as colonization by symbiotic bacteria begins. This colonization is often influenced strongly by the composition of the flora of the maternal vagina and gastrointestinal tract, but also by the general environment, and is believed to enhance the mucosal protective barrier, modify the systemic immune system, and exclude less desirable microbes by competition (for reviews, see Fanaro et al. [2003] and Millar et al. [2003]). Administration of the probiotic *Lactobacillus rhamnosus* has been shown to limit viral gastroenteritis and diarrhea in infants receiving antibiotics [Arvola et al. 1999]. There can be no doubt that enteric flora would influence gene transfer to these tissues, a strategy that might be considered in order to limit or prevent the gut pathology seen in cystic fibrosis. These influences remain undefined, however.

Several other factors dictate whether immune tolerance or sensitization prevails: for example, the age of intervention, as the logical extreme is the production of transgenic organisms by gene transfer before or just after conception. Indeed, in protein therapy, early intervention has been shown to improve the chances of achieving immune tolerance to, for example, human factor VIII by hemophilia A mice after neonatal administration [Madoiwa et al. 2004]. For secreted transgenic proteins. another important factor appears to be their circulating concentration, For example, Zhang and colleagues [2004] demonstrated that high or intermediate but not low doses of retrovirus resulted in sufficiently high expression of human factor IX to achieve immune tolerance to the xenoprotein. There also appears to be a need for *persistent* expression. When we injected fetal mice with adenovirus to deliver human factor IX, protein expression fell exponentially until around 8 weeks of age, where it tended to plateau. Mice that express the protein, albeit at low concentrations ($\approx 0.5\%$) were tolerant of immune challenge with purified human factor IX protein combined with adjuvant. However, in mice that had initially very high factor IX concentrations that eventually became undetectable

($<0.1\%$), and which were not producing anti-hFIX antibodies, immune challenge provoked an anti-hFIX immune response (unpublished observations).

It is also evident that just as in gene transfer to the adult, the nature of the transgenic protein is also a determinant of the immune response. Immune tolerance to xenogeneic factor IX has been shown after fetal or neonatal administration in numerous studies [Waddington et al. 2003a, 2004; Zhang et al. 2004; Xu et al. 2007]. In contrast, a more variegated profile is seen with early gene transfer of hFVIII, where it has been observed that a proportion of animals develop anti-hFVIII antibodies after neonatal gene transfer [VandenDriessche et al. 1999]. This may relate to the above-mentioned issue concerning amounts of circulating antigen, since factor VIII is synthesized in relatively low amounts compared to factor IX following gene transfer. In fact, a very marked dose-dependent effect was observed for retrovirus-mediated gene transfer of human factor VIII (hFVIII) to neonatal mice. Those mice receiving the high retroviral dose synthesized relatively high concentrations of hFVIII and were resistant to subsequent challenge with protein or adjuvant challenges in that they continued to synthesize hFVIII and few developed an anti-hFVIII immune response. In contrast, those receiving medium or low retroviral doses, when challenged with FVIII and adjuvant, developed anti-hFVIII antibodies [Xu et al. 2007].

7.3 LONG-TERM EXPRESSION AFTER FETAL GENE TRANSFER

In the following two sections we summarize the majority of studies using gene transfer in the fetal and neonatal period. In the final section, specific comments are made on some of the papers, which shed light on the nature of fetal and immune tolerization after gene transfer. Buoyed by a combination of improvements in vector technology, administration technique, and sensitivity and breadth of analysis, a plethora of studies have been published this decade showing long-term transgene expression after fetal or neonatal delivery. Notably, and in contrast to many studies reporting on adult gene transfer, these results were achieved without any form of immune suppression.

Byrne's group used AAV2/1 to achieve expression of human α-glucosidase in the diaphragm of mice deficient in this enzyme. Human patients often die from respiratory failure [Rucker et al. 2004]. Here, restoration of normal contractile function was observed for up to six months after birth. In 2005, Bennett's group also used AAV2/1 to deliver human RPE65 to the retinal pigmented epithelium of Rpe65$^{-/-}$ mice and demonstrated restoration of visual function [Dejneka et al. 2004]. Very recently, AAV2/1 were also used, by Karolewski and Wolfe [2006], to treat a mouse model of mucopolysaccharidosis type VII. This vector carrying the human β-glucuronidase cDNA was injected into the ventricle of the fetal brain, resulting in widespread gene expression in the brain and spinal cord, and survival was significantly improved at one year. All three studies used nonintegrating vectors for gene delivery to tissues that undergo minimal cell cycling in adult life. In contrast, HIV-based vectors pseudotyped with VSV-G were used to correct three disease models after fetal administration. This vector integrates into the recipient's genome and may therefore provide long-term expression if delivered to appropriate progenitor cells. For treatment of factor IX hemophilia, Coutelle's group injected the vector into the fetal vitelline vessels, which resulted in predominant expression of human factor IX in the mouse liver (the site of endogenous synthesis) and achieved lifelong correction of the bleeding diathesis [Waddington et al. 2004]. For treatment of a rat model of Crigler–Najjar type I disease [bilirubin UDP-glucuronyltransferase (UGT1A1) deficiency], intraperitoneal and hepatic delivery of the transgene was achieved from direct intrahepatic vector injection by Seppen et al. [2003]. This ameliorated the metabolic defect significantly for at least one year. In both studies, long-term detection of clusters of transduced cells in liver and intestine, respectively, indicated that organ-specific progenitors had been transduced and become a source of transgene-expressing cells over a rodent's lifetime. Interestingly, a later study by Seppen et al. [2005] documents the development of a nonablative immune response against the transgenic protein.

7.4 LONG-TERM EXPRESSION AFTER NEONATAL GENE TRANSFER

Studies demonstrating long-term therapeutic effects have been more numerous following neonatal rather than fetal intervention, probably because neonatal vector administration is technically easier. Several studies from the laboratories of Ponder and Haskins have centered on correction of mucopolysaccharidoses I and VII and hemophilias A and B using retroviral vectors. They observed long-term expression and therapeutic benefit following neonatal administration of β-glucuronidase delivered by retroviral vectors in mice [Xu et al. 2002] and dogs [Mango et al. 2004; Sleeper et al. 2004]. Similarly, long-term prevention of disease was documented following retroviral delivery of α-L-iduronidase to mucopolysaccharidosis I mice [Liu et al. 2005; Chung et al. 2006].

Ponder and colleagues also used retroviral vectors to deliver human factor IX to neonatal hemophilia B mice and dogs, resulting in long-term expression and immune tolerance to the transgenic protein [Zhang et al. 2004]. In a wider-ranging study, the group examined the immune response after neonatal gene therapy in mice, cats, and dogs after retroviral human factor IX delivery. Treated dogs, mice, and three out of four cats were tolerant to, and persistently expressed, the human transgene. The fourth cat lost expression, and this was believed to be a consequence of a cytotoxic T-lymphocyte response. A similar phenomenon was subsequently demonstrated after retroviral delivery of B domain–deleted human factor VIII to hemophilia A mice [Xu et al. 2007]. This study was valuable, as it demonstrated tolerization to factor VIII, which has been shown to be more immunogenic than factor IX when used in the context of either gene or protein therapy. It provided evidence that the greater the level of gene expression, the more likely it would be to achieve immune tolerance.

This group also provided evidence that acquisition of immune tolerance to human factor IX by neonatal administration of retroviral vector was dependent on clonal deletion (i.e., the elimination of T-cell clones which are responsible for mediating immune response to the transgenic protein) [Xu et al. 2007]. However, in our laboratory we have observed adoptive transfer of tolerance to human factor IX. When naive mice received spleen and lymph node cells from mice that had been injected with factor IX adenovirus in utero, they showed a blunted anti-hFIX antibody response compared with mice that had received spleen and lymph node cells from naive donors [Nivsarkar 2006]. Tolerization after fetal or neonatal gene transfer probably involves both clonal deletional and regulatory T cells, and the relative dominance of each may depend on the mode of delivery, vector, and antigen.

A study by Kohn's group demonstrated near-total reversal of disease phenotype in MPS I after neonatal administration, but only partial improvement after treatment of young adults [Kobayashi et al. 2005]. Ma and colleagues [2007] clearly demonstrated that immune suppression during treatment of adults with retroviral vectors improved the phenotype of MPS I mice in some organ systems. This illustrates that neonatal administration crucially utilizes an environment predisposed to immune tolerance but also takes advantage of increased vector spread and organ penetration.

Gamma-retroviral and lentiviral vectors, used in the studies noted above, lead to integration of the transgene into the host's genome, thus providing stable, permanent expression of the transgenic protein. Nevertheless, numerous other studies have described prolonged correction and immune tolerance in mucopolysaccharidoses even following application of nonintegrating vectors such as adenovirus and adeno-associated virus (AAV). Kamata, Kanaji, and colleagues described long-term normalization of defects in the skeleton [Kanaji et al. 2003], central nervous system, and eyes [Kamata et al. 2003] after a single neonatal intravenous injection of adenovirus. This is not the first time that immune tolerance to transgenic protein has been achieved after early adenovirus gene transfer as Zepeda and colleagues demonstrated that intranasal adenovirus administration produced long-term marker gene expression in the lungs of cotton rats [Zepeda and Wilson 1996] and Waddington and co-workers [2003b] showed that fetal intravenous adenovirus resulted in prolonged human factor IX expression in mice. Nevertheless, it emphasizes that even with a relatively potent immunogen such as adenovirus, tolerance can be achieved. In the study by Zepeda et al., lymphocytes harvested following neonatal adenovirus administration were not activated when stimulated in vitro by exposure to the vector. In contrast, adult administration resulted in brief in vivo expression and antibody production; harvested lymphocytes produced a robust in vitro response to inactivated vector.

Several studies from Sands' laboratory and one from Elliger and colleagues demonstrate long-term improvement in the phenotype of MPS VII mice after neonatal intravenous [Daly et al. 1999, 2001], intracranial [Frisella et al. 2001], or intrathecal [Elliger et al. 1999] AAV injection.

Another disease that has proved tractable to neonatal gene therapy is bilirubin UDP-glucuronosyltransferase deficiency. One of the earliest examples of effective neonatal gene transfer was that of Takahasi and colleagues in 1995.

They demonstrated long-term partial correction in the serum bilirubin load and also demonstrated that rats treated in the neonatal period produced much lower antibody titers than did those receiving vector as adults. Intriguingly, they also demonstrated that T cells from neonatally treated rats had a greatly reduced killing effect against vector-infected hepatocytes. Although the rats were, nevertheless, capable of eliminating a wild-type adenovirus infection, it does provide credibility to the concern that immunity toward the originating virus serotype may be compromised. This study is one of the few to provide evidence for tolerization to *vector* as well as transgenic protein [Takahashi et al. 1996]. In our laboratory, we, too, have observed preliminary evidence for tolerization to adenovirus vector after fetal gene transfer to BALB/c mice. Some of those that received intravascular adenovirus vector did not produce anti-adenovirus antibodies when, as adults, they received one or even two additional doses of adenovirus vector of the same serotype. In contrast, all naive adult mice produced anti-adenovirus antibodies after a single vector administration [Nivsarkar 2006].

Nguyen, Bellodi-Privato, and colleagues demonstrated long-term complete phenotypic correction of the Gunn rat using HIV-based vector [Nguyen et al. 2005] and gamma retrovirus vector [Bellodi-Privato et al. 2005]. In the latter study, they sought antibody response against the transgenic protein but detected none.

A miscellany of other studies has shown long-term correction of diseases after neonatal gene transfer. Sun et al. [2002] demonstrated improved survival and long-term expression of glucose-6-phosphate (G6Pase) in the liver and kidney of a mouse model of glycogen storage disease type Ia. Following combined administration of adenovirus and AAV2 to deliver mouse G6Pase to G6Pase$^{-/-}$ recipients, they measured no anti-G6Pase antibodies. The same group then demonstrated a similar effect using repeated administration of AAV2/1, again with no detectable immune response against the mG6Pase [Ghosh et al. 2006]. Broekman et al. [2007] showed complete correction of GM1-gangliosidosis in a mouse model of β-galactosidase deficiency by injecting AAV2/1 into the brain ventricles to deliver mouse lysosomal acid β-galactosidase. Similarly, intraventricular injection of AAV2/1 carrying galactocerebrosidase into a mouse model of the lysosomal disease human globoid cell leukodystrophy slightly improved survival [Shen et al. 2001].

An interesting study by Allamand et al. [2000] used early generation adenovirus to deliver α-sarcoglycans (α-SGs) to the muscles of 4-day-old mice lacking this gene. Long-term expression was achieved and there was no evidence of inflammation or immunologic response. No humoral response developed against either the α-SG or adenoviral proteins, as assessed by ELISA.

7.5 STUDIES HIGHLIGHTING FAILURE TO ACHIEVE IMMUNE TOLERANCE

Although the studies noted above have shown long-term transgene expression after fetal or neonatal delivery, only a few have specifically investigated the nature and mechanisms of immune tolerization. Intriguing are those in which the outcome was immune sensitization rather than tolerization. For example, as mentioned earlier, Seppen and colleagues [2005] observed that rats injected as fetuses or neonates with lentiviral vector encoding UGT1A1 all developed antibodies against the transgenic protein, whereas none arose against GFP delivered by the control vector. This is surprising given that UGT1A1 is a mammalian protein, whereas GFP is derived from the jellyfish *Aequorea victoria*. However, there should be homologs to neither in UGT1A1-deficient rats. Therefore, it may be an aspect of intracellular protein processing and presentation, of availability of immunogenic epitopes, or once again, related to the amount of protein produced.

A study by Liu et al. [2006] demonstrated long-term expression of human factor VIII in hemophilic mice after neonatal gene transfer using nonviral technology and a Sleeping Beauty transposon to achieve expression in lung endothelium. Anti-hFVIII antibodies appeared but slowly disappeared over 168 days in the low-expressing group. However, in those with higher expression, anti-hFVIII antibodies persisted. Rechallenge with additional gene transfer in the low-expressing group caused a large increase in inhibitory antibodies. Although the antibody levels were much lower than had been observed after adult gene transfer, Liu et al. describe several paradoxical observations. First, why did the high-FVIII group but not the low-FVIII group also produce high concentrations of antibody? Second, the fact that FVIII plasmid rechallenge boosted antibody production suggests that immune tolerance had not been achieved [Liu et al. 2006]. There are numerous factors that may account for this. For example, expression of FVIII from this plasmid versus viral vectors may be slower, so onset of expression may be beyond the neonatal "window of tolerization." Also, the plasmid may result in strong expression in lung antigen-presenting cells. Additionally, lung endothelium may not be the principal site of FVIII expression—this may be ascribed to the liver endothelium. Therefore, incorrect protein processing might result in excess failure of quality control and may trigger an immune response.

Although fetal and neonatal gene transfer frequently results in immune tolerance (or at least, ignorance), in many preclinical models it is yet to be seen whether this would be observed in humans. Certainly, the immune system of a newborn baby is much more mature than that of a newborn mouse; however, there are relatively few data on fetal or neonatal gene transfer in the closest model, nonhuman primates. Such studies will be critical in informing us of what might be expected in humans, and are timely given the burgeoning volume of data in preclinical studies using smaller-animal models.

REFERENCES

Adkins B, Williamson T, et al. 2003. Murine neonatal lymphocytes show rapid early cell cycle entry and cell division. *J Immunol* 170:4548–4556.

Allamand V, Donahue KM, et al. 2000. Early adenovirus-mediated gene transfer effectively prevents muscular dystrophy in alpha-sarcoglycan-deficient mice. *Gene Ther* 7:1385–1391.

Arck P, Hansen PJ, et al. 2007. Progesterone during pregnancy: endocrine-immune cross talk in mammalian species and the role of stress. *Am J Reprod Immunol* 58:268–279.

Arvola T, Laiho K, et al. 1999. Prophylactic *Lactobacillus* GG reduces antibiotic-associated diarrhea in children with respiratory infections: a randomized study. *Pediatrics* 104:e64.

Ayatollahi M, Geramizadeh B, et al. 2007. Effect of the immunoregulatory cytokines on successful pregnancy depends upon the control of graft rejection mechanisms. *Transplant Proc* 39:244–245.

Bastian A and Schafer H. 2001. Human alpha-defensin 1 (HNP-1) inhibits adenoviral infection in vitro. *Regul Pept* 101:157–161.

Bellodi-Privato M, Aubert D, et al. 2005. Successful gene therapy of the Gunn rat by in vivo neonatal hepatic gene transfer using murine oncoretroviral vectors. *Hepatology* 42:431–438.

Benincasa M, Skerlavaj B, et al. 2003. In Vitro and in vivo antimicrobial activity of two alpha-helical cathelicidin peptides and of their synthetic analogs. *Peptides* 24:1723–1731.

Berkhout B, van Wamel JL, et al. 2002. Characterization of the anti-HIV effects of native lactoferrin and other milk proteins and protein-derived peptides. *Antiviral Res* 55:341–355.

Broekman ML, Baek RC, et al. 2007. Complete correction of enzymatic deficiency and neurochemistry in the GM1-gangliosidosis mouse brain by neonatal adeno-associated virus-mediated gene delivery. *Mol Ther* 15:30–37.

Buckley SMK, Waddington SN, et al 2005. Factors influencing adenovirus-medated airway transduction in fetal mice. *Mol Ther* 12:484–492.

Buisine MP, Devisme L, et al. 1999. Developmental mucin gene expression in the human respiratory tract. *Am J Respir Cell Mol Biol* 20:209–218.

Bullard KM, Longaker MT, et al. 2003. Fetal wound healing: current biology. *World J Surg* 27:54–61.

Chung S, Ma X, et al. 2006. Effect of neonatal administration of a retroviral vector expressing alpha-l-iduronidase upon lysosomal storage in brain and other organs in mucopolysaccharidosis I mice. *Mol Genet Metab*.

Cole AM, Hong T, et al. 2002. Retrocyclin: a primate peptide that protects cells from infection by T- and M-tropic strains of HIV-1. *Proc Natl Acad Sci U S A* 99:1813–1818.

Dakic A, Shao QX, et al. 2004. Development of the dendritic cell system during mouse ontogeny. *J Immunol* 172:1018–1027.

Daly TM, Vogler C, et al. 1999. Neonatal gene transfer leads to widespread correction of pathology in a murine model of lysosomal storage disease. *Proc Natl Acad Sci U S A* 96:2296–2300.

Daly TM, Ohlemiller KK, et al. 2001. Prevention of systemic clinical disease in MPS VII mice following AAV-mediated neonatal gene transfer. *Gene Ther* 8:1291–1298.

De Wit D, Olislagers V, et al. 2004. Blood plasmacytoid dendritic cell responses to CpG oligodeoxynucleotides are impaired in human newborns. *Blood* 103:1030–1032.

Dejneka NS, Surace EM, et al. 2004. In utero gene therapy rescues vision in a murine model of congenital blindness. *Mol Ther* 9:182–188.

Di Biase AM, Pietrantoni A, et al. 2003. Heparin-interacting sites of bovine lactoferrin are involved in anti-adenovirus activity. *J Med Virol* 69:495–502.

Dorschner RA, Lin KH, et al. 2003. Neonatal skin in mice and humans expresses increased levels of antimicrobial peptides: innate immunity during development of the adaptive response. *Pediatr Res* 53:566–572.

Douar AM, Themis M, et al. 1996. Effect of amniotic fluid on cationic lipid mediated transfection and retroviral infection. *Gene Ther* 3:789–796.

Duggan PJ, Maalouf EF, et al. 2001. Intrauterine T-cell activation and increased proinflammatory cytokine concentrations in preterm infants with cerebral lesions. *Lancet* 358:1699–1700.

Elliger SS, Elliger CA, et al. 1999. Elimination of lysosomal storage in brains of MPS VII mice treated by intrathecal administration of an adeno-associated virus vector. *Gene Ther* 6:1175–1178.

Fanaro S, Chierici R, et al. 2003. Intestinal microflora in early infancy: composition and development. *Acta Paediatr Suppl* 91:48–55.

Frisella WA, O'Connor LH, et al. 2001. Intracranial injection of recombinant adeno-associated virus improves cognitive function in a murine model of mucopolysaccharidosis type VII. *Mol Ther* 3:351–358.

Garvy BA and Qureshi MH. 2000. Delayed inflammatory response to *Pneumocystis carinii* infection in neonatal mice is due to an inadequate lung environment. *J Immunol* 165:6480–6486.

Ghosh A, Allamarvdasht M, et al. 2006. Long-term correction of murine glycogen storage disease type Ia by recombinant adeno-associated virus-1–mediated gene transfer. *Gene Ther* 13:321–329.

Huard J, Lochmuller H, et al. 1995. Differential short-term transduction efficiency of adult versus newborn mouse tissues by adenoviral recombinants. *Exp Mol Pathol* 62:131–143.

Huard J, Feero WG, et al. 1996. The basal lamina is a physical barrier to herpes simplex virus–mediated gene delivery to mature muscle fibers. *J Virol* 70:8117–8123.

Kamata Y, Tanabe A, et al. 2003. Long-term normalization in the central nervous system, ocular manifestations, and skeletal deformities by a single systemic adenovirus injection into neonatal mice with mucopolysaccharidosis VII. *Gene Ther* 10:406–414.

Kanaji A, Kosuga M, et al. 2003. Improvement of skeletal lesions in mice with mucopolysaccharidosis type VII by neonatal adenoviral gene transfer. *Mol Ther* 8:718–725.

Karolewski BA and Wolfe JH. 2006. Genetic correction of the fetal brain increases the lifespan of mice with the severe multisystemic disease mucopolysaccharidosis type VII. *Mol Ther* 14:14–24.

Kniesel U, Risau W, et al. 1996. Development of blood–brain barrier tight junctions in the rat cortex. *Brain Res Dev Brain Res* 96:229–240.

Kobayashi H, Carbonaro D, et al. 2005. Neonatal gene therapy of MPS I mice by intravenous injection of a lentiviral vector. *Mol Ther* 11:776–789.

Laurema A, Vanamo K, et al. 2004. Fetal membranes act as a barrier for adenoviruses: gene transfer into exocoelomic cavity of rat fetuses does not affect cells in the fetus. *Am J Obstet Gynecol* 190:264–267.

Lee-Huang S, Huang PL, et al. 1999. Lysozyme and RNases as anti-HIV components in beta-core preparations of human chorionic gonadotropin. *Proc Natl Acad Sci U S A* 96:2678–2681.

Liu L, Mah C, et al. 2006. Sustained FVIII expression and phenotypic correction of hemophilia A in neonatal mice using an endothelial-targeted Sleeping Beauty transposon. *Mol Ther* 13:1006–1015.

Liu Y, Xu L, et al. 2005. Liver-directed neonatal gene therapy prevents cardiac, bone, ear, and eye disease in mucopolysaccharidosis I mice. *Mol Ther* 11:35–47.

Ma X, Liu Y, et al. 2007. Improvements in mucopolysaccharidosis I mice after adult retroviral vector-mediated gene therapy with immunomodulation. *Mol Ther* 15:889–902.

Madison KC. 2003. Barrier function of the skin: "la raison d'etre" of the epidermis. *J Invest Dermatol* 121:231–241.

Madoiwa S, Yamauchi T, et al. 2004. Induction of immune tolerance by neonatal intravenous injection of human factor VIII in murine hemophilia A. *J Thromb Haemost* 2:754–762.

Mallow EB, Harris A, et al. 1996. Human enteric defensins: gene structure and developmental expression. *J Biol Chem* 271:4038–4045.

Mango RL, Xu L, et al. 2004. Neonatal retroviral vector–mediated hepatic gene therapy reduces bone, joint, and cartilage disease in mucopolysaccharidosis VII mice and dogs. *Mol Genet Metab* 82:4–19.

Marchetti M, Trybala E, et al. 2004. Inhibition of herpes simplex virus infection by lactoferrin is dependent on interference with the virus binding to glycosaminoglycans. *Virology* 318:405–413.

Millar M, Wilks M, et al. 2003. Probiotics for preterm infants? *Arch Dis Child Fetal Neonatal Ed* 88:F354–F358.

Munk C, Wei G, et al. 2003. The theta-defensin, retrocyclin, inhibits HIV-1 entry. *AIDS Res Hum Retroviruses* 19:875–881.

Murphy SP, Fast LD, et al. 2005. Uterine NK cells mediate inflammation-induced fetal demise in IL-10-null mice. *J Immunol* 175:4084–4090.

Nalbantoglu J, Pari G, et al. 1999. Expression of the primary coxsackie and adenovirus receptor is downregulated during skeletal muscle maturation and limits the efficacy of adenovirus-mediated gene delivery to muscle cells. *Hum Gene Ther* 10:1009–1019.

Nguyen TH, Bellodi-Privato M, et al. 2005. Therapeutic lentivirus-mediated neonatal in vivo gene therapy in hyperbilirubinemic Gunn rats *Mol Ther* 12:852–859.

Nivsarkar M. 2006. Investigation of immune aspects of in utero gene therapy after intravascular vector delivery. Ph.D. dissertation, University of London.

Okoko BJ, Wesumperuma LH, et al. 2001. Materno–foetal transfer of *H. influenzae* and pneumococcal antibodies is influenced by prematurity and low birth weight: implications for conjugate vaccine trials. *Vaccine* 20:647–650.

Ota MO, Vekemans J, et al. 2004. Hepatitis B immunisation induces higher antibody and memory Th2 responses in new-borns than in adults. *Vaccine* 22:511–519.

Pravieux JJ, Poulet H, et al. 2007. Protection of newborn animals through maternal immunization. *J Comp Pathol* 137(Suppl 1):S32–S34.

Qureshi MH, Cook-Mills J, et al. 2003. TNF-alpha-dependent ICAM-1- and VCAM-1-mediated inflammatory responses are delayed in neonatal mice infected with *Pneumocystis carinii*. *J Immunol* 171:4700–4707.

Rastogi D, Wang C, et al. 2007. Antigen-specific immune responses to influenza vaccine in utero. *J Clin Invest* 117:1637–1646.

Rucker M, Fraites TJ Jr, et al. 2004. Rescue of enzyme deficiency in embryonic diaphragm in a mouse model of metabolic myopathy: Pompe disease. *Development* 131:3007–3019.

Rybka K, Orzechowska B, et al. 2003. Age related natural antiviral non-specific immunity of human leukocytes. *Med Sci Monit* 9:BR413–417.

Schneider H, Adebakin S, et al. 1999. Therapeutic plasma concentrations of human factor IX in mice after gene delivery into the amniotic cavity: a model for the prenatal treatment of haemophilia B. *J Gene Med* 1:424–432.

Schultz C, Temming P, et al. 2004. Immature anti-inflammatory response in neonates. *Clin Exp Immunol* 135:130–136.

Seppen J, van der Rijt R, et al. 2003. Long-term correction of bilirubin UDP-glucuronyltransferase deficiency in rats by in utero lentiviral gene transfer. *Mol Ther* 8:593–599.

Seppen J, van Til NP, et al. 2005. Immune response to lentiviral bilirubin UDP-glucuronosyltransferase gene transfer in fetal and neonatal rats. *Gene Ther*.

Shen JS, Watabe K, et al. 2001. Intraventricular administration of recombinant adenovirus to neonatal twitcher mouse leads to clinicopathological improvements. *Gene Ther* 8:1081–1087.

Shirafuji Y, Oono T, et al. 1999. Detection of cryptdin in mouse skin. *Clin Diagn Lab Immunol* 6:336–340.

Sleeper MM, Fornasari B, et al. 2004. Gene therapy ameliorates cardiovascular disease in dogs with mucopolysaccharidosis VII. *Circulation* 110:815–820.

Stonestreet BS, Patlak CS, et al. 1996. Ontogeny of blood–brain barrier function in ovine fetuses, lambs, and adults. *Am J Physiol* 271:1594–601.

Sun MS, Pan CJ, et al. 2002. Sustained hepatic and renal glucose-6-phosphatase expression corrects glycogen storage disease type Ia in mice. *Hum Mol Genet* 11:2155–2164.

Szekeres-Bartho J, Par G, et al. 1997. The antiabortive effect of progesterone-induced blocking factor in mice is manifested by modulating NK activity. *Cell Immunol* 177:194–199.

Takahashi M, Ilan Y, et al. 1996. Long term correction of bilirubin-UDP-glucuronosyltransferase deficiency in Gunn rats by administration of a recombinant adenovirus during the neonatal period. *J Biol Chem* 271:26536–26542.

Tasker L and Marshall-Clarke S. 2003. Functional responses of human neonatal B lymphocytes to antigen receptor cross-linking and CpG DNA. *Clin Exp Immunol* 134:409–419.

Thormar H and Hilmarsson H. 2007. The role of microbicidal lipids in host defense against pathogens and their potential as therapeutic agents. *Chem Phys Lipids* 150:1–11.

VandenDriessche T, Vanslembrouck V, et al. 1999. Long-term expression of human coagulation factor VIII and correction of hemophilia A after in vivo retroviral gene transfer in factor VIII–deficient mice. *Proc Natl Acad Sci U S A* 96:10379–10384.

Waddington SN, Buckley SMK, et al. 2003a. In utero gene transfer of human factor IX to fetal mice can induce postnatal tolerance of the exogenous clotting factor. *Blood* 101:1359–1366.

Waddington SN, Mitrophanous KA, et al. 2003b. Long-term transgene expression by administration of a lentivirus-based vector to the fetal circulation of immuno-competent mice. *Gene Ther* 10:1234–1240.

Waddington SN, Nivsarkar M, et al. 2004. Permanent phenotypic correction of haemophilia B in immunocompetent mice by prenatal gene therapy. *Blood* 104: 2714–2721.

Weitkamp JH, Kallewaard N, et al. 2003. Infant and adult human B cell responses to rotavirus share common immunodominant variable gene repertoires. *J Immunol* 171:4680–4688.

Xu L, Mango RL, et al. 2002. Evaluation of pathological manifestations of disease in mucopolysaccharidosis VII mice after neonatal hepatic gene therapy. *Mol Ther* 6:745–758.

Xu L, Mei M, et al. 2007. Immune response after neonatal transfer of a human factor IX–expressing retroviral vector in dogs, cats, and mice. *Thromb Res* 120:269–280.

Xu L, Mei M, et al. 2007. High expression reduces an antibody response after neonatal gene therapy with B domain–deleted human factor VIII in mice. *J Thromb Res* 5:1805–1812.

Yorty JL, Schultz SA, et al. 2004. Postpartum maternal corticosterone decreases maternal and neonatal antibody levels and increases the susceptibility of newborn mice to herpes simplex virus–associated mortality. *J Neuroimmunol* 150:48–58.

Yoshio H, Tollin M, et al. 2003. Antimicrobial polypeptides of human vernix caseosa and amniotic fluid: implications for newborn innate defense. *Pediatr Res* 53:211–216.

Zepeda M and Wilson JM. 1996. Neonatal cotton rats do not exhibit destructive immune responses to adenoviral vectors. *Gene Ther* 3:973–979.

Zhang J, Xu L, et al. 2004. Neonatal gene transfer with a retroviral vector results in tolerance to human factor IX in mice and dogs. *Blood* 103:143–151.

Zhang L, Yu W, et al. 2002. Contribution of human alpha-defensin 1, 2, and 3 to the anti-HIV-1 activity of CD8 antiviral factor. *Science* 298:995–1000.

Zhao Y, Dai ZP, et al. 2002. Phenotypic and functional analysis of human T lymphocytes in early second- and third-trimester fetuses. *Clin Exp Immunol* 129:302–308.

8

IMMUNOLOGY OF HEPATIC GENE TRANSFER

Brad E. Hoffman, Ph.D., and Roland W. Herzog, Ph.D
Department of Pediatrics, University of Florida, Gainesville, Florida

8.1 INTRODUCTION

The liver is being investigated increasingly as a target organ for gene replacement therapy. In addition to being the site of many metabolic processes and vital for detoxification, the liver appears to have an idiosyncratic immunological role that makes it an attractive, although complex target for the in vivo correction of inherited or acquired single-gene metabolic and endocrine disorders. The success of liver-directed gene therapy depends largely on the ability of the gene transfer

Gene Therapy Immunology, Edited by Roland Herzog

vehicle to deliver a therapeutic gene to hepatocytes with sufficient efficacy while minimizing deleterious immunological side effects [Bessis et al. 2004]. Immune responses directed against the viral vector backbone and/or the transgene product have the potential to severely impair the gene transfer efficiency, abrogate long-term transgene expression, and prevent readministration of the same vector. However, depending on the choice of viral vector, the dose at which it is given, and the therapeutic protein it encodes, liver-directed gene replacement could also result in the induction of peripheral tolerance, enabling long-term therapeutic protein expression.

The fundamental purpose of this chapter is to examine our current understanding of the unique immunological role the liver plays in gene replacement therapy, focusing primarily on the immune response to adenovirusal, adeno-associated viral (AAV), and lentiviral vectors, and the potential for inducing immune tolerance to therapeutic proteins. The unique structure and cellular architecture in the liver, as it relates, will be discussed briefly, and the reader is referred to several reviews for a more detailed description of hepatic immunobiology [Mackay 2002; Wick et al. 2002; Crispe 2003].

8.2 ANATOMY OF THE "LYMPHOID" LIVER

Historically, the liver has been considered relatively immunologically inert in its normal, noninflamed state. However, within the last decade or so, an increasing body of evidence suggests that the liver is an integral and unique component of the immune system that possesses a distinctive microenvironment [Wajahat et al. 2001; Wick et al. 2002]. From an immunological point of view, this would seem self-evident given that the liver receives blood directly from the digestive system, where the majority of antigens gain access to the organism. Hence, the immunological milieu of the liver has to maintain a delicate balance between producing an immune response and generating a state of tolerance to self and nonself molecules and microorganisms. Fortunately, especially in the context of gene therapy, the hepatic microenvironment generally favors the development of immune tolerance over that of immunity.

As an intrinsic lymphoid organ, the liver harbors immune cells that subserve innate and adaptive immune responses and has been shown to support the primary activation of naive T cells [Bertolino et al.]. Moreover, it has been suggested that antigens expressed in situ or that are delivered to the liver via the portal vein are more likely to be tolerogenic than those received from the periphery [Knolle et al. 1999].

Whether an exogenous antigen delivered to the liver results in the induction of immunity or tolerance is influenced by the source of the antigen, the cell type presenting the antigen, and the local environment. Therefore, it is important to discuss briefly the cellular composition and architecture of the liver (Fig. 8-1) to appreciate the intricate mechanisms directing the immune responses in situ as it relates to gene therapy.

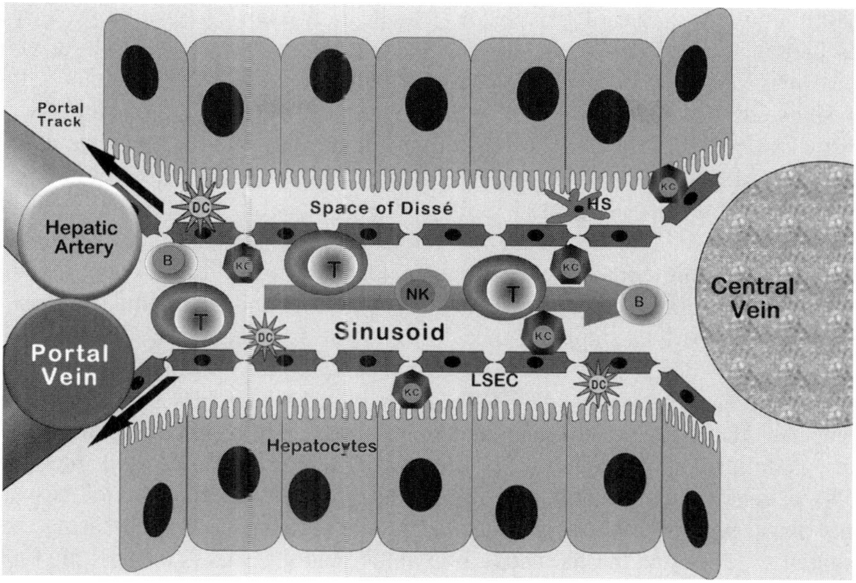

Figure 8-1 Anatomy of the hepatic sinusoid. The sinusoid is lined by a fenestrated layer of LSECs. KCs and DCs patrol the sinusoid and can pass into the space of Dissé, where they can interact with the hepatocytes. B, B cell; DC, dendritic cell; HS, hepatic stellate cell; KC, Kupffer cell; LSEC, liver endothelial cell; T, T cell.

The liver's anatomical location and structural organization suggest that it has a uniquely important role in the regulation of immune responses. Approximately 30% of total blood volume passes through a network of sinusoids every minute, delivering about 10^8 peripheral blood lymphocytes in 24 hours [Sheth and Bankey 2001; Wick et al. 2002]. Blood from the portal vein (about 80%) and the hepatic artery (about 20%) mix as it passes through the tight network of sinusoids before leaving the parenchyma via the central hepatic vein. The parenchyma consists primarily of hepatocytes that are organized into sheets, which are oriented to form vascular sinusoids [Markiewski et al. 2006]. The hepatic sinusoids are lined with a monolayer of fenestrated, or discontinuous, liver sinusoidal endothelial cells (LSECs), forming a sieve plate that demarcates the space of Dissé. Microvilli of the hepatocytes protrude into this subendothelial space, potentially allowing passing cells to make direct contact. Such contact by lymphocytes and antigen-presenting cells (APCs) is further enhanced by the small diameter of the sinusoids, reduced venous pressure, and the occasional blockade by Kupffer cells (KCs) [Racanelli and Rehermann 2006].

8.2.1 Hepatocytes

Hepatocytes, which constitute 60 to 80% of parenchymal cells, are responsible for the synthesis and secretion of numerous biological molecules. In the past, the immunological role of hepatocytes has generally been neglected because it was thought that naive T cells are unable to gain access to these cells in vivo. However, Warren and co-workers have demonstrated that naive T cells within the sinusoids can indeed interact with hepatocytes through cytoplasmic extensions that penetrate the LSEC fenestrations, suggesting that hepatocytes can be active participants in immune responses and/or tolerance [Bertolino et al. 1998; Bowen et al. 2004; Warren et al. 2006]. Hepatocytes have also been shown to express various immunomodulary molecules on their perisinusoidal hepatocyte membrane. Resting hepatocytes express major histocompatibility complex class (MHC) I molecules [Bumgardner et al. 1990], CD1, and intercellular adhesion molecule-1 (ICAM-1), implying that they can act as an APC for CD1 or MHC class I–restricted $CD8^+$ T cells [Bertolino et al. 2002]. Although hepatocytes lack constituent expression of CD40L and various MHC class I co-stimulatory molecules, these can be up-regulated upon stress. Under inflammatory conditions, certain cytokines, such as interleukin (IL)-2, IL-6, IL-12, and interferon (IFN)-γ, can stimulate hepatocytes to produce pro-inflammatory cytokines and acute-phase proteins such as C-reactive protein (CRP), thereby increasing their potential to recruit additional active host inflammatory cells [Lieber et al. 1997; Schnell et al. 2001; Zhang et al. 2001; Zaiss et al. 2002]. In addition to being able to modulate a variety of pro-inflammatory cytokines in response to infectious stimuli, it has also been demonstrated that a change in hepatocyte phenotype can be induced by peripherally activated $CD8^+$ T cells that precipitate the production of anti-inflammatory cytokines (e.g., IL-4 and IL-10) [Dikopoulos et al. 2004].

In a series of reports, Bertolino et al. [1995, 1998] demonstrated using both in vitro and in vivo systems that hepatocytes are indeed capable of activating naive $CD8^+$ T cells without prior priming in the lymph nodes. However, T cells activated in the sinusoids subsequently undergo apoptosis because of inadequate co-stimulation as compared to fully activated T cells in the hepatic lymph nodes, all of which suggests further that interactions between naive T cells and hepatocytes in the sinusoids typically results in tolerance [Bowen et al. 2004; Warren et al. 2006].

8.2.2 Kupffer Cells

KCs are the liver's resident macrophages and are responsible for the clearance of pathogens, including viral vectors, received from the portal circulation. They represent the largest population (about 80%) of bone marrow–derived monocyte/macrophages in the body and about 20% of the nonparenchymal cells (NPCs) of the liver [Mackay 2002]. Restricted primarily to the lumen of the sinusoids, they are in close contact with the sinusoidal endothelium and may reach or transcytose into the space of Dissé. KCs constituently express MHC class II molecules, ICAM-1, and low levels of CD80 and CD86, which distinguishes them differentially from extrahepatic macrophages [Lohse et al. 1996; Leifeld et al. 1999; Mehal et al. 1999]. Upon phagocytosis, activated KCs can initiate and meditate immune responses via the production and release of pro-inflammatory cytokines that act as a paracrine signals on hepatocytes and enhance chemotaxis and recruitment of neutrophils [Lieber et al. 1997; Markiewski et al. 2006].

There are several mechanisms by which KCs may also be involved in the down-regulation of immune reactivity and tolerance. In response to stimulation by lipopolysaccharide (LPS), they will secrete IL-10, transforming growth factor (TGF)-β, and prostanoids, which promote tolerance [Knolle and Gerken 2000]. Cross-presentation of antigen to dendritic cells (DCs) and the synthesis of nitric oxide has also been shown to suppress T-cell activation in vitro [Roland et al. 1994; Crispe 2003; Crispe et al. 2006]. In an in vitro system, LPS-stimulated KCs were shown to induce apoptosis in nonspecific T-cell hybridomas [Muschen et al. 1998]. From this it is apparent that KCs are capable of exerting multiple modalities of immune modulation. However, the hepatic DC population is still considered to be the main initiator of liver-induced tolerance.

8.2.3 Dendritic Cells

Although intrahepatic DCs comprise the smallest subset of liver nonparenchymal cells (<1%), when mature they are recognized as being the most potent APCs. They are also considered responsible for induction immune tolerance, especially following transplantation [Khanna et al. 2000; Bowen et al. 2002]. In a noninflamed liver, intrahepatic DCs are typically found in the portal triads and central veins. Akin to DCs in other peripheral sites, they are able to capture, process, and transport antigen efficiently to regional lymphoid tissues [Lau and Thomson 2003]. In the mouse, three major subsets of DCs have been identified that exhibit distinct functional capabilities for promoting the induction of tolerance or inducing immunity: myeloid DCs, lymphoid DCs, and plasmacytoid DCs. The myeloid and lymphoid subsets are referred to as conventional DCs and are located primarily at the periportal fields, whereas the plasmacytoid subset is generally located in the liver parenchyma.

Additionally, the maturation state of DCs is important with respect to their capacity to trigger immune responses. It has been suggested that the tolerogenic nature of the liver is largely attributed to the preponderance of immature hepatic DCs. In fact, it has been demonstrated that freshly isolated hepatic DCs from healthy (noninflamed) livers predominately exhibit a functionally immature phenotype and are poor activators of naive allogeneic T cells [Khanna et al. 2000]. Additionally, it is generally accepted that the microenvironment in which APCs are activated will modify their function and effects on T-cell populations. Taken collectively, it seems likely that hepatic DCs are somewhat functionally and phenotypically different from DCs in other tissues. Indeed, it has been shown that intrahepatic DCs are less immunogenic and more tolerogenic than other peripheral DCs, such as those in the skin or the spleen. On the other hand, it is plausible (especially under inflammatory conditions) that immature hepatic DCs may take up an antigen and emigrate the hepatic microenvironment to the draining lymph nodes. Here, upon maturation the DCs can present the antigen to T cells in the context of MHC. In turn, the T cells will clonally expand and migrate back to the liver in full effector mode.

8.2.4 Liver Sinusoidal Endothelial Cells

Antigens entering through the hepatic sinusoids will encounter the strategically located LSECs. LSECs line the sinusoids linking the portal tracts with the central veins and have a distinct morphology compared to the vascular endothelial cells that line arterial branches and central and portal veins. They form a fenestrated barrier that may allow cells in the sinusoid to make direct contact with hepatocytes. The lack of a proper basement membrane, which is unique to the hepatic sinusoid vascular system, and restricted blood flow facilitate the extravasation of T cells without the need for selectin involvement.

Antigen uptake by LSECs has been demonstrated to be highly efficient in several experimental systems and may even be more efficient than KCs in certain circumstances [Knolle and Gerken 2000]. Similar to DCs, antigen uptake by LSECs is mediated by specific receptors, such as the mannose and scavenger receptors [Lohse et al. 1996; Crispe 2003]. In the mouse, LSECs constituently express MHC classes I and II, CD54 (ICAM-I), CD106 (VCAM-I), and the co-stimulatory markers CD80, CD86, and CD40, suggesting that LSECs are fully equipped to be immunologically active APCs, capable of presenting antigen to both $CD4^+$ and $CD8^+$ T cells. Despite this, the most common consequence of T-cell priming by LSECs is antigen-specific tolerance, not immunity [Knolle et al. 1999; Limmer et al. 2000; Crispe 2003].

8.2.5 Lymphocytes

The noninflamed liver also contains a large population of intrahepatic lymphocytes that are distributed through the sinusoidal spaces as small lymphoid aggregates in the portal tracts [Crispe et al. 2006] as well as scattered throughout the parenchyma [Racanelli and Rehermann 2006]. As part of the adaptive immune system, conventional $CD4^+$ and $CD8^+$ display a diverse repertoire of T-cell receptors (TCRs) that can recognize antigen when it is presented in MHC class II or I complexes, respectively. Differing from the peripheral blood and lymphoid organs, $CD8^+$ T cells are generally more abundant than $CD4^+$ cells. However, in both subsets, activated T cells are more frequent in the lymph nodes and spleens of mice and in the blood of humans [Norris et al. 1998]. As part of the innate immune system, the liver also contains two major populations of unconventional T cells: classical (NK) and nonclassical natural killer T (NKT) cells, which represent up to 30% of the intrahepatic lymphocyte population [Racanelli and Rehermann 2006]. NK cells are activated in response to various chemokines and cytokines and serve to contain viral infections while the adaptive immune response is generating antigen-specific CTLs. NKT cells respond to lipid antigen presented by the atypical MHC class I molecule, CD1d, and express intermediate levels of TCR. Once activated, NKT cells can rapidly release cytokines (such as IL-2, IFN-γ, TNF-α, and IL-4) that promote or suppress different immune responses.

8.3 INTRAHEPATIC IMMUNE RESPONSES TO VIRAL VECTORS

Inherently, the use of viruses as a vehicle to achieve efficient hepatic gene transfer has a significant risk for inducing a deleterious immune response. For that reason, circumventing, redirecting, or suppressing the immune response is critical for successful clinical applications and has been a constant challenge in the field of gene replacement therapy. The immune response following administration of a viral vector can be broken down into two broad classifications: innate or nonspecific responses and adaptive or specific responses. The innate response represents the first line of defense, occurring almost immediately, and is essential for controlling the extent of infection. More important, the innate response provides antigen-specific determinants and drives the antigen-specific adaptive response. The adaptive immunity develops afterward and is responsible for the induction of long-term immunity or memory. In either case, an effectively mounted immune response directed against a viral vector or its product could inevitably reduce transduction efficiency, eliminating the vector and/or the transduced cells.

Innate immune responses involve various soluble and cellular components, such as cytokines, chemokines, neutrophils, NK cells, DCs, and macrophages (KCs in the liver) to initiate and maintain hepatic inflammation. The initial non-MHC-specific interaction of viral particles following vector administration is dependent on recognition or engagement of conserved molecular structures known as *pathogen-associated molecular patterns* (PAMPs) through various Toll-like receptors (TLRs) expressed on immune cells, hepatocytes, and endothelial cells [Guidotti and Chisari 2001; Medzhitov 2001; Girardin et al. 2002]. The ligand-induced engagement of TLRs triggers a series of overlapping downstream signaling cascades, culminating with the production of various immunomodulatory factors that are responsible for the elimination of pathogens and setting the stage for subsequent immune responses.

8.3.1 Adenoviral Vectors

In the early 1990s, adenoviral vectors gained considerable attention and have been studied extensively as a vehicle for gene delivery to the liver due to their high transfection efficiency, their ability to transduce both quiescent and dividing cells, and their high tropism for hepatocytes [Jaffe et al. 1992; Li et al. 1993]. Unfortunately, there has been only limited clinical success with these vectors. It has been well established in various animal models and human clinical trials that systemically injected adenoviral vectors trigger a rapid and potent innate immune response by the host. The response is dose dependent and is characterized by the expression of numerous pro-inflammatory serum factors, resulting in significant hepatic inflammation, rapid vector elimination, transient transgene expression, and the initiation of an immune response against viral capsid proteins [Wolff et al. 1997; Worgall et al. 1997; Tao et al. 2001].

Adenoviral vectors injected into the systemic circulation are rapidly endocytosed as they enter the hepatic sinusoids by KCs patrolling lumen, leaving only a fraction of them viable to transduce hepatocytes [Zhang et al. 2002; van Til et al. 2005]. Similar sequestering by the liver has been shown for other viruses, including lentiviral vectors [van Til et al. 2005]. Demonstrating this initially, Worgall and co-workers [1997] reported that upon intravenous administration of a first-generation E1-deleted adenoviral vector expressing β-galactosidase to immunocompetent mice, 90% of the viral genome was eliminated from the liver by KCs within the first 24 hours. The phagocytosis of vector particles in rodents and nonhuman primates has been shown to result in the production of pro-inflammatory cytokines such as IL-6, IL-12, IL-10, IL-8, tumor necrosis factor alpha (TNF)-α, IFN-γ, chemokines such as MIP-1 and MIP-2, and prostaglandin E2 (PGE2) [Decker 1990; Crettaz et al. 2006].

The early sequestration and loss of adenoviral vector DNA by KCs results in a nonlinear dose response. At lower vector doses, adenoviral vectors are quickly taken up and degraded by KCs, ultimately resulting in failure to transduce hepatocytes. It is only after the concentration of vector is more than can be sequestered that the adenoviral vectors are able to transduce hepatocytes efficiently [Tao et al. 2001; Zhang et al. 2001]. However, such vector doses also lead to a spillover effect, with vector particles being delivered to the lymph nodes and/or the spleen, where they initiate systemic innate response. Providing evidence supporting this, it has been established in nonhuman primates that intraportal injection of adenoviral vector results in the rapid activation of splenic macrophages and a significant increase in systemic IL-6 levels [Schnell et al. 2001]. These results have been underscored by the death of a patient participating in a clinical trial of gene replacement therapy for ornithine transcarbamylase (OTC) deficiency. Forty-eight hours after intrahepatic administration of 6×10^{13} adenoviral vector particles expressing the gene for OTC, the patient experienced an acute inflammatory response characterized by high serum IL-6 levels [Schnell et al. 2001; Tao et al. 2001].

Additional evidence that KCs are responsible for, or at least play a significant role in, the rapid elimination of adenoviral vectors, induction of pro-inflammatory mediators, and transient transgene expression, a series of experiments were performed aimed at depleting these cells. Depletion of KCs from the liver, by either dichloromethylene bisphosphate (Cl_2MBP) or gadolinium chloride ($GdCl_3$), resulted in a significantly attenuated vector elimination, prolonged persistence of vector DNA, and transgene expression in the liver [Kuzmin et al. 1997; Wolff et al. 1997]. In fact, the long-term expression of factor VIII has been achieved following macrophage/KC depletion in hemophilia A/factor VIII-knockout mice [Bristol et al. 2000; Chuah et al. 2003].

Finally, as with any other professional APCs, KCs not only present vector particles in MHC class I molecules but can also present them in class II molecules via cross presentation, thus activating $CD4^+$ T-helper cells and $CD8^+$ cytotoxic T lymphocytes (CTLs), respectively. In sum, it is unquestionable that hepatic macrophages are indeed participants in limiting hepatocyte transduction, elimination of transduced cells, or development of the adaptive immune response following adenoviral vector administration.

8.3.2 Adeno-Associated Viral Vectors

In stark contrast to adenoviral vectors, AAV vectors do not initiate a potent innate or adaptive immune response. The absence of any appreciable inflammatory response has been attributed to the inability of AAV to infect DCs or macrophages. Although in a recent study it was demonstrated that within 1 hour of intravenous infusion of an AAV vector there was an increase in mRNA transcripts for several chemokines (e.g., MIP-1β, MIP-2, MCP-1, IP-10, and RANTES) [Zaiss et al. 2002], this rise was only transient, lasting less than 6 hours, and did not result in any significant increase in serum cytokines or chemokines.

Intrahepatic delivery of AAV vectors to mice, dogs, and nonhuman primates results in long-term hepatic expression of the therapeutic gene. Importantly, hepatocyte transduction is achieved without any noticeable vector-related toxicity or immune responses [Herzog et al. 1997, 1999; Snyder et al. 1997, 1999; Mount et al. 2002; Nathwani et al. 2002]. As a result, AAV vectors have gained significant popularity in recent years and are rapidly becoming the vector of choice for liver-directed gene therapy. As promising as these vectors are, they are not without limitations. AAV-based gene therapy has been impeded by factors such as their limited packaging capacity, low efficiency of gene transfer, delayed transgene expression, and the high prevalence of preexisting immunity to the viral capsid proteins among the human population. It has been reported that 35 to 80% of the human population, depending on age and demographic location, have preexisting anti-AAV2 antibodies, which has a neutralizing effect that adversely affects the efficiency of vector transduction in the liver [Halbert et al. 1997; Erles et al. 1999; Bessis et al. 2004].

In fact, a recent clinical trial of liver-directed AAV2-based gene transfer was unsuccessful because of an unprecedented host immune response against the transduced hepatocytes. In contrast to the long-term transgene expression seen in dogs and nonhuman primates, expression at therapeutic levels in humans was short lived, lasting only about 4 weeks, at which time transaminase levels became transiently elevated (indicative of liver damage) concomitantly with decreasing transgene product. Results from a series of experiments attempting to identify the mechanism responsible for the failure suggested that in humans, a $CD8^+$ T-cell-mediated immune response to AAV capsid antigens caused the destruction of AAV2-transduced hepatocytes [Manno et al. 2006]. Notably, unlike many of the experimental animals used to evaluate AAV vectors, humans are a natural host for AAV infections. Therefore, it is likely that during a natural infection, in combination with a helper virus such as adenovirus, the immune response generated against the helper virus also produced antigen-specific $CD8^+$ T cells for AAV capsid. Resolution of the initial infection would inevitably result in a small pool of memory cells which through homeostatic proliferation could be maintained and/or restimulated throughout one's lifetime. Current efforts are focused on development of alternative serotype vectors, modifications of viral capsid sequences, and immune modulation and suppression protocols to solve immunological hurdles derived from preexisting immunity and memory responses, such as T-cell- and antibody-mediated responses to AAV capsid sequences.

8.3.3 Lentiviral Vectors

Lentiviral vectors (LVs), derived from proviral DNA of human immunodeficiency virus (HIV) or related viruses, represent yet another vector system capable of transferring genes to nondividing target cells such as hepatocytes (see Chapter 5). In contrast to adenovirus or AAV, LVs are unlikely to encounter preexisting neutralizing antibodies or memory lymphocyte responses in HIV-negative subjects. These enveloped viral particles can be pseudotyped with envelope proteins that confer efficient infection of hepatocytes and to which the human immune system should be naive. Potential drawbacks of these vectors are the difficulty of manufacturing sufficient quantities for in vivo gene transfer in humans and risks related to insertional mutagenesis following integration of the reversed transcribed genome into host chromosomal DNA, an event that is required for LV gene transfer.

A major obstacle for liver-directed gene transfer with LV has been a robust adaptive immune response to the transgene product, which includes antibody- and CTL-mediated elimination of gene expression. This immune response is the consequence of two events: an early innate response to the enveloped virus and a subsequent antigen-specific response to the transgene product [Follenzi et al. 2004; Brown et al. 2007]. The single-stranded RNA genome of HIV is recognized by TLR7 as a PAMP, which leads to activation of plasmacytoid dendritic cells [Diebold et al. 2004; Fonteneau et al. 2004; Beignon et al. 2005]. As a result, this subset of DCs produces a strong antiviral type I interferon response characterized by secretion of high levels of INF-αβ. Furthermore, DC maturation following TLR7 activation leads to antigen processing and presentation to T cells. In the context of LV gene transfer, the ensuing interferon production has two consequences. First, it severely limits the efficacy of LV gene transfer to hepatocytes. Second, INF-αβ is required for the subsequent transgene product-specific CTL response to be effective [Brown et al. 2007].

Elegant work by Naldini and colleagues has shown that in addition to the innate response to the viral genome, a second event is required for the immune response to the transgene product: transgene expression in professional, bone marrow–derived APCs [Follenzi et al. 2004; Brown et al. 2006]. Lentiviral vectors can, particularly if pseudotyped with vesicular stomatitis virus G (VSV-G) envelop protein, efficiently infect nonparenchymal liver cells, including resident APCs such as Kupffer cells. Furthermore, dissemination of vector to the spleen results in infection of splenic APCs, including DCs and macrophages. The resulting transgene expression in these cell types directs antigen presentation to and activation of $CD4^+$ and $CD8^+$ T cells followed by lymphocytic inflammatory infiltrates in the liver and destruction of LV-transduced hepatocytes by cytolytic $CD8^+$ T cells. It is therefore critical to de-target expression from APCs. In the case of LV, use of a hepatocyte-specific promoter may not be sufficient to achieve this goal [Follenzi et al. 2004]. One strategy is use of an envelope protein that does not direct infection of APCs [Kang et al. 2005]. Studies by Brown and Naldini describe a powerful alternative approach, which is to incorporate a sequence target for a hematopoietic lineage-specific micro-RNA into the transcript of the transgene [Brown et al. 2006]. This maneuver results in degradation of the transcript, specifically in infected hematopoietic cells such as professional APCs, thereby efficiently preventing transgene expression in these cell types. Without transgene expression in bone marrow–derived APCs, liver-directed LV gene transfer is stable without deleterious immune responses. These studies are also important from a second mechanistic point of view, in that the data illustrate the importance of directing expression away from the lymphoid and toward the hepatic environment (see below for further discussion).

8.4 HEPATIC GENE THERAPY AND TOLERANCE

Immunological tolerance is the failure to form an immune response to a specific antigen. In the setting of gene replacement therapy, the ability to induce tolerance to a therapeutic protein delivered by in vivo gene transfer would provide new potential to the field. The tolerogenic properties of the liver were first realized by Calne and colleagues in 1969 when they reported the acceptance of a liver allograft across an MHC mismatch in a pig. Since then, an increasing body of evidence suggests that hepatic antigens expressed in situ or that are delivered to the liver via the portal circulation are more likely to be tolerogenic than are those received from the periphery [Knolle et al. 1999]. Although the mechanism(s) that determine the balance between intrahepatic immunity and tolerance in hepatic gene therapy are poorly understood, the concept of hepatic control of the immune response by resident T cells provides an explanation for a number of observations in which a difference between systemic and local immune response has been documented [Lee et al. 1998; Knolle et al. 1999]. Generation of antigen-specific tolerance within the liver is an active process and not the result of a generalized immunosupression [Bertolino et al. 2002]. Thus, the induction of intrahepatic tolerance is due, at least in part, to the ability of the resident liver APCs to process and present antigen to naive T cells, independently of lymphoid organs [McAvoy and Kubes 2006].

In general, mechanisms leading to T-cell unresponsiveness include T-cell anergy (a state of unresponsiveness associated with lack of IL-2 cytokine expression), clonal deletion of antigen-specific T-cells (e.g. by Fas/FasL-induced cell death) or activation of regulatory T cells (Tregs). Upon activation, $CD4^+$ T cells mature and differentiate into various T helper (Th) cells. The subtype of Th cell that is being activated depends on various factors, including, but not limited to, the cytokine milieu present during the initial interaction between the T cell and the antigen-presenting cells. The subsets of Th cells are differentiated by their cytokine expression pattern and are referred to as Th1, Th2, Th3, and type 1 T regulatory (Tr1) cells. Characteristically, Th1 cells produce IFN-γ, TNF-α, and IL-2, and promote IgG2a formation in mice (equivalent to IgG1 in humans). In contrast, Th2 cells produce IL-4, IL-5, IL-10, and transforming growth factor (TGF)-β and direct B-cell formation of IgG1 in mice (IgG4 in humans). Th3 cells produce high amounts of TGF-β, and Tr1 cells produce large amounts of IL-10 and are immune suppressive. Additionally, $CD4^+$ Th1 cells provide help for $CD8^+$ T-cell differentiation into cytotoxic T lymphocytes (CTL) upon activation. This is of significant concern in gene-based treatment, because activation of CTLs could lead to destruction of cells expressing the therapeutic protein [Fields et al. 2000]. In fact, in a recent human clinical trial of hepatic gene therapy for the treatment of the blood disorder hemophilia B [or coagulation factor IX (hF.IX) deficiency], two patients developed a self-limiting transient hepatitis after administration of AAV vector in which subsequent analysis of blood samples revealed the presence of AAV capsid–specific $CD8^+$ T cells [Manno et al. 2006].

Various laboratories have demonstrated the induction of immune tolerance by hepatocyte-restricted transgene expression following in vivo gene transfer [Mingozzi et al. 2003; Ziegler et al. 2004; Dobrzynski and Herzog 2005; Franco et al. 2005]. However, the precise mechanism by which the hepatic environment permits the establishment of tolerance, as compared to other target tissue that often direct a local immune response to gene transfer, is not entirely understood. Nonetheless, the current evidence suggests that $CD4^+$ Tregs exert their suppressive functions in both a cell contact–dependent manner (possible via granzyme B or CTLA-4) and in a cytokine-dependent fashion (probably through IL-10 or possibly TGF-β) [Annacker et al. 2001; Gondek et al. 2005; Fallarino et al. 2006; Miyara and Sakaguchi 2007].

The specific mechanism(s) underlying the induction of tolerance toward transgene products was first investigated by our laboratory in a series of experiments. Initially using an ovalbumin (OVA)-specific TCR transgenic mouse, we obtained evidence for the induction of antigen-specific $CD4^+$ T-cell anergy and deletion [Dobrzynski et al. 2004]. Specifically, we reported a reduction in the proportion of TCR^+ $CD4^+$ T cells isolated from the spleens and lymph nodes of mice that received AAV2-OVA intrahepatically. In subsequent studies using a mouse model for hemophilia B, we demonstrated that mice expressing human factor IX (hF.IX) following hepatic AAV2-mediated gene transfer continued to express the protein and maintained immune tolerance even after subsequent administration of the hF.IX protein in adjuvant or by secondary gene transfer with an immunogenic adenoviral vector (Ad-hF.IX). Additionally, we found that tolerance induction to hF.IX was associated with the induction of Tregs capable of suppressing antibody and CTL formation against hF.IX that would otherwise lead to the immune-mediated destruction of hepatocytes [Mingozzi et al. 2003; Dobrzynski et al. 2004, 2006]. To demonstrate experimentally the in vivo suppressive function of Tregs directly, we adoptively transferred $CD4^+$ splenocytes isolated from mice previously tolerized by hepatic gene transfer of AAV2-hF.IX, to naive mice that were subsequently systemically challenged with an adenoviral vector expressing hF.IX (Ad-hF.IX). All of the mice receiving the $CD4^+$ splenocytes showed prolonged hF.IX expression with 1 to 2% of the hepatocytes staining positive for hF.IX. In contrast, without exception, mice that received $CD4^+$ lymphocytes from nontolerized (control) mice lost systemic and hepatic hF.IX expression. Interestingly, the livers of mice that received $CD4^+$ cells from tolerized animals showed normal morphology without the presence of $CD8^+$ CTL infiltrates at two months post-transfer, whereas the livers from the control groups all had substantial inflammation and hepatocellular damage [Dobrzynski et al. 2006]. These data demonstrated that $CD4^+$ Tregs were able to suppress both humoral and cellular immune responses to the transgenic hF.IX protein as well as to the Ad-hF.IX–transduced hepatocytes. Although it should be noted that we did observe, in vitro, cytokine production and cytolytic activity to adenoviral antigens, this response did not result in loss of transgene expression.

Previous studies demonstrated the induction of immune tolerance to F.IX by hepatic AAV gene transfer. Using a Treg-deficient transgenic model provided the first definitive evidence for induction of transgene product-specific Tregs by in vivo gene transfer. Analysis of the splenocyte population from mice tolerized by hepatic AAV-hF.IX gene transfer suggests a complex pattern of $CD4^+$ T-cell activation, which includes a measurable increase in Tregs that have a phenotype similar to that of "naturally occurring" regulatory T cells that are generated through stimulation with self-antigens [Cao et al. 2007]. Such $CD4^+$ $CD25^+$ T cells constitutively express the α chain of the IL-2 receptor (CD25) and are critical for prevention of autoimmune disease [Sakaguchi et al. 2001]. Hepatic gene transfer induced Tregs that express FoxP3, GITR, and CTLA4, and that are capable of suppressing $CD4^+$ $CD25^-$ T cells. Additionally, adoptively transferred lymphocytes from mice tolerized to human F.IX by hepatic AAV gene transfer suggest induction of $CD4^+$ $CD25^+$ $GITR^+$ Tregs that are able to suppress antibody formation to F.IX. Moreover, in vivo depletion of $CD4^+$ $CD25^+$ Tregs resulted in the formation of antibodies against F.IX following hepatic gene transfer. All of this strongly suggests a vital role for $CD4^+$ $CD25^+$ Tregs in establishing and maintaining tolerance to the transgene product in liver-directed gene transfer [Cao et al. 2007].

In a recent paper, our lab further demonstrated that immune tolerance to hF.IX established by hepatic gene transfer could be maintained after secondary gene transfer to skeletal muscle. These results showed that a sustained and marked increase in systemic hF.IX expression without antibody formation could be achieved following supplementary IM gene transfer using AAV serotype-1 (AAV1) vector. More important, even when hepatically transduced/tolerized mice received intramuscular (IM) injections of the substantially more immunogenic and pro-inflammatory adenoviral vector (Ad-hF.IX) for secondary gene transfer, the established tolerance to hF.IX was maintained. Specifically, tolerized mice failed to form antibodies to hF.IX and essentially lacked $CD8^+$ T-cell responses in the liver.

Although $CD4^+$ and $CD8^+$/CTL responses to adenoviral antigens were detectable ex vivo, they were not sufficient to mount an effective CTL response to virally transduced hepatocytes in vivo, probably as a result of immunosuppressive regulatory $CD4^+$ T cells that had been induced by hepatic hF.IX transgene expression. An even more interesting and unexpected observation was that even though a brisk $CD8^+$ inflammatory infiltrate limited the duration of transgene expression in muscle tissue following IM Ad-hF.IX administration, there was no hepatocellular damage or loss of transgene expression from hepatocytes, despite the adenoviral vector being disseminated to the liver [Hoffman et al. 2007]. The results suggest that effector T-cell responses to adenoviral antigens in the muscle, as opposed to AAV1, are indeed sufficient to eliminate transduced myocytes but are unable to overcome hepatic tolerance. The reasons for these differences between muscle and liver tissues are unclear but may relate to differences in the context of antigen presentation to regulatory and effector T cells or in homing of Tregs.

8.5 ANTIGEN PRESENTATION

A great deal of research has been performed focusing on intrahepatic antigen presentation and the role it plays both in the innate and adaptive immune systems and in inducing tolerance. Resting T cells are typically restricted to lymphatic tissue and require two independent signals to develop into fully activated effector T cells. The classic scenario for primary activation of naive T cells involves professional APCs, such as bone morrow–derived immature DCs, which acquire antigen at the site of infection, migration to secondary lymphoid tissues, and undergo differentiation. The first activation signal is provided by the MHC–peptide complex to a specific TCR. The second, or co-stimulation signal is independent of the antigen/TCR receptor but is critical for full activation and functional differentiation of naive T cells [Knolle et al. 1999; Jenkins et al. 2001; Racanelli and Rehermann 2006].

Although tolerance is in all probability determined by multiple events targeting both $CD4^+$ and $CD8^+$ T cells, primary T-cell activation within the liver by resident APCs appears to be an important step in the process [Mehal et al. 2001]. The induction of an immune response, or tolerance, in the liver toward soluble antigens requires an APC that efficiently scavenges and takes up antigen. The APC then has to be able to express the antigen within MHC class I or II molecules for presentation to T cells [Limmer et al. 2000]. A number of reports have demonstrated that there are various cell types within the liver capable of functioning as an APC. Each has a varying proficiency in capturing, processing, and presenting antigen to immune effector cells in situ [Bertolino et al. 1998, 2001; Knolle et al. 1999; Limmer et al. 2000; Limmer and Knolle 2001, 2005; Bagley et al. 2002]. The three most important liver resident APCs are the DCs, LSECs, and KCs. They are all capable of internalizing antigen either by phagocytosis, receptor-mediated endocytosis, or pinocytosis and are known to participate in the induction of hepatic immune tolerance, even though they differ significantly in phenotype and immunomodulatory mechanisms [Lau et al. 2003; Wiegard et al. 2005].

Some studies have suggested that under certain conditions, liver resident DCs may contribute to the induction of tolerance [Thomson and Lu 1999]. However, it has also been shown that antigen presented to T cells by hepatic DCs can occur in lymphatic tissue, where mature DCs migrate upon inflammation [Kudo et al. 1997]. This implies that the biological activity of DCs following hepatic gene transfer can be either effective T-cell priming and/or induction of T-cell tolerance. The factors determining which will occur are dependent on the antigen dose, maturation state, and the immunological milieu of the liver at the time.

The currently accepted hypothesis is that the presence of preexisting hepatic inflammation is the critical determinate [Crispe 2003]. For example, Zhang et al. demonstrated that within 6 hours following administration of an adenoviral vector to mice, the liver exhibits an inflamed state with high amounts of IL-6, IL-12, and TNF-α present. This pro-inflammatory microenvironment resulted in a potent CTL response and complete loss of transgene expression. The authors went on to show that depletion of DCs and macrophages restricted the expression of these inflammatory cytokines and prevented subsequent CTL response against the transgene-expressing cells in the liver. Similar findings were obtained when an adenoviral vector was given to nonhuman primates [Zhang et al. 2001; Schagen et al. 2004]. The results in this study, however, could not rule out the possibility that activated hepatic DCs, which may have an increased capacity to migrate through the space of Dissé and enter the lymphatics via the portal tracts, eventually traveled to hepatic lymph nodes and induced immunity upon maturation and activation of T cells [Kudo et al. 1997; Racanelli and Rehermann 2006]. In either case, it seems apparent that DCs are responsible, at least in part, for the failure to obtain sustained gene transfer to the liver using adenoviral vectors.

In contrast to the inflamed liver, the microenvironment of the noninflamed liver is rich in the immunosuppressive cytokines IL-10 and TGF-β, both of which are produced by KCs and LSECs in response to physiologic concentrations of lipopolysaccharide (LPS) and can render DCs tolerogenic by inhibiting the production of the Th1 driving cytokine IL-12, preventing their maturation and blocking T-cell stimulatory function by down-regulating receptor-mediated antigen uptake and MHC class I expression [Liu 2001; Lau and Thomson 2003; Fainboim et al. 2007]. Additionally, these cytokines can also affect T helper (Th) cell differentiation by skewing them directly from Th1 to Th2, Th0, or Treg [Hsu et al. 2007]. To this, Yamaguchi and colleagues demonstrated that in the presence of IL-10 or TGF-β, replicating DC progenitors produce DCs that are suppressive or tolerogenic [Yamaguchi et al. 1997]. Interestingly, IL-10 has also been implicated in interfering with the homing ability of DCs to secondary lymphatic tissues [Takayama et al. 2001].

Another possible mechanism for the induction of tolerance is the generation of Tregs by immature liver DCs. It is thought that the presence of activated Tregs can down-regulate MHC class I and co-stimulatory molecules on DCs, maintaining them in an immature state [Lau et al. 2003]. In all, it would appear that the microenvironment, dominated by IL-10 and TGF-β produced by other liver resident cells, is ideal to promote or sustain a tolerogenic/immature phenotype on hepatic DCs.

The second liver resident cell that has the capacity to function as an APC and influence the immune response are the endothelial cells lining the sinusoids. LSECs are strategically positioned to interact with leukocytes and antigens as they traverse the liver sinusoids several hundred times per day. Similar to DCs, LSECs avidly take up antigen for processing via specific surface receptors, such as the mannose receptor, making them highly efficient liver-resident APCs. Importantly, unlike other endothelial cells, they are able to present exogenous soluble antigen passing through the sinusoids to naive T cells in the absence of additional stimulation by pro-inflammatory cytokines such as IFN-γ or TNF-α [Selmi et al. 2007].

It has been suggested that in the absence of hepatic inflammation, antigen presentation by LSECs preferentially promotes immune tolerance over a T-cell-mediated immune response. Supporting this, Knolle et al. demonstrated that the activation of naive $CD4^+$ T-cells by LSECs does not promote their differentiation into pro-inflammatory Th1 effectors cells expressing IFN-γ and IL-2, but instead, directs them toward regulatory Th0 cells, synthesizing IFN-γ, IL-4, and IL-10, but not TGF-β [Knolle et al. 1999]. Interestingly, this divergent pathway appears to be restricted to LSECs and may be due to the constitutive expression of TGF-β by LSECs [Bertolino et al. 2002].

It has also been demonstrated that LSECs are proficient at cross-presenting soluble antigen on MHC class I molecules to $CD8^+$ T-cells in vivo [Limmer et al. 2000]. Such presentation of antigen to $CD8^+$ cells results in the induction of systemic antigen-specific immune tolerance through clonal deletion and anergy [Limmer et al. 2000, 2005; Limmer and Knolle 2001]. Specifically, $CD8^+$ T cells that are primed by LSECs may be initially activated and even proliferate; they are, however, functionally inert, lack cytotoxic effector function, exhibit poor cytokine release, and eventually undergo apoptosis [Limmer et al. 2000].

Similar to other APCs, antigen presentation by LSECs is modulated by various cytokines present at the time that antigen is encountered. For example, in the presence of PGE_2, TNF-α, or elevated IL-10, murine LSECs have been shown to reduce their expression of MHC class I, co-stimulatory molecules and mannose receptor–mediated antigen uptake, resulting in diminished T-cell activation [Lohse et al. 1996; Knolle et al. 1998; Knolle and Gerken 2000; Lau and Thomson 2003]. Additionally, LSECs can express pro-apoptotic molecules such as Fas ligand, TNF receptor apoptosis-inducing ligand (TRAIL), and TNF-α that can contribute to T-cell apoptosis [Muschen et al. 1998]. In fact, a recent study provided evidence that LSECs may have a key role in liver-mediated peripheral tolerance via apoptosis. The authors demonstrated that upon in vitro co-culturing of activated T cells and LSECs, about 30% of activated T-cells underwent apoptosis [Karrar et al. 2007].

KCs located within the hepatic sinusoids represent the first line of defense against viral particles delivered from the portal circulation. Phagocytosis of systemically or intrahepatic administered viral vectors (e.g., adenoviral and lentiviral vectors) by KCs initiates T-cell responses, stimulates the production of pro-inflammatory cytokines (e.g., TNF-α, IFN-γ, IL-6, and IL-12) and chemokines [e.g., IFN-γ inducible protein (IP-10), macrophage inflammatory protein 1 and 2, MCP, RANTES], and stimulates up-regulation of MHC class II expression [Lieber et al. 1997; Schnell et al. 2001; Zhang et al. 2001; Zaiss et al. 2002; van Til et al. 2005]. The release of such serum factors can act as a paracrine signal for activation and recruitment of additional cells. For example, Brunetti-Pierri and co-workers demonstrated that IL-6, induced by virus particles or by IL-1 and TNF-α, stimulates the production of acute-phase proteins (e.g., C-reactive protein) by hepatocytes [Brunetti-Pierri et al. 2004]. Moreover, the resulting intrahepatic inflammation is likely to enhance subsequent adaptive immune responses by increasing antigen presentation, continued secretion of soluble mediators, and recruitment of additional inflammatory cells. Indeed, it has been established that the pro-inflammatory cytokines and chemokines produced in response to adenoviral vectors is associated with leukocyte recruitment mediated by E-selectin, P-selectin, and α4-integrin [Li et al. 2002].

Similar to DCs, KCs also appear to play a role in the induction of tolerance via mechanisms such as cross presentation of antigen derived from ingested apoptotic cells to either resident DCs or those traversing the liver. On the other hand, KCs may be deemed deactivated or tolerogenic if antigen uptake occurs under noninflammatory conditions or an immunosuppressive environment. In fact, it has been shown for other peripheral macrophages that stimulation by anti-inflammatory cytokines such as IL-10 and TGF-β inhibits their ability to secrete pro-inflammatory factors (e.g., IL-12, IFN-γ), down-regulate MHC class II expression, induce PGE_2 production, and promote paracrine and autocrine secretion of IL-10 and TGF-β [Gordon 2003].

Even though the liver harbors several cells that have been shown to function efficiently as APCs, there is only limited evidence supporting the idea that direct antigen presentation can occur efficiently in the liver. The concept that primary activation explicitly in the liver challenges the long-standing immunological dogma that naive T-cell activation in lymphoid tissue occurs only following tissue damage or inflammation [Bertolino et al. 2001]. In an interesting series of experiments, Bowen and colleagues examined this controversy. For this study the authors used two different transgenic mouse models, in which antigen was either expressed exclusively by hepatocytes or only within the lymph nodes. When they adoptively transferred antigen-specific TCR-transgenic $CD8^+$ T cells, they demonstrated that hepatitis is induced when primary activation occurs in the draining lymph nodes. However, when the initial T-cell activation occurred in the liver, the $CD8^+$ T cells transferred not only failed to induce hepatic inflammation but also exhibited defective cytotoxic functions and shortened half-life [Bowen et al. 2004; Racanelli and Rehermann 2006]. Another important finding reported by the authors was that activated $CD8^+$ T cells within the liver began to exhibit CTL activity and cell division and to recirculate after 24 hours. In contrast, $CD8^+$ T cells activated in the lymph nodes were retained for at least two days before recirculating in the blood [Bertolino et al. 2001]. In other words, compared to the lymph nodes, the variation in signals induced from the various hepatic APCs during the initial activation of naive T cells appears to drive the T-cells to an alternative outcome.

In addition to the site of primary activation, the level of transgene expression also appears to be an important factor influencing induction of T-cell immunity or tolerance, perhaps reflecting differences in the mode or context of antigen presentation. In a series of experiments using AAV-mediated hepatic gene transfer, our laboratory demonstrated that higher levels of transgene expression promoted a shift from a Th1 to a Th2 response or tolerance, with tolerance being favored at higher expression levels [Mingozzi et al. 2003]. It should be noted that although tolerance induction was successful in several different inbred and outbred strains of mice, a threshold level of expression was required, and success rates varied depending on the strain–genotype combination [Mingozzi et al. 2003; Wang et al. 2005].

8.6 CONCLUSIONS

Hepatic gene transfer is a promising approach to the treatment of genetic diseases. Ideally, the goal for in vivo gene transfer should be the induction of tolerance to the therapeutic protein. Recent evidence suggests that the liver has a unique tolerogenic microenvironment compared to that of lymphoid tissues. Even though the complex cellular interactions that determine the balance between immunity and tolerance in hepatic gene therapy are only now being investigated, it appears that the level of transgene expression and the location of antigen presentation are of critical importance and require further examination. The exploitation of these differences may hold the key to obtaining a clinically safe and feasible treatment.

Overall, there have been many advances and successes in animal models of liver direct gene transfer. Specifically, AAV and lentiviral vector systems have demonstrated the ability to induce immune tolerance to the transgene product. It is essential for future research to focus on the unique immunological properties of the liver and the role these play in hepatic gene transfer.

REFERENCES

Annacker O, Pimenta-Araujo R, et al. 2001. $CD25^+CD4^+$ T cells regulate the expansion of peripheral CD4 T cells through the production of IL-10. *J Immunol* 166:3008–3018.

Bagley J, Tian C, et al. 2002. Induction of T-cell tolerance to an MHC class I alloantigen by gene therapy. *Blood* 99:4394–4399.

Beignon AS, McKenna K, et al. 2005. Endocytosis of HIV-1 activates plasmacytoid dendritic cells via Toll-like receptor-viral RNA interactions. *J Clin Invest* 115:3265–3275.

Bertolino P, Heath WR, et al. 1995. Peripheral deletion of autoreactive CD8^{+} T cells in transgenic mice expressing H-2Kb in the liver. *Eur J Immunol* 25:1932–1942.

Bertolino P, Trescol-Biemont MC, et al. 1998. Hepatocytes induce functional activation of naive CD8^{+} T lymphocytes but fail to promote survival. *Eur J Immunol* 28:221.

Bertolino P, Bowen DG, et al. 2001. Antigen-specific primary activation of CD8^{+} T cells within the liver. *J Immunol* 166:5430–5438.

Bertolino P, McCaughan GW, et al. 2002. Role of primary intrahepatic T-cell activation in the "liver tolerance effect". *Immunol Cell Biol* 80:84–92.

Bessis N, GarciaCozar FJ, et al. 2004. Immune responses to gene therapy vectors: influence on vector function and effector mechanisms. *Gene Ther* 11 (Suppl 1):S10–S17.

Bowen DG, Warren A, et al. 2002. Cytokine-dependent bystander hepatitis due to intrahepatic murine CD8T-cell activation by bone marrow–derived cells. *Gastroenterology* 123:1252–1264.

Bowen DG, Zen M, et al. 2004. The site of primary T cell activation is a determinant of the balance between intrahepatic tolerance and immunity. *J Clin Invest* 114:701–712.

Bristol JA, Shirley P, et al. 2000. In vivo dose threshold effect of adenovirus-mediated factor VIII gene therapy in hemophiliac mice. *Mol Ther* 2:223–232.

Brown BD, Venneri MA, et al. 2006. Endogenous microRNA regulation suppresses transgene expression in hematopoietic lineages and enables stable gene transfer. *Nat Med* 12:585–591.

Brown BD, Sitia G, et al. 2007. In vivo administration of lentiviral vectors triggers a type I interferon response that restricts hepatocyte gene transfer and promotes vector clearance. *Blood* 109:2797–2805.

Brunetti-Pierri N, Palmer DJ, et al. 2004. Acute toxicity after high-dose systemic injection of helper-dependent adenoviral vectors into nonhuman primates. *Hum Gene Ther* 15:35–46.

Bumgardner GL, Matas AJ, et al. 1990. Comparison of in vivo and in vitro immune response to purified hepatocytes. *Transplantation* 49:429.

Calne RY, Sells RA, et al. 1969. Induction of immunological tolerance by porcine liver allografts. *Nature* 223:472–476.

Cao O, Dobrzynski E, et al. 2007. Induction and role of regulatory CD4^{+}CD25^{+} T cells in tolerance to the transgene product following hepatic in vivo gene transfer. *Blood* 110:1132–1140.

Chuah MK, Schiedner G, et al. 2003. Therapeutic factor VIII levels and negligible toxicity in mouse and dog models of hemophilia A following gene therapy with high-capacity adenoviral vectors. *Blood* 101:1734–1743.

Crettaz J, Berraondo P, et al. 2006. Intrahepatic injection of adenovirus reduces inflammation and increases gene transfer and therapeutic effect in mice. *Hepatology* 44:623–632.

Crispe IN. 2003. Hepatic T cells and liver tolerance. *Nat Rev Immunol* 3:51–62.

Crispe IN, Giannandrea M, et al. 2006. Cellular and molecular mechanisms of liver tolerance. *Immunol Rev* 213:101–118.

Decker K. 1990. Biologically active products of stimulated liver macrophages (Kupffer cells). *Eur J Biochem* 192:245–261.

Diebold SS, Kaisho T, et al. 2004. Innate antiviral responses by means of TLR7-mediated recognition of single-stranded RNA. *Science* 303:1529–1531.

Dikopoulos N, Wegenka U, et al. 2004. Recently primed $CD8^+$ T cells entering the liver induce hepatocytes to interact with naive $CD8^+$ T cells in the mouse. *Hepatology* 39:1256–1266.

Dobrzynski E and Herzog RW. 2005. Tolerance induction by viral in vivo gene transfer. *Clin Med Res* 3:234–240.

Dobrzynski E, Mingozzi F, et al. 2004. Induction of antigen-specific $CD4^+$ T cell anergy and deletion by in vivo viral gene transfer. *Blood* 104:969–977.

Dobrzynski E, Fitzgerald JC, et al. 2006. Prevention of cytotoxic T lymphocyte responses to factor IX–expressing hepatocytes by gene transfer-induced regulatory T cells. *Proc Natl Acad Sci U S A* 103:4592–4597.

Erles K, Sebokova P, et al. 1999. Update on the prevalence of serum antibodies (IgG and IgM) to adeno-associated virus (AAV). *J Med Virol* 59:406–411.

Fainboim L, Chernavsky A, et al. 2007. Cytokines and chronic liver disease. *Cytokine Growth Factor Rev* 18:143.

Fallarino F, Grohmann U, et al. 2006. The combined effects of tryptophan starvation and tryptophan catabolites down-regulate T cell receptor zeta-chain and induce a regulatory phenotype in naive T cells. *J Immunol* 176:6752–6761.

Fields PA, Kowalczyk DW, et al. 2000. Role of vector in activation of T cell subsets in immune responses against the secreted transgene product factor IX. *Mol Ther* 1:225–235.

Follenzi A, Battaglia M, et al. 2004. Targeting lentiviral vector expression to hepatocytes limits transgene-specific immune response and establishes long-term expression of human antihemophilic factor IX in mice. *Blood* 103:3700–3709.

Fonteneau JF, Larsson M, et al. 2004. Human immunodeficiency virus type 1 activates plasmacytoid dendritic cells and concomitantly induces the bystander maturation of myeloid dendritic cells. *J Virol* 78:5223–5232.

Franco LM, Sun B, et al. 2005. Evasion of immune responses to introduced human acid alpha-glucosidase by liver-restricted expression in glycogen storage disease type II. *Mol Ther* 12:876–884.

Girardin SE, Sansonetti PJ, et al. 2002. Intracellular vs. extracellular recognition of pathogens: common concepts in mammals and flies. *Trends Microbiol* 10:193–199.

Gondek DC, Lu LF, et al. 2005. Cutting edge: contact-mediated suppression by $CD4^+CD25^+$ regulatory cells involves a granzyme B–dependent, perforin-independent mechanism. *J Immunol* 174:1783–1786.

Gordon S. 2003. Alternative activation of macrophages. *Nat Rev Immunol* 3:23–35.

Guidotti LG and Chisari FV. 2001. Noncytolytic control of viral infections by the innate and adaptive immune response. *Annu Rev Immunol* 19:65–91.

Halbert CL, Standaert TA, et al. 1997. Transduction by adeno-associated virus vectors in the rabbit airway: efficiency, persistence, and readministration. *J Virol* 71:5932–5941.

Herzog RW, Hagstrom JN, et al. 1997. Stable gene transfer and expression of human blood coagulation factor IX after intramuscular injection of recombinant adeno-associated virus. *Proc Natl Acad Sci U S A* 94:5804–5809.

Herzog RW, Yang EY, et al. 1999. Long-term correction of canine hemophilia B by gene transfer of blood coagulation factor IX mediated by adeno-associated viral vector. *Nat Med* 5:56–63.

Hoffman B, Dobrzynski E, et al. 2007. Muscle as a target for supplementary factor IX gene transfer. *Hum Gene Ther* 18:603–613.

Hsu W, Shu SA, et al. 2007. The current immune function of hepatic dendritic cells. *Cell Mol Immunol* 4:321–328.

Jaffe HA, Danel C, et al. 1992. Adenovirus-mediated in vivo gene transfer and expression in normal rat liver. *Nat Genet* 1:372–378.

Jenkins MK, Khoruts A, et al. 2001. In vivo activation of antigen-specific CD4T cells. *Annu Rev Immunol* 19:23–45.

Kang Y, Xie L, et al. 2005. Persistent expression of factor VIII in vivo following non-primate lentiviral gene transfer. *Blood* 106:1552–1558.

Karrar A, Broome U, et al. 2007. Human liver sinusoidal endothelial cells induce apoptosis in activated T cells: a role in tolerance induction. *Gut* 56:243–252.

Khanna A, Morelli AE, et al. 2000. Effects of liver-derived dendritic cell progenitors on Th1- and Th2-like cytokine responses in vitro and in vivo. *J Immunol* 164:1346–1354.

Knolle PA and Gerken G. 2000. Local control of the immune response in the liver. *Immunol Rev* 174:21–34.

Knolle PA, Schmitt E, et al. 1999. Induction of cytokine production in naive CD4(+) T cells by antigen-presenting murine liver sinusoidal endothelial cells but failure to induce differentiation toward Th1 cells. *Gastroenterology* 116:1428–1440.

Knolle PA, Uhrig, et al. 1998. IL-10 down-regulates T cell activation by antigen-presenting liver sinusoidal endothelial cells through decreased antigen uptake via the mannose receptor and lowered surface expression of accessory molecules. *Clin Exp Immunol* 114:427–433.

Kudo S, Matsuno K, et al. 1997. A novel migration pathway for rat dendritic cells from the blood: hepatic sinusoids-lymph translocation. *J Exp Med* 185:777–784.

Kuzmin AI, Finegold MJ, et al. 1997. Macrophage depletion increases the safety, efficacy and persistence of adenovirus-mediated gene transfer in vivo. *Gene Ther* 4:309–316.

Lau AH and Thomson AW. 2003. Dendritic cells and immune regulation in the liver. *Gut* 52:307–314.

Lau AH, de Creus A, et al. 2003. Liver tolerance mediated by antigen presenting cells: fact or fiction? *Gut* 52:1075–1078.

Lee KH, Panelli MC, et al. 1998. Functional dissociation between local and systemic immune response during anti-melanoma peptide vaccination. *J Immunol* 161:4183–4194.

Leifeld L, Trautwein C, et al. 1999. Enhanced expression of CD80 (B7-1), CD86 (B7-2), and CD40 and their ligands CD28 and CD154 in fulminant hepatic failure. *Am J Pathol* 154:1711–1720.

Li Q, Kay MA, et al. 1993. Assessment of recombinant adenoviral vectors for hepatic gene therapy. *Hum Gene Ther* 4:403–409.

Li Y, Muruve DA, et al. 2002. The role of selectins and integrins in adenovirus vector-induced neutrophil recruitment to the liver. *Eur J Immunol* 32:3443–3452.

Lieber A, He CY, et al. 1997. The role of Kupffer cell activation and viral gene expression in early liver toxicity after infusion of recombinant adenovirus vectors. *J Virol* 71:8798–8807.

Limmer A and Knolle PA. 2001. Liver sinusoidal endothelial cells: a new type of organ-resident antigen-presenting cell. *Arch Immunol Ther Exp (Warsz)* 49(Suppl 1): S7–S11.

Limmer A, Ohl J, et al. 2000. Efficient presentation of exogenous antigen by liver endothelial cells to $CD8^+$ T cells results in antigen-specific T-cell tolerance. *Nat Med* 6:1348–1354.

Limmer A, Ohl J, et al. 2005. Cross-presentation of oral antigens by liver sinusoidal endothelial cells leads to CD8T cell tolerance. *Eur J Immunol* 35:2970–2981.

Liu YJ. 2001. Dendritic cell subsets and lineages, and their functions in innate and adaptive immunity. *Cell* 106:259–262.

Lohse AW, Knolle PA, et al. 1996. Antigen-presenting function and B7 expression of murine sinusoidal endothelial cells and Kupffer cells. *Gastroenterology* 110:1175–1181.

Mackay IR. 2002. Hepatoimmunology: a perspective. *Immunol Cell Biol* 80:36–44.

Manno CS, Arruda VR, et al. 2006. Successful transduction of liver in hemophilia by AAV-factor IX and limitations imposed by the host immune response. *Nat Med* 12:342–347.

Markiewski MM, DeAngelis RA, et al. 2006. Liver inflammation and regeneration: two distinct biological phenomena or parallel pathophysiologic processes? *Mol Immunol* 43:45–56.

McAvoy EF and Kubes P. 2006. Holey endothelium: gateways for naive T cell activation. *Hepatology* 44:1083–1085.

Medzhitov R. 2001. Toll-like receptors and innate immunity. *Nat Rev Immunol* 1:135–145.

Mehal WZ, Juedes AE, et al. 1999. Selective retention of activated $CD8^+$ T cells by the normal liver. *J Immunol* 163:3202–3210.

Mehal WZ, Azzaroli F, et al. 2001. Antigen presentation by liver cells controls intrahepatic T cell trapping, whereas bone marrow–derived cells preferentially promote intrahepatic T cell apoptosis. *J Immunol* 167:667–673.

Mingozzi F, Liu Y-L, et al. 2003. Induction of immune tolerance to coagulation factor IX antigen by in vivo hepatic gene transfer. *J Clin Invest* 111:1347–1356.

Miyara M and Sakaguchi S. 2007. Natural regulatory T cells: mechanisms of suppression. *Trends Mol Med* 13:108–116.

Mount JD, Herzog RW, et al. 2002. Sustained phenotypic correction of hemophilia B dogs with a factor IX null mutation by liver-directed gene therapy. *Blood* 99:2670–2676.

Muschen M, Warskulat U, et al. 1998. Regulation of CD95 (APO-1/Fas) receptor and ligand expression by lipopolysaccharide and dexamethasone in parenchymal and non-parenchymal rat liver cells. *Hepatology* 27:200–208.

Nathwani AC, Davidoff AM, et al. 2002. Sustained high-level expression of human factor IX (hFIX) after liver-targeted delivery of recombinant adeno-associated virus encoding the hFIX gene in rhesus macaques. *Blood* 100:1662–1669.

Norris S, Collins C, et al. 1998. Resident human hepatic lymphocytes are phenotypically different from circulating lymphocytes. *J Hepatol* 28:84–90.

Racanelli V and Rehermann B. 2006. The liver as an immunological organ. *Hepatology* 43:S54–S62.

Roland CR, Walp L, et al. 1994. Outcome of Kupffer cell antigen presentation to a cloned murine Th1 lymphocyte depends on the inducibility of nitric oxide synthase by IFN-gamma. *J Immunol* 153:5453–5464.

Sakaguchi S, Sakaguchi N, et al. 2001. Immunologic tolerance maintained by $CD25^+CD4^+$ regulatory T cells: their common role in controlling autoimmunity, tumor immunity, and transplantation tolerance. *Immunol Rev* 182:18–32.

Schagen FHE, Ossevoort M, et al. 2004. Immune responses against adenoviral vectors and their transgene products: a review of strategies for evasion. *Crit Rev Oncol Hematol* 50:51.

Schnell MA, Zhang Y, et al. 2001. Activation of innate immunity in nonhuman primates following intraportal administration of adenoviral vectors. *Mol Ther* 3:708–722.

Selmi C, Mackay IR, et al. 2007. The immunological milieu of the liver. *Semin Liver Dis* 27:129–139.

Sheth K and Bankey P. 2001. The liver as an immune organ. *Curr Opin Crit Care* 7:99–104.

Snyder RO, Miao CH, et al. 1997. Persistent and therapeutic concentrations of human factor IX in mice after hepatic gene transfer of recombinant AAV vectors. *Nat Genet* 16:270–276.

Snyder RO, Miao C, et al. 1999. Correction of hemophilia B in canine and murine models using recombinant adeno-associated viral vectors. *Nat Med* 5:64–70.

Takayama T, Morelli AE, et al. 2001. Mammalian and viral IL-10 enhance C-C chemokine receptor 5 but down-regulate C-C chemokine receptor 7 expression by myeloid dendritic cells: impact on chemotactic responses and in vivo homing ability. *J Immunol* 166:7136–7143.

Tao N, Gao G-P, et al. 2001. Sequestration of adenoviral vector by Kupffer cells leads to a nonlinear dose response of transduction in liver. *Mol Ther* 3:28.

Thomson AW and Lu L. 1999. Are dendritic cells the key to liver transplant tolerance? *Immunol Today* 20:27–32.

van Til NP, Markusic DM, et al. 2005. Kupffer cells and not liver sinusoidal endothelial cells prevent lentiviral transduction of hepatocytes. *Mol Ther* 11:26–34.

Wajahat ZM, Francesco A, et al. 2001. Immunology of the healthy liver: old questions and new insights. *Gastroenterology* 120:250.

Wang L, Cao O, et al. 2005. Major role of local immune responses in antibody formation to factor IX in AAV gene transfer. *Gene Ther* 12:1453.

Warren A, Le Couteur DG, et al. 2006. T lymphocytes interact with hepatocytes through fenestrations in murine liver sinusoidal endothelial cells. *Hepatology* 44:1182–1190.

Wick MJ, Leithauser F, et al. 2002. The hepatic immune system. *Crit Rev Immunol* 22:47–103.

Wiegard C, Frenzel C, et al. 2005. Murine liver antigen presenting cells control suppressor activity of $CD4^+CD25^+$ regulatory T cells. *Hepatology* 42:193–199.

Wolff G, Worgall S, et al. 1997. Enhancement of in vivo adenovirus-mediated gene transfer and expression by prior depletion of tissue macrophages in the target organ. *J Virol* 71:624–629.

Worgall S, Wolff G, et al. 1997. Innate immune mechanisms dominate elimination of adenoviral vectors following in vivo administration. *Hum Gene Ther* 8:37–44.

Yamaguchi Y, Tsumura H, et al. 1997. Contrasting effects of TGF-beta 1 and TNF-alpha on the development of dendritic cells from progenitors in mouse bone marrow. *Stem Cells* 15:144–153.

Zaiss AK, Liu Q, et al. 2002. Differential activation of innate immune responses by adenovirus and adeno-associated virus vectors. *J Virol* 76:4580–4590.

Zhang L, Dailey PJ, et al. 2002. The liver is a major organ for clearing simian immunodeficiency virus in rhesus monkeys. *J Virol* 76:5271–5273.

Zhang Y, Chirmule N, et al. 2001. Acute cytokine response to systemic adenoviral vectors in mice is mediated by dendritic cells and macrophages. *Mol Ther* 3:697–707.

Ziegler RJ, Lonning SM, et al. 2004. AAV2 vector harboring a liver-restricted promoter facilitates sustained expression of therapeutic levels of alpha-galactosidase A and the induction of immune tolerance in fabry mice. *Mol Ther* 9:231–240.

9

IMMUNE RESPONSES TO ADENOVIRAL, ADENO-ASSOCIATED VIRAL, AND LENTIVIRAL VECTORS USED FOR GENE THERAPY OF BRAIN DISEASES: THE ROLE OF IMMUNOLOGICAL SYNAPSES AND THE CELL BIOLOGY OF NEUROIMMUNE INTERACTIONS

PEDRO R. LOWENSTEIN, M.D., PH.D.

Gene Therapeutics Research Institute, Cedars-Sinai Medical Center, and Departments of Medicine and Molecular and Medical Pharmacology, David Geffen School of Medicine, University of California–Los Angeles, Los Angeles, California

RONALD J. MANDEL, PH.D.

Department of Neuroscience, Powell Gene Therapy Center, McKnight Brain Institute, University of Florida College of Medicine, Gainesville, Florida

WEI-DONG XIONG, M.D., PH.D., KURT KROEGER, M.S., AND MARIA G. CASTRO, PH.D.

Gene Therapeutics Research Institute, Cedars-Sinai Medical Center, and Departments of Medicine and Molecular and Medical Pharmacology, David Geffen School of Medicine, University of California–Los Angeles, Los Angeles, California

Gene Therapy Immunology, Edited by Roland Herzog

9.1 INTRODUCTION

Gene therapy is an attractive and promising tool for the treatment for neurological disorders, many of which constitute major unmet medical needs. Viral vectors are versatile gene delivery vehicles to the central nervous system (CNS), due to the ability to produce vector stocks with concentrations high enough to use only doses small enough to be effective upon administration to the nervous system. Furthermore, the ability of some viral vectors to infect both dividing and nondiving cells, as would be encountered in the brain, makes viral vectors attractive therapeutic agents. Numerous preclinical and early-phase clinical trials have been performed using gene therapy strategies to treat human neurological disorders, including Parkinson's disease [During et al. 2001; Muramatsu et al. 2002; Wong et al. 2006; Kaplitt et al. 2007], Alzheimer's disease [Levi-Montalcini 1987; Eriksdotter Jonhagen et al. 1998; Tuszynski et al. 2005], and glioma [Chiocca et al. 2004; Immonen et al. 2004; Ali et al. 2005]. So far, however, the initial successes of preclinical animal gene therapy experiments have often failed to translate into equally impressive therapeutic outcomes in the clinic. A likely culprit for the diminished clinical efficacy is the impact of the patient's immune response on therapeutic gene expression. Here we examine the immune response against gene therapy vectors in the brain. A thorough review of the unique immunological status of the brain is followed by an examination of the innate and adaptive arms of the immune system in the brain vis-á-vis the therapeutic viral vectors. The consequences of activating the immune system on therapeutic gene expression in the brain mediated by first-generation, high-capacity, helper-dependent adenoviral vectors, adeno-associated vectors, and lentiviral vectors are discussed in detail.

9.2 THE IMMUNE COMPARTMENTS OF THE BRAIN

There are two main immune compartments in the brain. The intensity and duration of the antiviral vector–mediated immune responses are directly dependent on which compartment is targeted by the therapeutic viral vectors. One compartment, the brain ventricles, meninges, and choroid plexi, contain all cellular, vascular, and lymphatic elements of the immune system, as do most other organs in the body. Specifically, dendritic cells (DCs), the major cell type capable of inducing primary T-cell responses, are located within the meninges, choroid plexus, and cerebrospinal fluid (CSF) of the normal noninflamed brain [McMenamin 1999; Lowenstein 2002b; Pashenkov et al. 2003; Bechmann et al. 2007; Galea et al. 2007]. Strategically located to capture foreign or self-antigens throughout the brain ventricular system, DCs can migrate to the cervical draining lymph nodes (CLNs), the primary lymph nodes draining the brain, and CSF [Cserr and Knopf 1992]. The brain parenchyma, the "other" brain immune compartment, is separated from the general circulation by the blood–brain barrier, formed by tight intercellular endothelial junctions [Bechmann et al. 2007], and is devoid of lymphatics and DCs in the absence of inflammation. In addition, a large number of molecular mechanisms serve to dampen immune reactivity in the brain parenchyma itself (e.g., TGF-β).

What are the immune consequences of making antigens available to either of the brain immune compartments? Injection of a particulate antigen or infectious agent (e.g., live influenza virus, BCG, nonreplicative viral vectors) only into the brain parenchyma (avoiding any leakage to the brain ventricles) causes innate inflammatory responses but does not trigger systemic adaptive immune responses [Matyszak and Perry 1996; Stevenson et al. 1997b; Cartmell et al. 1999; Lowenstein 2002a;] that is, the systemic immune system remains unaware of the delivery of antigens into the brain. However, injection of the same particulate antigen or infectious agent into the brain ventricular system will stimulate an innate inflammatory and a systemic adaptive immune response [Matyszak and Perry 1996; Stevenson et al. 1997a; Matyszak 1998]. Conversly, the injection of a soluble diffusible antigen (e.g., ovalbumin) into either compartment does induce a systemic B-cell response [Knopf et al. 1998], due to the ability of the antigen to diffuse to the ventricular, reach the CLNs, and stimulate a systemic humoral immune response. Particulate antigens carefully delivered to the brain parenchyma fail to elicit a specific adaptive systemic immune response because they cannot diffuse out into the ventricular system to reach the CLNs.

Throughout the body, DCs localize predominantly to lymphoid tissue, where they take up antigen and mature to potent antigen-presenting cells (APCs). Alternatively, DCs acquire antigen at inflamed sites, from where they migrate to secondary lymphoid organs to activate naive T cells [Caux et al. 2000; Leon et al. 2007]. A possible reason underlying the different immune responses upon antigen delivery to either brain ventricles or parenchyma may be due to the inability of particulate antigen to move from the brain parenchyma to the CLNs, using either diffusion or cellular transport. When particulate antigens are injected into the brain parenchyma, they are not transported to the lymph nodes to prime a systemic adaptive immune response, although they may cause localized inflammation. On the other hand, soluble antigens can diffuse from the brain parenchyma into the ventricular system to eventually reach the lymph nodes and stimulate systemic adaptive immune responses.

Once the antigen has reached the CLNs, naive T cells are primed, expand, exit the lymph nodes, and migrate to the site of insult, where they will exert their effector function (such as secretion of IFN-γ or target cell killing) when the specific antigen is encountered. While DCs can enter the CNS parenchyma during inflammatory responses to sustain T-cell function, initial naive T-cell activation is most likely to occur in the CLNs. During chronic inflammation, however, brain-infiltrating DCs have been proposed to be able to present antigen to naive T cells [McMahon et al. 2005].

9.3 IMMUNE RESPONSES AGAINST VIRAL VECTORS USED IN GENE THERAPY

9.3.1 Innate Immune Responses in the Brain

As viral vector technology is at the very heart of many gene therapy strategies, the immunogenicity of the gene therapy vectors must be evaluated and characterized thoroughly. Administartion of viral vectors into the CNS induces acute inflammation, including microglial activation, macrophage recruitment, and antigen-nonspecific T-cell infiltration that is dose dependent, but these innate immune responses occur in both neuroimmune compartments. Due to their identical capsids, the immune system is unable to distinguish between a recombinant viral vector and a wild-type virus. In most cases the interaction between viral capsid proteins and specific innate immune receptors, such as Toll receptors, mediates initial inflammatory responses. Due to the compartmentalization of the brain's immune system, however, injection of viral vectors into the immune-privileged brain parenchyma stimulates innate inflammatory responses without necessarily inducing a linked systemic adaptive immune response. Substantial leakage of the vectors to the brain ventricular system will, however, stimulate an adaptive immune response.

In a detailed dose–response study, Thomas and co-workers assessed the short-term (3-day) and medium-term (30-day) inflammatory consequences of injecting increasing doses of adenoviral vectors delivered in small volumes directly into the mouse striatum (i.e., injections circumscribed to the brain parenchyma) [Thomas et al. 2001a]. Vector doses ranging from 10^6 to 10^9 infectious units (i.u.) were injected directly into the striatum. Both transgene expression and cellular inflammation, including microglia activation, macrophage infiltration, and antigen-nonspecific T-cell recruitment, were evaluated at 3 and 30 days after vector administration. β-Galactosidase expression was detected as early as 3 days post-vector injection in brains injected with 10^6 i.u. While expression levels increased with escalating doses, a plateau was reached following administration of 10^8 i.u. of vector. In addition, cytotoxicity also increased concomitantly with increasing doses of vectors injected. Minimal local cytotoxicity was observed at doses below 10^8 i.u., but immunoreactivity for the astrocyte marker GFAP and the neuronal marker NeuN suggested a substantial loss of astrocytes and neurons following the injection of 10^9 i.u. Importantly, administration of equally high doses of heat-inactivated adenoviral vectors (1×10^9 i.u.) failed to cause any significant inflammation and/or leukocyte infiltration into the brain, demonstrating that acute toxicity is indeed caused by intact viral particles, but not the viral proteins or vector genomes [Thomas et al. 2001a].

Importantly, 30 days post-intracranial vector injection, doses of vectors that elicited an *increased* inflammatory response consisting of increased markers for monocytes and lymphocytes at 3 days had a corresponding *elimination* of transgene expression at 30 days; that is, reduced transgene expression at doses of 10^8 and a complete loss of transgene expression following intracranial administration of 10^9 i.u. However, stable transgene expression at 30 days was observed at doses of 10^6 and 10^7. Thus, doses below 10^8 lead to stable and noninflammatory transgene expression.

An increase in apoptotic cells revealed by TUNEL staining indicated that cytotoxicity was caused by the acute inflammatory-induced cell death resulting from the dose of 10^9 i.u. Thomas et al. detected persistent brain inflammation and activation of microglia and the continued presence of monocytes and leukocytes corresponding to an increase in the brain cell loss. A direct correlation between acute cytotoxicity (at 3 days) and the long-term persistence (at 30 days) of macrophages, $CD8^+$ T cells, and increased expression of MHC class I in the CNS was observed. There was also a positive correlation between short- and medium-term (>30 days) brain cellular inflammation and long-term loss of transgene expression from adenoviral vectors. Inversely, 30 days after brains were injected with noncytotoxic doses (i.e., below 1×10^8) any early initial inflammatory mononuclear cell infiltration and microglia activation had resolved completely. These data indicate that intracranial injection of adenoviral vectors in naive animals elicits a dose-dependent, transient, and self-limiting acute innate inflammatory response. Doses below 1×10^8 provide therapeutically accepted levels of transgene expression without any long-term inflammation, monocyte recruitment, or cytotoxicity. The vector dose threshold further underscores the necessity of strong promoters to ensure that therapeutically acceptable levels of transgene expression are obtained from vector doses below the amounts that induce persistent inflammation and toxicity [Gerdes et al. 2000; Appleby et al. 2003].

In a follow-up work, we demonstrated that interferon-regulated and chemokine mRNAs were not up-regulated [Zirger et al. 2006a] at the noncytotoxic doses established in the work of Thomas et al. [2001a]. Using increasing doses of adenoviral vector from 10^5 to 10^8, Zirger et al. only observed an increase in αβ-interferon-regulated genes such as OAS, IRF-1, and PKR, and chemokines, such as RANTES, MCP-1, and IFN-γ-inducible protein 10, following injection of 10^8 i.u. above the threshold established for activation of local microglia, and recruitment of circulating mononuclear cells, established by us previously [Thomas et al. 2001a]. Moreover, even at this high vector dose, production of mRNAs for αβ-interferon-regulated genes and chemokines was transient, with expression of most mRNAs returning to baseline by 7 days post injection into the brain. This indicates that innate inflammatory responses to adenovirus (i.e., increase in expression of interferon-inducible genes, and chemokine genes) are dose dependent.

The injection of adenoviral vectors above a particular threshold increases the expression of chemokines and induces local cytotoxicity. Once this inflammatory threshold is crossed, long-term, potentially chronic (i.e., six months) brain inflammation can be expected [Dewey et al. 1999]. As with injections into the brain, when adenoviral vectors are injected into the periphery in preclinical and clinical trials, a dose-dependent inflammatory immune response ensues, preceding the development of an adaptive immune response [Crystal et al. 1994; Knowles et al. 1995; McCoy et al. 1995; Raper et al. 2002; Cotter and Muruve 2005]. It was shown previously that delivery of 10^9 to 10^{10} i.u. of adenoviral vectors to organs not considered immune-privileged (i.e., liver, lung) induced up-regulation of numerous inflammatory genes, including TNF-α, IFN-γ, IL1-1β, IL-6, IL-12, MIL1α, MIP-1β, MIP-2, MCP-1, IP-10, and RANTES within hours of vector transduction [Benihoud et al. 1998; Otake et al. 1998; Muruve et al. 1999; Schnell et al. 2001; Li et al. 2002]. Studies have shown that similar effects have been shown using ultraviolet (UV)–psoralen-inactivated adenoviral vectors, indicating that gene transcription is not required to activate this cellular host inflammatory response [Cotten et al. 1994]. Interestingly, data published by Thomas et al. demonstrated that systemic immunization with UV–psoralen-inactivated adenoviral vectors failed to mediate the elimination of adenoviral vector–mediated transgene expression in the brain. These data suggest that continued expression of viral proteins is needed to induce an immune reponse capable of eliminating transgene expression from the brain.

The Daniel Muruve group has described a biphasic time course of cytokines and chemokines in the liver corresponding to the immune response against the capsid proteins (phase 1, less than 24 hours) and immune response against viral gene products produced in situ (phase 2, 4 to 5 days post-transduction) [Liu et al. 2003; Cotter and Muruve 2005]. Whether a similar biphasic up-regulation of inflammatory genes following intrastriatal administration of adenoviral vector at noncytotoxic doses ($<1 \times 10^8$ i.u.) occurs in the brain remains to be studied.

9.3.2 Vector Dose Thresholds

The inflammatory threshold to intracranial delivery of adenoviral vectors is 1×10^8 i.u. If this immunological threshold is crossed, increased expression of interferon-inducible and chemokine-encoding genes, the activation of local microglia, and the recruitment of circulating monocytes and lymphocytes ensues. Injections of vector doses below this threshold do not induce any significant recruitment of inflammatory cells to the brain, do not cause glial or neuronal toxicity, do not cause an increase in expression of interferon-regulated genes or chemokine genes, and achieve long-term transgene expression of at least up to one year (Barcia et al. 2007b). The consequences of this work demonstrate the necessity to consider carefully the dose-dependent increased inflammatory gene expression or recruitment of inflammatory cells caused by adenoviral vectors when planning preclinical and/or clinical trials. A similar evaluation of the inflammatory threshold for intracranial delivery of lentiviral vectors was also performed by Abordo-Adesida et al. [2005]. In that study, increasing amounts of lentiviral vector were injected diluted in 3-μL volume into the brain. Maximum transgene expression was detected at a dose of 10^6 transducing units of lentiviral vector without an increase of either macrophages or $CD8^+$ T cells. A significant increase of $CD8^+$ T cells infiltrating the brain parenchyma was observed only in animals injected with 10^6 transducing units of lentiviral vector. A similar dose escalation study of AAV vectors in the brain has yet to be evaluated.

These studies highlight the importance of using high-quality, well-characterized viral vectors. Imprecise titration of these vectors and calculation errors in the amount of vectors administered will have serious, deleterious consequences for long-term therapeutic transgene expression in the brain. All vectors will be likely to be effective as therapeutic vehicles for gene therapy into the brain, *but only at the right dose*.

9.3.3 Adaptive Immune Responses Against Adenoviruses Injected into the Brain

As a result of the diverse compartments of the brain immune system, careful injection into the brain parenchyma of recombinant viral vectors at doses below the established immunological threshold provides long-term therapeutically effective levels of transgene expression in experimental models of neurological disorders. However, if the viral vectors escape to the peripheral organs or the lymphatic drainage, a systemic adaptive antiadenoviral T-cell immune response ensues that almost completely eliminates transgene expression from the brain. T cells are able to recognize as little as 1×10^3 i.u. of vector injected into the brain, an equivalent of 1000 transduced cells [Barcia et al. 2007a].

For example, transgene expression in the brain will be reduced by 50 to 90% when animals are immunized systemically against adenovirus 30 to 60 days after intracranial injection with adenovirus (Fig. 9-1). In the studies mentioned above, Barcia et al. [2007a] demonstrated that an adaptive immune response was able to eliminate transgene expression from as little as 1000 i.u. injected into the brain. For these experiments, a dose escalation of adenovirus was injected into the brain of naive animals, followed by systemic immunization against adenovirus. The resulting systemic immune response was able to eliminate transgene expression at doses from 10^7 i.u. to as low as 10^3 i.u. injected into the brain.

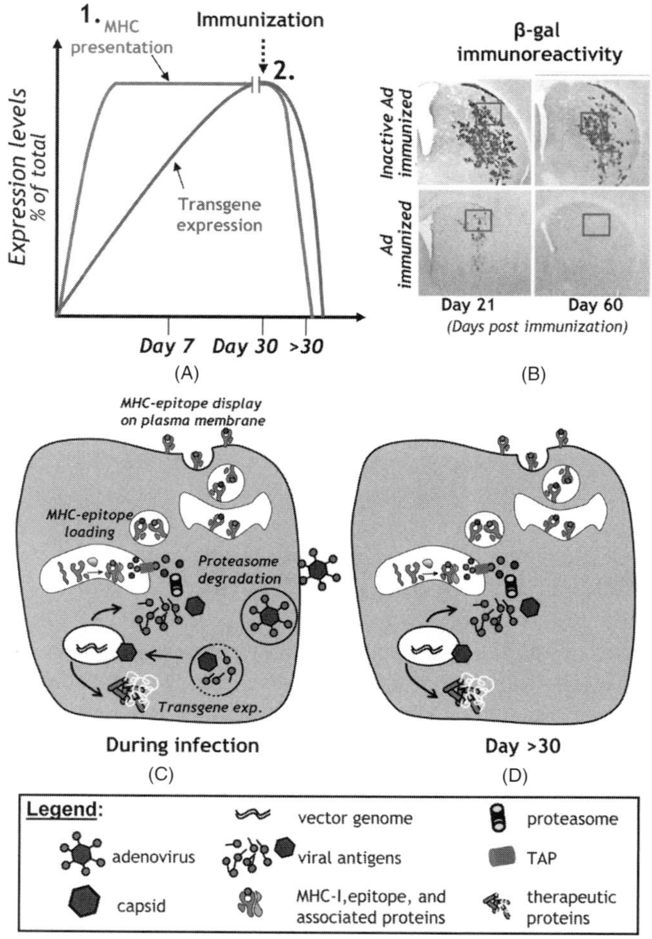

Figure 9-1 Antiadenoviral immune responses completely eliminate transgene expression from first-generation adenoviral vectors. (A) The levels of transgene expression and MHC presentation of viral epitopes in animals injected into the CNS with a first-generation adenoviral vector are illustrated. MHC class I presentation of viral epitopes peaks earlier, due to intracellular degredation and presentation of capsid-derived epitopes. Transgene expression (and consequent MHC antigen presentation) are completely abrogated following systemic immunization with adenovirus. (B) Immunoreactivity for β-galactosidase illustrates the effects of a systemic immune response against adenovirus on transgene expression from first-generation adenoviral vectors in the brains of rats immunized against inactivated adenovirus (top panels) or adenovirus (bottom panels). Short-term (21 days post-immunization, left panels) and medium-term (60 days post-immunization, right panels) expression of β-gal are shown. Note the sharp reduction of β-gal immunoreactivity in immunized animals compared to control animals immunized with inactivated adenovirus. Sixty days later, transgene expression is completely eliminated in immunized animals, while transgene expression is sustained in control immunized animals. (C) A schematic of first-generation vector infection, uncoating, nuclear transduction, production of transgene, and presentation of viral antigenic epitopes on MHC class I is shown shortly after and during vector infection. (D) A schematic of the same cells more than 30 days later. Note the continued expression of viral proteins from the first-generation adenoviral vector genomes and their presentation by MHC molecules on the cell surface.

Further experiments by Barcia et al. [2006], and Zirger and colleagues (in preparation), have shown that elimination of transgene expression from the brain of immunized animals is mediated by $CD8^+$ and $CD4^+$ T cells; it is also likely that B cells are needed for transgene expression loss [Zirger et al. 2006b; Barcia et al. 2007b]. We have also shown that the promoter used to drive transgene expression has no impact on the immune-mediated elimination of transgene expression. The immune system is able to eliminate transgene expression from all promoters tested, whether viral, housekeeping, or cell-type-specific promoters [Barcia et al. 2007a]. This indicates furher that the immune system can clear transgene expression from all transduced brain cells, including neurons.

9.3.4 Overcoming the Immune Response with High-Capacity Helper-Dependent adenoviruses

To overcome the immune challenges of first-generation adenoviral vectors, a new generation of adenoviral vectors, known as high-capacity helper-dependent adenoviruses (HC-Ads) were developed to evade detection the immune system. HC-Ad vectors are engineered to allow the insertion of up to 30 to 34 kb of transgenic sequences into the vector, but most important, the vector genomes do not encode any viral proteins. As a result, upon in vivo delivery, HC-Ad genomes do not produce any adenoviral proteins de novo that could be recognized as antigenic epitopes by the immune system (Fig. 9-2). A series of papers by Thomas et al. [2000, 2001a], Xiong et al. [2006], Barcia et al. [2007b], O'Neal et al. [2000], Mian et al. [2005], Parks et al. [1999], Maione et al. [2001], and others have now demonstrated that transgene expression from these viruses remained stable for up to one year. Further, Barcia and co-workers [2007b] recently demonstrated that HC-Ad-mediated transgene expression is sustained for up to one year, even in the presence of preexisting immune response against adenovirus (Fig. 9-2B). These data demonstrating prolonged transgene expression in the presence of systemic immune responses against adenovirus strongly suggest that HC-Ad vectors could be used in clinical trials to treat human patients that have been preexposed to adenovirus before being subjected to gene therapy, as would be the case in the vast majority of human patients undergoing experimental gene therapy using an adenoviral gene delivery system.

Before HC-Ad vectors infect their target cells in the brain, the viral capsid of these vectors could, in principle, be neutralized by anti-adenovirus antibodies either in the general circulation or in the brain extracellular space. However, data from Thomas et al. [2001b] and Barcia et al. [2007a] demonstrate that a preexisting immune response against adenovirus is insufficient to block vector transduction and resulting β-gal expression from either first-generation or HC-Ad vectors injected in the brain of immunized animals, as evidenced by transgene expression at early time points (i.e., 3 days post-injection). This indicates that circulating antibodies are unable to block transduction of brain cells. Further, Xiong and colleagues demonstrated that regulatable expression of β-gal was unaffected by a preexisting systemic anti-adenovirus immune response [Xiong et al. 2006].

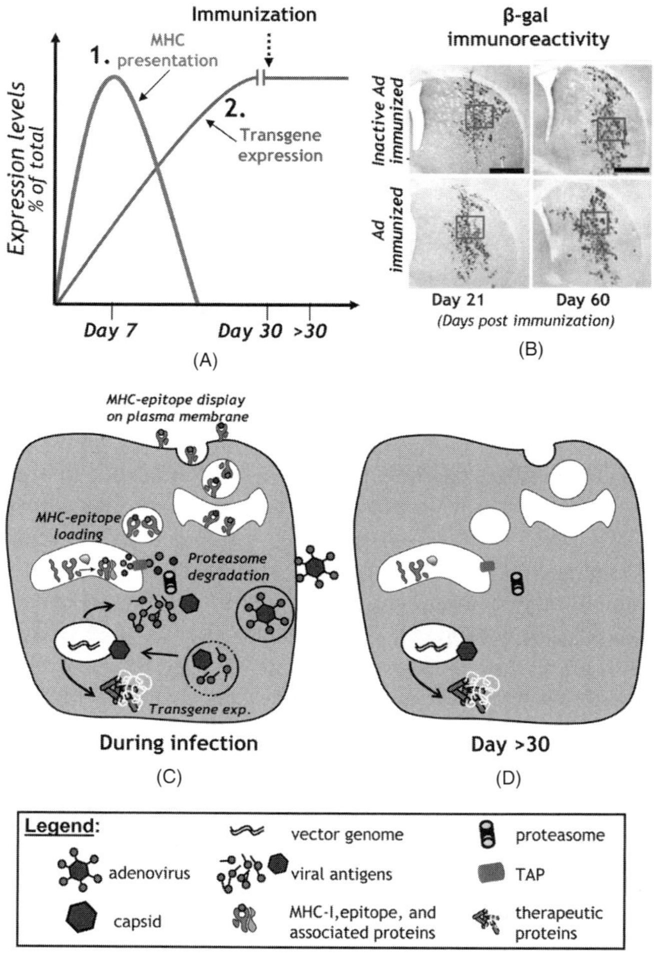

Figure 9-2 Antiadenoviral immune responses are incapable of eliminating transgene expression from HC-Ad vectors. (A) The levels of transgene expression and MHC presentation of viral epitopes in animals injected with an HC-Ad vector into the CNS are illustrated. MHC presentation of viral protein is short term because only capsid-derived epitopes can be presented during capsid degredation. Transgene expression in the brain is sustained even after systemic immunization against adenovirus. (B) Immunoreactivity for β-galactosidase illustrates the failure of a systemic immune response against adenovirus to eliminate transgene expression from HC-Ad vectors in the brain of rats immunized against adenovirus (top panels) or saline alone (bottom panels). Short-term (21 days post-immunization, left panels) and medium-long-term (60 days post-immunization, right panels) expression of β-gal are shown. Note the sustained expression of β-gal in both adenovirus-immunized animals and controls animals immunized with saline alone at 14 and 60 days immunization. (C) A schematic of HC-Ad vector infection, uncoating, nuclear transduction, production of transgene, and presentation of viral antigenic epitopes on MHC class I is shown after vector infection. (D) A schematic of the same cells more than 30 days later. Note the absence of expression of viral proteins from the HC-Ad vector and the lack of presentation of viral epitopes by MHC molecules on the cell surface.

Very recently, King et al. used a syngeneic intracranial model of glioma [Ali et al. 2005] to demonstrate that therapeutic gene expression of HSV1-thymidine kinase (TK) encoded from either first-generation or HC-Ad vectors injected into the brain was unaffected by a preexisting systemic anti-adenovirus immune response at 1 week following intracranial injection [King et al. 2008]. These data add further support to the conclusion that circulating anti-adenovirus immune responses fail to block transduction of both first-generation and HC-Ad vectors when injected carefully into the brain in small volumes. However, King demonstrated that only intratumoral treatment with HSV1-TK encoded from an HC-Ad vector was effective in eradicating intracranial glioma in the presence of a preexisting systemic anti-adenovirus immune response, while intratumoral TK therapy completely fails to improve survival when encoded on first-generation adenoviral vector. This indicates that even in the presence of a systemic immune response against adenoviral vectors, transduction, regulated transgene expression, and therapeutic efficacy of HC-Adv are maintained.

From the perspective of the adaptive arm of the immune system, T cells would have a very short period of time during which they can recognize cells that have been infected with HC-Ad vectors. Antigens derived from HC-Ad capsid proteins could be transiently presented on MHC class I molecules. However, such "input" proteins could only be provided by the disassembly of the vector originally injected, because the HC-Ad genome does not encode for any viral proteins. Once these input virion proteins from the viral capsid have been metabolized and turned over, the HC-Ad-vector-transduced cells effectively become invisible to the antiadenovirus-specific T cells. Once the genome of these viruses has reached the nucleus, HC-Ad-vector-transduced cells are completely impervious to the adaptive arm of the immune system (Fig. 9-2D). Therefore, further engineering of these vectors demonstrates that adenoviruses are indeed effective vehicles for long-term sustained therapeutic transgene expression in the brain. However, transgene-specific immune responses must also be taken into consideration and are described in the next section.

9.3.5 Administering Gene Therapy to Preimmunized Animals: A Clinically Relevant Paradigm

To mimic the preexisting antiadenovirus immunization status of human patients undergoing clinical trials using adenoviral vectors, Thomas et al. [2001b], Xiong et al. [2006], and Barcia et al. [2007b] performed experiments to assess the longevity of transgene expression in animals that had been preimmunized against adenovirus before intracranial delivery of adenoviral vectors. This clinically relevant paradigm was used to determine the effects of a preexisiting systemic antiadenoviral immune response on intracranial transgene expression in rats for up to 60 days post-intracranial delivery [Thomas et al. 2001b] and also in mice for up to one year after intracranial delivery [Barcia et al. 2007b] (Fig. 9-3A). In systemically immunized animals of both species, intracranial transgene expression mediated by first-generation adenoviral vectors was nearly abolished (mouse) or totally abolished (rats) within 60 days of vector delivery compared to control saline-immunized animals (Fig. 9-3B). As expected, HC-Ad sustained intracranial transgene expression in both rats and mice, even in the presence of an antiadenoviral immune response. High levels of HC-Ad-mediated transgene expression was detected in the brains of animals at the longest time point tested (i.e., 60 days in rats and 365 days in mice) (Fig. 9-3C). In fact, statistical analysis revealed that the levels of HC-Ad-mediated transgene expression were indistinguishable between mice immunized with adenovirus or saline alone for all points tested between 14 and 365 days [Barcia et al., 2007b]. These data further support implementing HC-Ad vectors in upcoming clinical trials for neurological disorders.

We also utilized the preimmunization paradigm to examine the effects of a systemic immune response against the vector-encoded transgene. To do so, Xiong and co-workers [2007] used a systemic administration of a mammalian expression plasmid containing the transgene lacZ to immunize naive mice. Animals then received an intracranial administration of an HC-Ad vector encoding β-gal. Animals were euthanized 7 weeks later and thee brains were analyzed for β-gal immunoreactivity (Fig. 9-3C). Quantitative stereology revealed a statistically significant decrease in β-gal immunoreactivity in animals preimmunized against β-gal compared to mice immunized with saline alone (Fig. 9-3D). These data and data from other groups [Molnar-Kimber et al. 1998; Favre et al. 2002; Lena et al. 2005; Di Domenico et al. 2006; Shi et al. 2006] suggest that transgene-specific immune responses must also be taken into consideration when planning and implementing a gene therapy clinical trial. Notably, Chenuaud and co-workers [2004] observed that systemic delivery of homologous erythropoietin (Epo) via an adeno-associated viral vector to nonhuman primates elicited circulating neutralizing antibodies against endogenous Epo. The resulting profound anemia that ensued was the first example of the development of an autoimmune disease in nonhuman primates following delivery of a viral vector. This indicates that even overexpression of endogenous proteins, or expression of endogenous proteins, from a novel transduced cell type can lead to immune responses. Whether the mechanisms that reduce transgene expression in the brain and peripheral organs are the same remains to be determined.

9.3.6 Immune Responses Against AAV and Lentiviral Vectors Injected into the Brain

Adeno-associated virus (AAV) is a small single-stranded DNA virus that was originally discovered as a contaminant in cell lines used to study adenovirus [Muzyczka and Berns 2001]. Similar to HC-Ad, all the viral encoding genes have been removed from the recombinant AAV (rAAV) and replaced with a transgene and transcriptional elements inserted between two ITRs [Muzyczka and Berns 2001]. Wild-type AAV has no known association with any known human disease and requires helper functions from adenovirus or other cytotoxic viruses in order to replicate and infect new host cells [Muzyczka and Berns

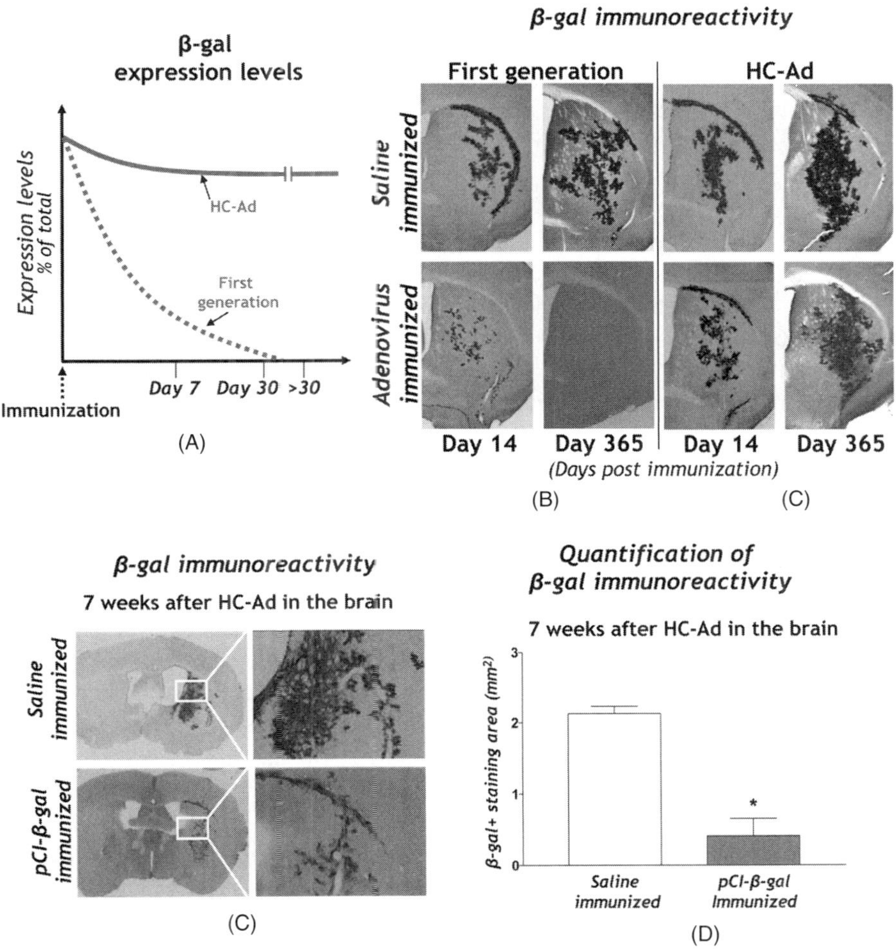

Figure 9-3 Comparison of preexisting responses against first-generation adenovirus, high-capacity adenovirus, and transgene. (A) The levels of intracranial transgene expression in the presence of a preexisting systemic antiadenovirus immune response are shown. Note the sharp reduction of transgene expression following intracranial delivery of first-generation adenovirus compared to HC-Ad transgene expression. (B) First-generation adenovirus and (C) HC-Ad-mediated transgene expression in the mouse brain are visualized by β-gal immunoreactivity at 21 days and one year post-intracranial vector delivery. Note the sustained expression of β-gal from both vectors in control immunized animals and the persistence of expression in animals injected with HC-Ad even at one year post-vector injection compared to the complete ablation of transgene expression in animals injected with first-generation adenoviral vectors. (C) β-gal immunoreactivity in the brain of animals preimmunized with saline (top panels) or with β-gal (bottom panels) is shown 7 weeks post-intracranial vector delivery. Right panels depict high-magnification images of immuoreactive area. (D) Quantitative stereology of β-gal immunocytochemistry reveals a statistically significant decrease in β-gal immunoreactivity in animals preimmunized with β-gal compared to animals immunized with saline alone.

2001]. Also, like Ad5, the majority of the human population has been exposed to the most common AAV serotype (AAV2), resulting in circulating preexisting neutralizing antibodies specific to AAV2 capsids [Blacklow et al. 1968, 1971; Chirmule et al. 1999; Erles et al. 1999]. Immune responses to rAAV2 have been reported following systemic administration to the periphery [Zaiss and Muruve 2005; Mingozzi et al. 2007a,b].

rAAV has been used extensively in the brain [Mandel et al. 2006] and is currently in several clinical trials for neurological disorders [Mandel and Burger 2004; Kaplitt et al. 2007]. Due to the immune compartmentalization of the brain and lack of an adaptive immune response as discussed above [Matyszak and Perry 1996; Stevenson et al. 1997b; Cartmell et al. 1999; Lowenstein 2002a], administration of rAAV into the brain parenchyma has been thought to result in minimal immune responses, especially when injected only once in the striatum of naive animals [Mandel et al. 1998; Lo et al. 1999; Mastakov et al. 2002; Peden et al. 2004].

As with both first-generation adenovirus and HC-Ad vectors, transient, innate inflammatory responses to highly purified rAAV also occur when higher doses are administered into the naive brain parenchyma [Reimsnider et al. 2007]. The discrepancy regarding the innate inflammatory responses between earlier reports from our lab [Mandel et al. 1998] and our recent data [Reimsnider et al. 2007] is most likely due to the increased amount of rAAV injected. While a formal study of the dose-dependant innate immune response to rAAV has yet to be performed, there was little or no detectable innate immune response when injecting lower titers of rAAV2 vectors (2×10^8 particles [Mandel et al. 1998], 4×10^8 particles [Peden et al. 2004]) 4 weeks after postintracranial delivery. However, when injecting higher titers rAAV2 vectors ($\approx 4 \times 10^{10}$ particles) [Reimsnider et al. 2007], a significant transient $GFAP^+$ (glial fibrillary acidic protein) astrogliosis was observed. Thus, the observation of an increased striatal inflammatory response to increasing titers of rAAV2 could be considered similar to the observation that intrastriatal injections of increasing titers of adenoviral vectors also leads to an innate immune response once a threshold adenovirus titer is reached [Thomas et al. 2001a].

In addition to single injections of rAAV2 into naive rats, readministration of rAAV2 vectors in the opposite hemisphere either 2 or 4 weeks apart induces a significantly greater inflammatory response in the second injection site [Mastakov et al. 2002; Peden et al. 2004] (Fig. 9-4A). Mastakov and colleagues [2002] also reported reduced expression of the rAAV2-mediated luciferase transgene in the second injection site, whereas Peden et al. [2004] did not observe reduced transgene expression when using human glial cell line–derived neurotrophic factor (GDNF) as the transgene. However, we have subsequently replicated the loss of rAAV2-mediated transgene expression in the second injection site when using GFP as the transgene [Peden and Mandel, unpublished observations].

Upon first consideration, the absence of viral genes encoding viral proteins, the lack of in situ expression of viral proteins after rAAV transduction makes the immune response following readministration rAAV in the brain difficult to

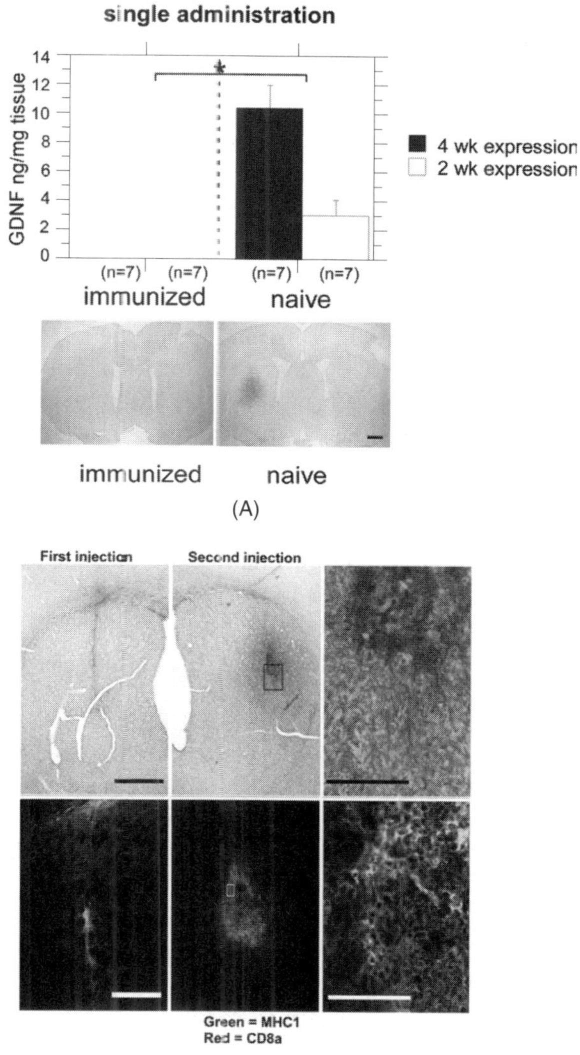

Figure 9-4 Preexisting responses against AAV vectors. (A) Intrastriatal GDNF expression as determined by ELISA (top panels) and immunohistochemistry (bottom panels). Immunization with wtAAV2 completely blocked GDNF expression at both the 2- and 4-week time points following rAAV2-GDNF striatal transduction as evidenced in the striatum by both ELISA and ICC compared to naive animals. Injection of rAAV2 in the right striatum completely blocked GDNF expression when AAV2-GDNF was readministered in the left striatum (bottom left panel). The bottom right panel shows a representative section from a naive animal 4 weeks after rAAV2-GDNF injection in the right striatum, with no further treatment. (B) Striatal sections were immunostained with for MHC class I and CD8α in animals injected with rAAV. Note the increase of CD8α immunoreactivity in the brains of animals that received a second injection (middle panel) compared to animals receiving only a single injection (left panel). The right panel is a higher-magnification image of the middle panel.

explain. However, rAAV2 vectors have been reported to uncoat slowly, thus potentially allowing processed capsid peptides to be presented via MHC class I to specific antiviral T cells for prolonged periods of time compared to adenoviral vectors [Lowenstein 2004; Thomas et al. 2004; Herzog 2007]. Increased MHC class I expression observed in the second injection site after intrastriatal delivery of rAAV2 vectors supports the hypothesis that extended presentation of AAV2 capsid peptides mediates an increased inflammatory response in the second injection site [Peden et al. 2004] (Fig. 9-4B). Another possibility is a transgene-specific inflammatory response. However, when rAAV5 expressing GFP, a different serotype but identical transgene, is readministered in the second injection site, no enhanced inflammation or reduction of rAAV-transduced GFP^+ neurons was observed [Reimsnider, Manfredsson, and Mandel, unpublished observations]. Furthermore, Mastakov et al. [2002] reported that following readministration of rAAV2 three months after the first intrastriatal injection, after the conclusion of capsid peptide presentation, AAV-mediated transgene expression was unaffected. We have also recently replicated the phenomenon that a longer delay between rAAV2 administrations allows high levels of transgene expression following readministration of the vector [Reimsnider, Manfredsson, and Mandel, unpublished observations]. Finally, we have shown that acute readministration of rAAV5 vectors, which uncoat more rapidly than rAAV2 capsids, does not result in increased inflammation or transgene reduction at the second injection site.

All of the foregoing experiments were carried out in animals that were not preimmunized against AAV, as wtAAV does not ordinarily infect rodents. However, it is important to study any potential immune response against delivery of rAAV into the brains of preimmunized animals because a significant portion of the human population has been exposed to AAV [Blacklow et al. 1968, 1971; Chirmule et al. 1999; Erles et al. 1999]. Thus, two studies demonstrated that intrastriatal rAAV2-mediated transduction was blocked completely by systemic preimmunization against wtAAV2 [Peden et al. 2004] or against rAAV2 [Sanftner et al. 2004]. In both studies, high levels of circulating specific anti-AAV2-neutralizing antibodies were observed, as transduction with rAAV5 was unaffected [Peden et al. 2004]. Unlike with neutralizing antibodies against adenovirus, these studies clearly established that circulating neutralizing antibodies could block transduction of rAAV in the brain. Any potential role of T cells in the these responses, however, needs to be formally excluded.

Moreover, when Peden and co-workers [2004] readministered rAAV2 to preimmunized rats, an enhanced greater immune response was seen at the second injection site than at the second injection site in nonimmunized rats. These data suggest that the adaptive arm of the immune system be primed by intracranial administration of rAAV2. This consideration is especially important because Mingozzi and co-workers [2007b] have demonstrated that memory T-cell responses to AAV1, AAV2, and AAV8 are present in healthy individuals. Moreover, as mentioned above, it has been proposed that dendritic cells may enter the brain in response to parencyhmal inflammation and present antigen to naive T cells [McMahon et al. 2005]. Therefore, although the naive brain is relatively immunoprivileged, especially with regard to its incapacity to prime T cells, $CD8^+$ T cells can be found in the brain in preimmunized animals inoculated with intrastriatal rAAV2 [Peden et al. 2004]. Thus, utilizing careful in vitro assays to detect preexisting $CD8^+$ T-cell responses to AAV capsid proteins such as those described by Mingozzi et al. [2007a] prior to rAAV administration might be useful in rAAV clinical trials for neurological disorders. This may be especially important when using AAV2 vectors. Because of their smaller size they may be able to diffuse out of the brain, even following careful delivery into the brain parenchyma; this does not occur following the injection of the larger adenoviral vectors.

In a recent phase I clinical trial for Parkinson's disease using a 50-μL injection of AAV2 vector expressing glutamic acid decarboxlyase into the subthalamic nucleus (total of 5×10^{10} vector genomes), there was no change in the levels of preexisting anti-AAV2 circulating antibodies and/or neutralizing at any of the time points tested following treatment (1, 3, 6, and 12 months) compared to baseline levels. The work published by Kaplitt and co-workers [2007] suggests that careful administration of small volumes of AAV2 into the brain did not induce a measurable systemic antibody immune response against AAV2. Moreover, neutralizing antibodies against the therapeutic protein were not detected for up to one year following administration of the viral vector. The existence of T-cell responses, much more difficult to detect, but potentially more deleterious remain to be explored in gene therapy brain clinical trials. In a clinical trial for Canavan disease using 900 μL of AAV2 expressing aspartocylase (ASPA) split among six injection sites (total of 4.5×10^{12} vector genomes), investigators found low to moderately high levels of neutralizing antibodies to AAV2 in 3 out of 10 patients compared to pre–gene therapy levels [McPhee et al. 2006]. The differences in the neutralizing antibody responses between these two clinical trials could be attributed to differences in vector dose, intracerebral injection volumes, anatomical site of injection, and the underlying brain pathology. These issues remain to be monitored in future ongoing studies.

As Xiong and co-workers demonstrated with in vivo gene transfer using adenoviral vectors, the group of Herzog et al. demonstrated an immune response specific against transgenes encoded in an AAV vector. Using an AAV2 vector expressing ovalbumin (OVA), Wang et al. [2005] showed that OVA-specific helper $CD4^+$ T cells had been activated in the draining lymph nodes within 10 days of systemic AAV administration. Cytotoxic $CD8^+$ T cells then destroyed OVA-expressing muscle fibers, a response that was not prevented using a muscle-specific promoter. This study demonstrates that expression of a secreted protein transferred by AAV2 vectors is eliminated by a local, transgene-specific immune response.

Interestingly, Herzog's group also demonstrated the regulatory T-cell (Treg)–mediated induction of immune tolerance to the transgene product delivered by AAV vectors; in this case, coagulation factor IX [Dobrzynski et al. 2006]. In a recent continuation of their studies, Herzog's group provided the first definitive evidence of transgene product–specific Tregs ($CD4^+$ $CD25^+$) following in vivo delivery of an AAV vector. Cao and colleagues [2007] used adoptive transfer and in vivo depletion studies to show that transgene product–specific Tregs were observed as early as 2 weeks following gene transfer and effectively suppress antibody formation to FIX. These data indicate that Tregs are required for transgene product–specific induction of tolerance following systemic AAV-mediated gene transfer.

In summary, in contrast to adenovirus, there have been few studies of the adaptive immune response after rAAV administration in the brain. However, the studies that exist indicate that there can be rAAV-induced immune reactions, especially when using high-titer viruses [Reimsnider et al. 2007]. The existence of a dose threshold above which inflammation is caused indicates the need to monitor the dose and purity of the vector carefully to keep within safe, nontoxic parameters. Thus, it is clear that more careful analysis of rAAV-mediated immune responses in the brain, similar to the studies that have been carried out with adenovirus, should be undertaken.

9.3.7 Immune Responses Against Lentiviral Vectors in the Brain

Lentivirus is a subclass of the retrovirus family of viruses comprizing single-stranded RNA viruses. Unlike adenovirus and adeno-associated virus, lentivirus integrates its genome into the genome of the host cell. When transgenes are embedded in lentiviral vectors, vector integration establishes a permanent presence of the transgene in the host cell genome. Unlike their retrovirus cousins, lentiviral vectors also have the added advantage of the ability to infect nondividing cells, which makes them an attractive candidate for gene therapy for targets in the nervous system. Another major advantage of lentivial vectors is the almost complete removal of all viral encoding genes from the vector. As with the HC-Ad vector system, the "gutted" configuration of the lentiviral vector limits the host immune response due to the absence of in situ expression of viral proteins [Breckpot et al. 2007].

Relatively few studies characterizing the immune response against lentiviral vectors have been carried out. In 2005, Abordo-Adesida et al. published a study detailing the effects of both systemic anti-lentiviral and anti-transgene immune responses of transgene expression in the brain. To do so, a lentoviral vector expressing GFP was injected intracranially, followed by systemic immunization with either the same vector or with a lentiviral vector expressing an unrelated transgene (factor IX). Interestingly, the levels of intracranial transgene expression were affected only in animals receiving a systemic immunization with the identical vector, while transgene expression was sustained in animals immunized with the lentiviral vector expressing an unrelated transgene. These data indicate that systemic immunization with viral epitopes alone is insufficient to induce an immune response capable of eliminating lentiviral vector–mediated transgene expression in the brain. These data also underscore the potential immunogenicity of transgenes encoded within viral vectors as demonstrated by [Xiong et al.

2007] and discussed above. Recently, the group of Luigi Naldini demonstrated that systemic immunization with a lentiviral vector induces rapid and transient up-regulation of the cytokine IFN-αβ in both the liver and the spleen. Brown et al. [2007] postulate that innate immune response involving IFN-αβ inhibits the transduction capacity of the lentiviral vector in liver cells and contributes to the clearance of transduced cells. The IFN-αβ response did not occur when animals were injected with noninfectious lentiviral particles, suggesting that the vector-mediated activation of the innate immune is dependent on viral entry into the host cell. Whether this phenomenon occurs in lentiviral treatments of the brain remains to be evaluated.

9.4 CAUSES OF THE LOSS OF TRANSGENE EXPRESSION

Although the case has clearly been made that the adaptive immune response is able to eliminate transgene expression from the brain, the mechanisms by which transgene expression are eliminated is not yet fully understood. Moreover, the consequences or "fate" of the cell infected by the viral vector has yet to be elucidated. In theory, two main possibilities could account for the loss of transgene expression. On the one hand, through the secretion of effector molecules such as IFN-γ, T cells could selectively turn off or silence transgene expression from transduced cells of the CNS while maintaining the presence of the vector genome [Guidotti and Chisari 2001]. Alternatively, T cells could be able to eliminate transgene expression by killing transduced cells by cytotoxic pathways. The consequences of the particular mechanism of clearance of virally transfused cells are of paramount important. If T cells are able to silence expression from the viral genome, no anatomical damage is being done. Moreover, it could be possible to restart transgene expression from the quiescent vector genome. However, if cytotoxic T cells eliminate transgene expression by killing transduced cells, the consequences to gene therapy clinical trials would be more severe. So far, work done in various laboratories has been inconclusive on this issue.

Discovering if the immune system can kill transduced brain cells directly in vivo has been difficult to determine beyond a reasonable doubt. If CTLs could kill brain cells, these would need to express MHC class I. Although emphasis has been placed on determining whether astrocytes and neurons express MHC class I, it is unknown whether the full complement of the intracellular machinery necessary to load antigenic peptides onto MHC class I is present. Strong evidence that neuronal MHC class I can actually bind the TCR of CTLs remains to be uncovered. It is also highly likely that the ability of the immune system to eliminate brain cells will depend on the antigens presented by the brain APCs, which virus they are derived from, and the nature of the immune response that was stimulated to detect infected cells in the brain. Dissecting these issues is part of important ongoing investigations by several laboratories. Of course, indirect killing of mechanisms would not necessitate that neurons express MHC class I.

Some limitations in detecting brain cell death relate to the number of infected cells in target brain areas. Because the number of transduced cells is low (i.e., generally below 5% for the total number of brain cells in any particular brain region), loss of such a relatively small percentage of brain cells can be very difficult to detect, much less quantify experimentally. Moreover, dead brain cells are quickly phagocytosed by local microglial cells (and possibly incoming macrophages), thereby keeping brain inflammation at a reasonable minimum.

For the long-term success of clinically effective and safe neurological gene therapy, the ultimate outcomes of the elimination of transgene expression are of crucial importance. If the immune system uses inhibitory transcriptional mechanisms simply to turn off transgene expression, no permanent anatomical damage will ensue. However, if the immune system kills transduced cells, the underlying disease could worsen as transduced cells are eliminated. Therefore, the detailed mechanisms by which the immune system abolishes transgene expression from transduced brain cells need to be determined in order to develop alternative ways to escape, manipulate, or hide from the immune system.

A potential solution would be short-term immunosuppression while the viral capsid epitopes are displayed on MHC class I during vector uncoating [Herzog et al. 2001; Lowenstein 2005; Mingozzi et al. 2007b]. As discussed above (Figs. 9-1 and 9-2), the duration of viral capsid antigen presentation on MHC class I, and consequent necessary immunosuppression, would be determined by the half-life of the viral capsid proteins (i.e., first-generation adenoviruses, HC-Ads or AAV vectors). Interestingly, despite their long uncoating process, AAV2 vectors fail to stimulate the systemic anti-AAV2 immune response when administered into the brain in small doses (50 μL) [Kaplitt et al. 2007], yet when 900 μL was delivered, increased levels of neutralizing antibodies to AAV2 were observed in 3 out of 10 patients compared to pre–gene therapy levels [McPhee et al. 2006]. Whether this immune response was caused by the increased vector titer or increased volume of injection, or was due to the underlying neuropathology, remains to be determined. These data suggest, nevertheless, that an immune suppression regime could potentially be applicable during the period of vector uncoating in clinical indications for which large-volume doses of AAV2 vector are required to be therapeutically effective.

9.5 THE CELLULAR SUBSTRATE OF BRAIN IMMUNE RESPONSES: IMMUNOLOGICAL SYNAPSES

Recent advances in microscopy and molecular methods now allow us to study the interactions between T cells and their targets at the single-cell level. Thus, in addition to analysis of the function of large populations of immune cells studied using methods such as CTL and ELISPOT assays, the biology of immune responses can now be studied at the level of single-cell interactions in vivo. Over the last 10 years, stereotyped structural rearrangements of proteins at the interfaces of interacting immune cells have been observed. These areas of contact between T cells and various types of antigen-presenting cells have been described as immunological synapses and consist of a reorganization of membrane proteins [i.e., intercellular adhesion molecules (e.g., ICAM-1), TCR, intracellular

TCR-induced signaling tyrosine kinase cascades as well as cytoskeletal structures, and intracellular organelles of the secretory pathway of T cells] [Monks et al. 1998; Grakoui et al. 1999; Dustin and Cooper 2000; Lee et al. 2002; Huppa and Davis 2003; Friedl et al. 2005; Huse et al. 2006; Cemerski et al. 2007]. Immunological synapses are thought to facilitate the intracellular communication between T cells and APCs.

Mature immunological synapses consist of a characteristic peripheral supramolecular activation cluster (pSMAC) consisting of a ring of adhesion molecules that anchor the membrane of the T cell to the membrane of the APC, surrounding a central SMAC (cSMAC), consisting of a higher concentration of TCR and signaling molecules. Immunological synapses have been described for both $CD4^+$ and $CD8^+$ T cells and NK cells in contact with various types of APCs (e.g., dendritic cells, B cells, or target cells). Most studies on immunological synapses have studied the interactions between T and APCs in vitro, or the interaction of T cells with artificial bilayer membranes.

The particular arrangement of proteins at the immunological synapses depends on the nature of the cells engaged in the contact. Recently, the first existence of in vivo mature immunological synapses between a virally infected astrocyte and a $CD8^+$ CTL was described in the rat brain during an immune-mediated elimination of transgene expression in the brain. Barcia and co-workers [2006, 2007] found that anti-adenoviral $CD8^+$ T cells infiltrate the brain and form Kupfer-type mature immunological synapses with astrocytes that express MHC class I. Immunological synapses in vivo displayed the typical organizational hallmarks of immunological synapses originally described by the group of Abraham Kupfer (i.e., segregation of TCR and LFA-1 into c-SMAc and p-SMAC, respectively) (Fig. 9-5).

Our experimental model to characterize the cellular and molecular biology of adaptive immune responses against a nonreplicating adenoviral gene therapy vector consists of several unique characteristics that facilitated the first-ever in vivo evidence of immunological synapses. A first-generation adenoviral vector was used to target astrocytes in the rat brain. This virus is replication defective and thus unable to kill infected cells directly. As described above, a parenchymal CNS infection with adenoviral vectors below the immunological threshold does not induce significant inflammation nor a systemic anti-adenoviral immune response. Animals were immunized systemically with a different adenoviral vector injected subcutaneously. Systemic anti-adenoviral immunization triggered a systemic antiadenoviral immune response, leading to brain infiltration of antiviral T cells and brain inflammation. Brain inflammation consisted mainly of CD8 T cells and macrophages that homed into the area occupied by infected astrocytes and a perivascular infiltration of $CD4^+$T cells.

As would be expected if the lymphocytes were killing infected brain cells, the systemic anti-adenoviral immune response resulted in a significant reduction in the number of brain astrocytes transduced and a reduction in the number of viral genome copy numbers present in the CNS. The presence of $CD8^+$T cells within the brain parenchyma suggested the operation of direct cytotoxicity,

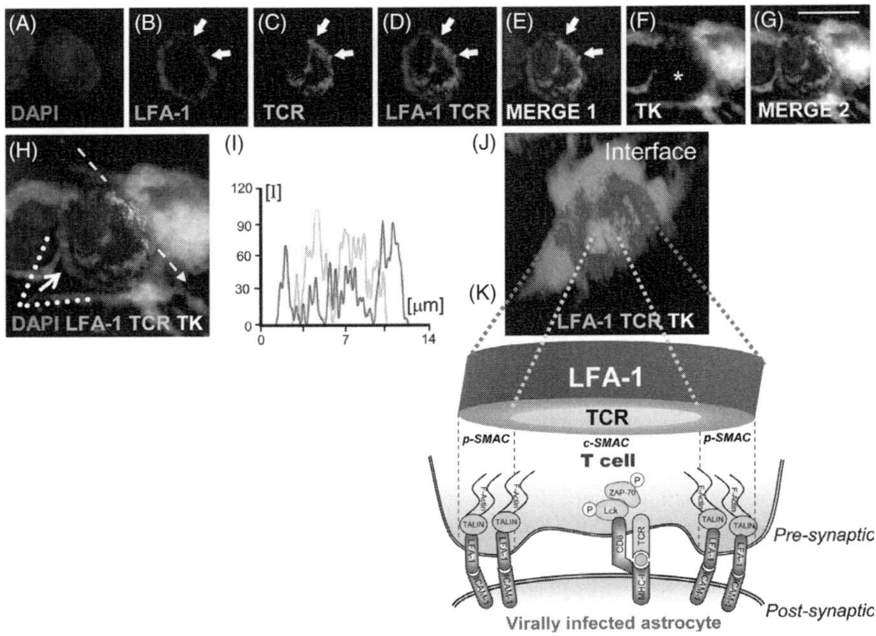

Figure 9-5 SMAC formation at immunological synapses in vivo between T cells and infected astrocytes in the brain. Upper panels (A–F) illustrate confocal images of: DAPI, LFA-1, TCR, and the virally infected cell (TK; in white). Scale bars = 15 µm. The asterisk in image F indicates the location of the T cell. Low (G) and high (H) magnifications of the synapse are illustrated. Three-dimensional reconstructed image J illustrates the characteristic structure of the p-SMAC (outer LFA-1 ring) and c-SMAC (inner TCR cluster) of the immunological synapse. Image J was rotated so that the plane of the interface of the immunological synapse (dashed arrow in **H**) could be observed from above (the white arrow in H shows the angle of vision of the three-dimensional reconstruction in J). Panel I illustrates the intensity of fluorescence measured at the interface (line in H) of the immunological synapse. The graph shows the relative intensity values of fluorescence of LFA-1 and TCR, showing the expected distribution, with more intense LFA-1 staining toward the outside p-SMAC and stronger TCR in the c-SMAC. (K) Diagrammatic view of a T cell contacting an infected astrocyte, illustrating the localization of molecules involved in the immunological synapse, as well as polarized phosphorylated tyrosine kinases. LFA-1 transduces signals to the cytoskeleton through talin, and binds to ICAM-1 on the target cells.

although no direct evidence for apoptotic astrocytes was obtained. Nevertheless, macrophages containing remains of infected astrocytes were found, indicating that infected cells had been cleared by brain monocyte–derived cells.

We thus proposed that immunological synapses represent the microanatomical substrate underlying $CD8^{+}$T-cell effector functions in the brain, and mediate the clearing of infected astrocytes by $CD8^{+}$T cells. The in vivo description of immunological synapses in the context of an antiviral immune response highlights their physiological role as the structure underlying neuroimmune interactions in vivo. These data further demonstrate that $CD8^+$ T cells are able to interact directly with, and eliminate, infected astrocytes. If we consider immunological synapses as the substrate of T-cell interactions with target APCs in vivo, we can then use them to help us to dissect whether effector mechanisms are exerted through direct or indirect interactions. For example, the visualization of $CD8^+$ T cells interacting directly with target astrocytes argues for a direct cytotoxic mechanism underlying the elimination of infected astrocytes; however, if we would only be able to visualize $CD8^+$ T cells interacting with macrophages, we would have to postulate an indirect mechanism to account for the clearing of virally infected astrocytes. Study of the in vivo cell biology of effector immune mechanisms in the brain will allow us to dissect the detailed cellular pathways through which the immune system achieves its functions in vivo, in the context of antiviral, antitumor, and autoimmune interactions in the brain.

9.6 THE FUTURE OF NEUROIMMUNOLOGY

Intercellular interactions between $CD8^+$ T cells and resident cells of the CNS are highly sophisticated, yet our understanding of how these complex in vivo interactions lead to either viral clearing from the brain or brain cell death, and how these processes are regulated, is only now emerging. The difficulties of studying neuroimmune interactions include the complex brain neuroanatomy, large numbers of brain cell types and their interactions, and the challenges in understanding how brain-infiltrating immune cells communicate with resident brain cells to exert their functions. The complex interactions between the various brain cell types in vivo limit the relevance of results obtained from in vitro primary cells co-cultured with lymphocytes and often fail to predict results from in vivo experiments. The recent development of three-dimensional cell culture scaffolding technology has the potential to enhance the utility of in vitro experiments, but currently there is no substitute for an animal model. Although applied to other areas of immunology, in vitro three-dimensional cell cultures have not yet been applied to neuroimmunology paradigms. In many cases, lymphocyte function differs in vitro from in vivo (i.e., T cells being able to kill neurons in vitro but not in vivo) in certain experimental paradigms.

Determining the outcome of direct neuroimmune interactions has also proved challenging, as until very recently it has been impossible to observe the interaction between an immune cell and its target in the CNS in real time. For instance, the mode of $CD8^+$T-cell function and the outcome of its interaction with target APCs in the CNS has been determined largely via surrogate indicators such as loss of transgene expression, loss of viral genomes, demyelination, or tissue atrophy. The direct outcome of the specific interactions between T cells and target brain cells remains unsolved and will benefit from the application of in vivo imaging technologies. For example, T cells clear viral infections from the CNS. How they do so, however, has been difficult to determine.

How lymphocytes clear viral infections from the brain depends on many factors, including the type of virus or viral vector, the viral life cyle, the type of brain cell infected, the anatomical region of the infected cells, and the level of T-cell activation as well as the age and gender of the host. To understand how T cells clear brain viral infections is essential not just for gene therapy but to understand immunity to natural viral infections of the brain, such as HIV, CMV, HSV-1, and others.

9.7 DETERMINING BRAIN CELL DEATH IN VIVO: CYTOTOXIC VERSUS NONCYTOTOXIC MECHANISMS IN THE LOSS OF TRANSGENE EXPRESSION

Whether the elimination of transgene expression from the brain of immunized animals is accomplished via cytolytic or noncytolytic mechanisms remains to be determined. Direct contact or even proximity of class I expressing cells and $CD8^{+}$T cells in situ has been demonstrated only in isolated reports. However, how significant such contacts are is currently unclear. It has also been proposed that T cells can eliminate viruses through noncytolytic mechanisms, referred to as curative. However, the notion of curative rather than cytolytic virus clearance should be regarded critically, as demonstration of apoptotic or dead CNS resident cells in situ is technically challenging, especially if the infected cell numbers are sparse. Therefore, until we can observe and follow the process of T-cell clearing of virally infections in vivo, we will be unable to separate causal from contingent interactions.

Whether cell death occurs in vivo is crucial for understanding the consequences of immune-mediated responses to brain cells transduced by viral vectors. In vitro cell-killing studies have been used to determine the capacity of T cells to kill brain cells; however, these studies remove T cells from the brain and expose them to artificial target cells in vitro to demonstrate the capacity of T cells to kill preselected target cells ex vivo. Even if they are exposed to cultures of primary brain cells, such primary cells are not representative of adult mature brain cells. The application of in vivo killing assays using CFSE-labeled target cells to CNS tissue has not yet been achieved. While in vitro cell killing assays come closer to demonstrating the cytotoxic potential of T cells in vivo, whether T cells can directly kill brain target cells in situ remains to be explored further. The development of novel methods will probably need to examine the direct capacity of T cells to kill target APCs within the brain.

Novel microanatomical imaging techniques will probably facilitate discovery of the answers to these questions. Using two-photon microscopy should allow real-time examination of the complex in vivo interactions of T cells with target brain cells at the individual cellular level, allowing new perspectives on T-cell function in the CNS. Two-photon microscopy, and potentially fiber-optic fluorescence imaging [Mehta et al. 2004; Flusberg et al. 2005], along with further studies of the function of in vivo immunological synapses, could usher in complete descriptions of T-cell function in the brain in vivo during the clearing of viral infections, immunopathology in response to brain infection, or autoimmune attack. Furthermore, a novel system developed by the group of Tony Wyss-Coray utilizing SMAD binding elements–luciferase reporter transgenic mice to detect in vivo neurotoxicity could also contribute to the elucidation of the consequence of T-cell attack on virally infected astrocytes [Lin et al. 2005; Luo et al. 2006; Tesseur et al. 2006].

9.8 CONCLUSIONS

The deleterious impact of immune responses following delivery of viral vectors to the CNS has been documented by our group and others. T-cell responses have been implicated in the clearance of vector-mediated transgene expression in the brain. Evidence in both rats and mice strongly suggest that T cells can actually physically eliminate vector-transduced brain cells through effector mechanisms that are likely to include IFN-γ and cytotoxic granule release. The difficultly in comparing immune responses to gene therapy vectors in the brain across species and the variations in overall magnitude of the immune responses over time in different species and strains make definitive predictions on the implications of this work for human clinical trials elusive.

Animal models of preexisting immunity are unlikely to accurately reflect the strength of the immune response in humans, who may have been exposed to wild-type virus sometime during their lifetime before being treated with a gene therapy vector. However, should these data be correct (i.e., the immune system can kill infected brain cells), the logical conclusions would be to avoid the use of viral vectors in clinical gene therapy trials. The mechanisms of immune-mediated clearance of virally infected brain cells are likely to be virus-specific, and thus these phenomena should be examined for all types of viral vectors. Serious immune-adverse events in humans support this proposal [Manno et al. 2006].

Fortunately for the field of gene therapy, there are various options. Carefully crafted inclusion–exclusion criteria in clinical trials should be used to ensure that clinical trials are performed in humans never exposed to adenovirus during their lifetime or those in whom evidence of previous exposure cannot be detected. However, this would severely reduce the number of patients enrolled in protocols, and the detection of preexisting cellular immunity, as opposed to the humoral response, is difficult. This solution will not protect from exposure to wild-type virus and/or therapeutic vectors during the course of therapeutic treatment and the resulting immune response that may ensue. However, for some applications, such as gene therapy of brain tumors, short-term application could be sufficient to achieve therapeutic benefits; also, an immune response against tumor cells infected with viral vectors could be therapeutically beneficial.

The work described above regarding the existence of immunological thresholds in the dose of vector needed to cause inflammation indicates that a lower dose could avoid serious adverse events in the clinic. Clinical data suggest that similar thresholds exist potentially in patients, as evidenced by the lack of induction of a systemic antivector immune response upon intracranial delivery of

5×10^{10} vector genomes of AAV vector, whereas delivery of 5×10^{12} vector genomes of AAV vector resulted in a systemic anti-AAV response in 3 out of 10 patients [McPhee et al. 2006]. The drawback of this approach would be the decrease in the vector dose used to levels below those required to be therapeutically efficacious. The existence of dose-limiting toxicities highlights the need to develop stronger promoters to maximize therapeutic gene expression at lower vector doses. Immunosuppression should also be considered strongly for use during the clinical treatment regime, or at least during the time between vector administration and vector uncoating (Figs. 9-1 and 9-2). Modifications such as PEGylation of the viral vector capsids have also been employed to avoid elimination of vectors by circulating neutralizing antibodies prior to transduction with first-generation and high-capacity adenoviral vectors, AAV vectors, and lentoviral vectors [Croyle et al. 2002, 2004, 2005; Le et al. 2005]. Finally, yet importantly, the development of novel viral vectors with the ability to avoid priming a vector-specific immune response needs to be pursued and refined continually. The configuration of HC-Ad vectors eliminates the in situ expression of antigenic viral epitopes, allowing them to remain effectively invisible to the immune system once all input virions have been uncoated and their constituent proteins catabolized. Thus, a new generation of vectors devoid of viral protein coding sequences, such as AAV, retro-, and lentiviral vectors and the HC-Ad and HSV amplicon vectors, which in addition to lack of viral protein expression makes it possible to carry very large transgenic sequences, probably represent a major step toward the implementation of gene therapy for neurological diseases. These novel vectors will be especially important for therapeutic approaches that require stable, long-term, sustained expression of one or more therapeutic transgenes.

REFERENCES

Abordo-Adesida E, Follenzi A, et al. 2005. Stability of lentiviral vector–mediated transgene expression in the brain in the presence of systemic antivector immune responses. *Hum Gene Ther* 16:741–751.

Ali S, King GD, et al. 2005. Combined immunostimulation and conditional cytotoxic gene therapy provide long-term survival in a large glioma model. *Cancer Res* 65:7194–7204.

Appleby CE, Kingston PA, et al. 2003. A novel combination of promoter and enhancers increases transgene expression in vascular smooth muscle cells in vitro and coronary arteries in vivo after adenovirus-mediated gene transfer. *Gene Ther* 10:1616–1622.

Barcia C, Thomas CE, et al. 2006. In vivo mature immunological synapses forming SMACs mediate clearance of virally infected astrocytes from the brain. *J Exp Med* 203:2095–2107.

Barcia C, Gerdes C, et al. 2007a. Immunological thresholds in neurological gene therapy: highly efficient elimination of transduced cells may be related to the specific formation of immunological synapses between T cells and virus-infected brain cells. *Neuron Glial Biol* 2:309–327.

Barcia C, Jimenez-Dalmaroni M, et al. 2007b. One-year expression from high-capacity adenoviral vectors in the brains of animals with pre-existing anti-adenoviral immunity: clinical implications. *Mol Ther* 15(12):2154–2163.

Bechmann I, Galea I, et al. 2007. What is the blood–brain barrier (not)? *Trends Immunol* 28:5–11.

Benihoud K, Saggio I, et al. 1998. Efficient, repeated adenovirus-mediated gene transfer in mice lacking both tumor necrosis factor alpha and lymphotoxin alpha. *J Virol* 72:9514–9525.

Blacklow NR, Hoggan MD, et al. 1968. Serologic evidence for human infection with adenovirus-associated viruses. *J Natl Cancer Inst* 40:319–327.

Blacklow NR, Hoggan MD, et al. 1971. A seroepidemiologic study of adenovirus-associated virus infection in infants and children. *Am J Epidemiol* 94:359–366.

Breckpot K, Aerts JL, et al. 2007. Lentiviral vectors for cancer immunotherapy: transforming infectious particles into therapeutics. *Gene Ther* 14:847–862.

Brown BD, Sitia G, et al. 2007. In vivo administration of lentiviral vectors triggers a type I interferon response that restricts hepatocyte gene transfer and promotes vector clearance. *Blood* 109:2797–2805.

Cao O, Dobrzynski E, et al. 2007. Induction and role of regulatory $CD4^+CD25^+$ T cells in tolerance to the transgene product following hepatic in vivo gene transfer. *Blood* 110:1132–1140.

Cartmell T, Southgate T, et al. 1999. Interleukin-1 mediates a rapid inflammatory response after injection of adenoviral vectors into the brain. *J Neurosci* 19:1517–1523.

Caux C, Ait-Yahia S, et al. 2000. Dendritic cell biology and regulation of dendritic cell trafficking by chemokines. *Springer Semin Immunopathol* 22:345–369.

Cemerski S, Das J, et al. 2007. The stimulatory potency of T cell antigens is influenced by the formation of the immunological synapse. *Immunity* 26:345–355.

Chenuaud P, Larcher T, et al. 2004. Autoimmune anemia in macaques following erythropoietin gene therapy. *Blood* 103:3303–3304.

Chiocca EA, Abbed KM, et al. 2004. A phase I open-label, dose-escalation, multi-institutional trial of injection with an E1B-attenuated adenovirus, ONYX-015, into the peritumoral region of recurrent malignant gliomas, in the adjuvant setting. *Mol Ther* 10:958–966.

Chirmule N, Propert K, et al. 1999. Immune responses to adenovirus and adeno-associated virus in humans. *Gene Ther* 6:1574–1583.

Cotten M, Baker A, et al. 1994. Lipopolysaccharide is a frequent contaminant of plasmid DNA preparations and can be toxic to primary human cells in the presence of adenovirus. *Gene Ther* 1:239–245.

Cotter MJ and Muruve DA. 2005. The induction of inflammation by adenovirus vectors used for gene therapy. *Front Biosci* 10:1098–1105.

Croyle MA, Chirmule N, et al. 2002. PEGylation of E1-deleted adenovirus vectors allows significant gene expression on readministration to liver. *Hum Gene Ther* 13:1887–1900.

Croyle MA, Callahan SM, et al. 2004. PEGylation of a vesicular stomatitis virus G pseudotyped lentivirus vector prevents inactivation in serum. *J Virol* 78:912–921.

Croyle MA, Le HT, et al. 2005. PEGylated helper-dependent adenoviral vectors: highly efficient vectors with an enhanced safety profile. *Gene Ther* 12:579–587.

Crystal RG, McElvaney NG, et al. 1994. Administration of an adenovirus containing the human CFTR cDNA to the respiratory tract of individuals with cystic fibrosis. *Nat Genet* 8:42–51.

Cserr HF and Knopf PM. 1992. Cervical lymphatics, the blood–brain barrier and the immunoreactivity of the brain: a new view. *Immunol Today* 13:507–512.

Dewey RA, Morrissey G, et al. 1999. Chronic brain inflammation and persistent herpes simplex virus 1 thymidine kinase expression in survivors of syngeneic glioma treated by adenovirus-mediated gene therapy: implications for clinical trials. *Nat Med* 5:1256–1263.

Di Domenico C, Di Napoli D, et al. 2006. Limited transgene immune response and long-term expression of human alpha-L-iduronidase in young adult mice with mucopolysaccharidosis type I by liver-directed gene therapy. *Hum Gene Ther* 17:1112–1121.

Dobrzynski E, Fitzgerald JC, et al. 2006. Prevention of cytotoxic T lymphocyte responses to factor IX–expressing hepatocytes by gene transfer-induced regulatory T cells. *Proc Natl Acad Sci U S A* 103:4592–4597.

During MJ, Kaplitt MG, et al. 2001. Subthalamic GAD gene transfer in Parkinson disease patients who are candidates for deep brain stimulation. *Hum Gene Ther* 12:1589–1591.

Dustin ML and Cooper JA. 2000. The immunological synapse and the actin cytoskeleton: molecular hardware for T cell signaling. *Nat Immunol* 1:23–29.

Eriksdotter Jonhagen M, Nordberg A, et al. 1998. Intracerebroventricular infusion of nerve growth factor in three patients with Alzheimer's disease. *Dement Geriatr Cogn Disord* 9:246–257.

Erles K, Sebokova P, et al. 1999. Update on the prevalence of serum antibodies (IgG and IgM) to adeno-associated virus (AAV). *J Med Virol* 59:406–411.

Favre D, Blouin V, et al. 2002. Lack of an immune response against the tetracycline-dependent transactivator correlates with long-term doxycycline-regulated transgene expression in nonhuman primates after intramuscular injection of recombinant adeno-associated virus. *J Virol* 76:11605–11611.

Flusberg BA, Cocker ED, et al. 2005. Fiber-optic fluorescence imaging. *Nat Methods* 2:941–950.

Friedl P, den Boer AT, et al. 2005. Tuning immune responses: diversity and adaptation of the immunological synapse. *Nat Rev Immunol* 5:532–545.

Galea I, Bechmann I, et al. 2007. What is immune privilege (not)? *Trends Immunol* 28:12–18.

Gerdes CA, Castro MG, et al. 2000. Strong promoters are the key to highly efficient, noninflammatory and noncytotoxic adenoviral-mediated transgene delivery into the brain in vivo. *Mol Ther* 2:330–338.

Grakoui A, Bromley SK, et al. 1999. The immunological synapse: a molecular machine controlling T cell activation. *Science* 285:221–227.

Guidotti LG and Chisari FV. 2001. Noncytolytic control of viral infections by the innate and adaptive immune response. *Annu Rev Immunol* 19:65–91.

Herzog RW. 2007. Immune responses to AAV capsid: Are mice not humans after all? *Mol Ther* 15:649–650.

Herzog RW, Mount JD, et al. 2001. Muscle-directed gene transfer and transient immune suppression result in sustained partial correction of canine hemophilia B caused by a null mutation. *Mol Ther* 4:192–200.

Huppa JB and Davis MM. 2003. T-cell-antigen recognition and the immunological synapse. *Nat Rev Immunol* 3:973–383.

Huse M, Lillemeier BF, et al. 2006. T cells use two directionally distinct pathways for cytokine secretion. *Nat Immunol* 7:247–255.

Immonen A, Vapalahti M, et al. 2004. AdvHSV-tk gene therapy with intravenous ganciclovir improves survival in human malignant glioma: a randomised, controlled study. *Mol Ther* 10:967–972.

Kaplitt MG, Feigin A, et al. 2007. Safety and tolerability of gene therapy with an adeno-associated virus (AAV) borne GAD gene for Parkinson's disease: an open label, phase I trial. *Lancet* 369:2097–2105.

King GD, Muhammad AK, et al. 2008. High-capacity adenovirus vector-mediated antiglioma gene therapy in the presence of systemic antiadenovirus immunity. *J Virol* 82(9):4680–4684.

Knopf PM, Harling-Berg CJ. et al. 1998. Antigen-dependent intrathecal antibody synthesis in the normal rat brain: tissue entry and local retention of antigen-specific B cells. *J Immunol* 161:692–701.

Knowles MR, Hohneker KW, et al. 1995. A controlled study of adenoviral-vector-mediated gene transfer in the nasal epithelium of patients with cystic fibrosis. *N Engl J Med* 333:823–831.

Le HT, Yu QC, et al. 2005. Utility of PEGylated recombinant adeno-associated viruses for gene transfer. *J Control Release* 108:161–177.

Lee KH, Holdorf AD, et al. 2002. T cell receptor signaling precedes immunological synapse formation. *Science* 295:1539–1542.

Lena AM, Giannetti P, et al. 2005. Immune responses against tetracycline-dependent transactivators affect long-term expression of mouse erythropoietin delivered by a helper-dependent adenoviral vector. *J Gene Med* 7:1086–1096.

Leon B, Lopez-Bravo M, et al. 2007. Monocyte-derived dendritic cells formed at the infection site control the induction of protective T helper 1 responses against *Leishmania*. *Immunity* 26:519–531.

Levi-Montalcini R. 1987. The nerve growth factor 35 years later. *Science* 237:1154–1162.

Li Y, Muruve DA, et al. 2002. The role of selectins and integrins in adenovirus vector-induced neutrophil recruitment to the liver. *Eur J Immunol* 32:3443–3452.

Lin AH, Luo J, et al. 2005. Global analysis of Smad2/3-dependent TGF-beta signaling in living mice reveals prominent tissue-specific responses to injury. *J Immunol* 175:547–554.

Liu Q, Zaiss AK, et al. 2003. The role of capsid–endothelial interactions in the innate immune response to adenovirus vectors. *Hum Gene Ther* 14:627–643.

Lo WD, Qu G, et al. 1999. Adeno-associated virus-mediated gene transfer to the brain: duration and modulation of expression. *Hum Gene Ther* 10:201–213.

Lowenstein PR. 2002a. Dendritic cells and immune responses in the central nervous system. *Trends Immunol* 23:70.

Lowenstein PR. 2002b. Immunology of viral-vector-mediated gene transfer into the brain: an evolutionary and developmental perspective. *Trends Immunol* 23:23–30.

Lowenstein PR. 2004. Input virion proteins: cryptic targets of antivector immune responses in preimmunized subjects. *Mol Ther* 9:771–774.

Lowenstein PR. 2005. The case for immunosuppression in clinical gene transfer. *Mol Ther* 12:185–186.

Luo J, Lin AH, et al. 2006. Bioluminescence imaging of Smad signaling in living mice shows correlation with excitotoxic neurodegeneration. *Proc Natl Acad Sci U S A* 103:18326–18331.

Maione D, Della Rocca C, et al. 2001. An improved helper-dependent adenoviral vector allows persistent gene expression after intramuscular delivery and overcomes preexisting immunity to adenovirus. *Proc Natl Acad Sci U S A* 98:5986–5991.

Mandel RJ and Burger C. 2004. Clinical trials in neurological disorders using AAV vectors: promises and challenges. *Curr Opin Mol Ther* 6:482–490.

Mandel RJ, Rendahl KG, et al. 1998. Characterization of intrastriatal recombinant adeno-associated virus mediated gene transfer of human tyrosine hydroxylase and human GTP-cyclohydroxylase I in a rat model of Parkinson's disease. *J Neurosci* 18:4271–4284.

Mandel RJ, Manfredsson FP, et al. 2006. Recombinant adeno-associated viral vectors as therapeutic agents to treat neurological disorders. *Mol Ther* 13:463–483.

Manno CS, Pierce GF, et al. 2006. Successful transduction of liver in hemophilia by AAV-factor IX and limitations imposed by the host immune response. *Nat Med* 12:342–347.

Mastakov MY, Baer K, et al. 2002. Immunological aspects of recombinant adeno-associated virus delivery to the mammalian brain. *J Virol* 76:8446–8454.

Matyszak MK. 1998. Inflammation in the CNS: balance between immunological privilege and immune responses. *Prog Neurobiol* 56:19–35.

Matyszak MK and Perry VH. 1996. The potential role of dendritic cells in immune-mediated inflammatory diseases in the central nervous system. *Neuroscience* 74:599–608.

McCoy RD, Davidson BL, et al. 1995. Pulmonary inflammation induced by incomplete or inactivated adenoviral particles. *Hum Gene Ther* 6:1553–1560.

McMahon EJ, Bailey SL, et al. 2005. Epitope spreading initiates in the CNS in two mouse models of multiple sclerosis. *Nat Med* 11:335–339.

McMenamin PG. 1999. Distribution and phenotype of dendritic cells and resident tissue macrophages in the dura mater, leptomeninges, and choroid plexus of the rat brain as demonstrated in wholemount preparations. *J Comp Neurol* 405:553–562.

McPhee SW, Janson CG, et al. 2006. Immune responses to AAV in a phase I study for Canavan disease. *J Gene Med* 8:577–588.

Mehta AD, Jung JC, et al. 2004. Fiber optic in vivo imaging in the mammalian nervous system. *Curr Opin Neurobiol* 14:617–28.

Mian A, Guenther M, et al. 2005. Toxicity and adaptive immune response to intracellular transgenes delivered by helper-dependent vs. first generation adenoviral vectors. *Mol Genet Metab* 84:278–288.

Mingozzi F, Hasbrouck NC, et al. 2007a. Modulation of tolerance to the transgene product in a non-human primate model of AAV-mediated gene transfer to liver. *Blood* 110 (7): 2334–2341.

Mingozzi F, Maus MV, et al. 2007b. CD8(+) T-cell responses to adeno-associated virus capsid in humans. *Nat Med* 13:419–422.

Molnar-Kimber KL, Sterman DH, et al. 1998. Impact of preexisting and induced humoral and cellular immune responses in an adenovirus-based gene therapy phase I clinical trial for localized mesothelioma. *Hum Gene Ther* 9:2121–2133.

Monks CR, Freiberg BA, et al. 1998. Three-dimensional segregation of supramolecular activation clusters in T cells. *Nature* 395:82–86.

Muramatsu S, Fujimoto K, et al. 2002. Behavioral recovery in a primate model of Parkinson's disease by triple transduction of striatal cells with adeno-associated viral vectors expressing dopamine-synthesizing enzymes. *Hum Gene Ther* 13:345–354.

Muruve DA, Barnes MJ, et al. 1999. Adenoviral gene therapy leads to rapid induction of multiple chemokines and acute neutrophil-dependent hepatic injury in vivo. *Hum Gene Ther* 10:965–976.

Muzyczka N and Berns KI. 2001. Parvoiridae: the viruses and their replication. In *Fields Virology*, DM Knipe and PM Howley, Eds. Lippincott, Williams & Wilkins, New York, pp. 2327–2360.

O'Neal WK, Zhou H, et al. 2000. Toxicity associated with repeated administration of first-generation adenovirus vectors does not occur with a helper-dependent vector. *Mol Med* 6:179–195.

Otake K, Ennist DL, et al. 1998. Nonspecific inflammation inhibits adenovirus-mediated pulmonary gene transfer and expression independent of specific acquired immune responses. *Hum Gene Ther* 9:2207–2222.

Parks R, Evelegh C, et al. 1999. Use of helper-dependent adenoviral vectors of alternative serotypes permits repeat vector administration. *Gene Ther* 6:1565–1573.

Pashenkov M, Teleshova N et al. 2003. Inflammation in the central nervous system: the role for dendritic cells. *Brain Pathol* 13:23–33.

Peden CS, Burger C, et al. 2004. Circulating anti-wt-AAV2 antibodies inhibit rAAV2-, but not rAAV5-mediated gene transfer in the brain. *J Virol* 78:6344–6359.

Raper SE, Yudkoff M, et al. 2002. A pilot study of in vivo liver-directed gene transfer with an adenoviral vector in partial ornithine transcarbamylase deficiency. *Hum Gene Ther* 13:163–175.

Reimsnider S, Manfredsson FP, et al. 2007. Time course of transgene expression after intrastriatal pseudotyped rAAV2/1, rAAV2/2, rAAV2/5, and rAAV2/8 transduction in the rat. *Mol Ther* 15(8): 1504–1511.

Sanftner LM, Suzuki BM, et al. 2004. Striatal delivery of rAAV-hAADC to rats with preexisting immunity to AAV. *Mol Ther* 9:403–409.

Schnell MA, Zhang Y, et al. 2001. Activation of innate immunity in nonhuman primates following intraportal administration of adenoviral vectors. *Mol Ther* 3:708–722.

Shi Q, Wilcox DA, et al. 2006. Factor VIII ectopically targeted to platelets is therapeutic in hemophilia A with high-titer inhibitory antibodies. *J Clin Invest* 116:1974–1982.

Stevenson PG, Freeman S, et al. 1997a. Virus dissemination through the brain parenchyma without immunologic control. *J Immunol* 159:1876–1884.

Stevenson PG, Hawke S, et al. 1997b. The immunogenicity of intracerebral virus infection depends on anatomical site. *J Virol* 71:145–151.

Tesseur I, Zou K, et al. 2006. Deficiency in neuronal TGF-beta signaling promotes neurodegeneration and Alzheimer's pathology. *J Clin Invest* 116:3060–3069.

Thomas CE, Schiedner G, et al. 2000. Peripheral infection with adenovirus causes unexpected long-term brain inflammation in animals injected intracranially with first-generation, but not with high-capacity, adenovirus vectors: toward realistic long-term neurological gene therapy for chronic diseases. *Proc Natl Acad Sci U S A* 97:7482–7487.

Thomas CE, Birkett D, et al. 2001a. Acute direct adenoviral vector cytotoxicity and chronic, but not acute, inflammatory responses correlate with decreased vector-mediated transgene expression in the brain. *Mol Ther* 3:36–46.

Thomas CE, Schiedner G, et al. 2001b. Preexisting antiadenoviral immunity is not a barrier to efficient and stable transduction of the brain, mediated by novel high-capacity adenovirus vectors. *Hum Gene Ther* 12:839–846.

Thomas CE, Storm TA, et al. 2004. Rapid uncoating of vector genomes is the key to efficient liver transduction with pseudotyped adeno-associated virus vectors. *J Virol* 78:3110–3122.

Tuszynski MH, Thal L, et al. 2005. A phase 1 clinical trial of nerve growth factor gene therapy for Alzheimer disease. *Nat Med* 11:551–555.

Wang L, Dobrzynski E, et al. 2005. Systemic protein delivery by muscle-gene transfer is limited by a local immune response. *Blood* 105:4226–4234.

Wong LF, Goodhead L, et al. 2006. Lentivirus-mediated gene transfer to the central nervous system: therapeutic and research applications. *Hum Gene Ther* 17:1–9.

Xiong W, Puntel M, et al. 2007. Immune responses against tetracycline-dependent trans-activators do not affect long-term transgene expression delivered by a helper-dependent adenoviral vector (HC-Ad). *Mol Ther* 15:S96–S97.

Xiong W, Goverdhana S, et al. 2006. Regulatable gutless adenovirus vectors sustain inducible transgene expression in the brain in the presence of an immune response against adenoviruses. *J Virol* 80:27–37.

Zaiss AK and Muruve DA. 2005. Immune responses to adeno-associated virus vectors. *Curr Gene Ther* 5:323–331.

Zirger JM, Barcia C, et al. 2006a. Rapid upregulation of interferon-regulated and chemokine mRNAs upon injection of 108 international units, but not lower doses, of adenoviral vectors into the brain. *J Virol* 80:5655–5659.

Zirger JM, Liu C, et al. 2006b. Immune regulation of transgene expression in the brain: B cells regulate an early phase of elimination of transgene expression from adenoviral vectors. *Viral Immunol* 19:508–517.

10

IMMUNOLOGY OF CUTANEOUS GENE TRANSFER

SOOSAN GHAZIZADEH, PH.D.
Departments of Oral Biology and Pathology, and Dermatology, Stony Brook University, Stony Brook, New York

Gene Therapy Immunology, Edited by Roland Herzog

10.1 INTRODUCTION

Gene transfer to skin can generally be divided into two topics with opposing goals: gene transfer to induce an immunological reaction (such as DNA vaccination) and gene transfer to induce synthesis of a protein that has therapeutic value either within the skin or at some distant site. DNA vaccination through skin takes advantage of the immunological functions associated with skin and requires transient antigen expression in subsets of skin cells. However, when considering therapeutic gene transfer to correct an inherited skin or systemic disorder, the opposite applies (i.e., durable long-term gene expression is required), and the immunological functions of the skin could act to limit or restrict the therapeutic effects of gene transfer. Central to both purposes is the cutaneous immune system, which, although similar in many respects to immune reactions elsewhere in the body, has its own special features. The central purpose of this chapter is to examine the unique immunological features of skin and how these features affect therapeutic gene transfer to skin. The immunological events that take place in the skin during DNA vaccination are mentioned briefly; readers are referred to several reviews [He and Falo 2006; Hengge 2006; Larregina and Falo 2000] for a more detailed description.

10.2 CUTANEOUS GENE THERAPY FOR INHERITED DISORDERS

Two main groups of diseases can potentially be treated by long-term therapeutic cutaneous gene transfer: genetic skin disorders and systemic metabolic disorders.

10.2.1 Genetic Skin Disorders

There are a wide variety of debilitating and untreatable skin diseases for which the underlying molecular defects have been characterized [Uitto and Pulkkinen 2000]. Several of these, especially monogenic inherited skin disorders, are candidates for cutaneous gene therapy. Examples of these genetic skin disorders include a subset of blistering disorders called epidermolysis bullosa (EB), keratinization disorders such as ichthyosis, and xeroderma pigmentosum (XP), in which increased sensitivity to ultraviolet light leads to increased frequency of skin cancers. Preclinical studies indicate that these diseases could be treated by reintroducing a single normal copy of the affected gene into the diseased skin cells [Choate et al. 1996; Marchetto et al. 2004; Ferrari et al. 2005]. Most research efforts toward cutaneous gene therapy focused on treatment of two genodermatoses: junctional EB, an autosomal recessive disorder associated with mutations in the genes encoding one of the three components of hemidesmosomes, including laminin 5, type XVII collagen, and $\alpha6/\beta4$ integrins, and dystrophic EB, which is caused by mutations in the gene encoding collagen type VII, a large basement membrane component that plays a major role in epidermal–dermal adhesion and skin integrity. Preclinical studies have demonstrated the feasibility of phenotypic correction of these disorders by cutaneous gene transfer and have led to the first successful phase I–II trial for junctional EB (laminin 5 deficiency) based on autologous transplantation of genetically modified epidermis [Mavilio et al. 2006].

10.2.2 Genetic Systemic Disorders

Certain metabolic deficiency disorders may benefit from the production and release of recombinant proteins synthesized by a patch of genetically modified skin. Skin is accessible and highly vascularized, and skin-produced polypeptides have been shown to reach the circulation [Fenjves et al. 1989]. Examples of gene products produced by genetically modified skin cells are growth hormone, transferrin, erythropoietin, apolipoprotein E, α1-antitrypsin, leptin, and coagulation factors [Taichman 1999; Del Rio et al. 2004]. The levels of therapeutic gene products were, however, at best a few nanograms in the serum of recipient animals, depending on the graft size. These levels may be sufficient to correct for several hormone–cytokine deficiencies, but not for serum protein deficiencies, in which therapeutic levels must reach a range of hundreds of nanograms to micrograms.

10.3 IMMUNE RESPONSES IN THERAPEUTIC CUTANEOUS GENE TRANSFER

Despite major advances in cutaneous gene therapy for inherited diseases, a major issue in long-term cutaneous gene therapy for either skin or systemic disorders is how to circumvent potential host responses against the therapeutic but foreign gene product, especially in patients carrying null mutations. The nature of host responses in gene therapy depends on various factors, including the immunogenicity of the transgene product and the vector elements, the route of vector administration, and the type of cell or tissue producing the gene product [Bessis et al. 2004]. Many patients with recessive hereditary skin diseases such as EB carry null mutations, and therefore de novo expression of the transgene in skin will likely result in induction of transgene-specific immune responses and clearance of the corrected cells. To appreciate the unique aspects of the cutaneous immune responses in long-term gene therapy, we first need to highlight the cellular components of skin and its mode of renewal.

10.4 TARGET CELLS OF CUTANEOUS GENE TRANSFER

Skin structure determines in a direct way how gene transfer is accomplished, and this in turn is important in subsequent cutaneous immune responses. Skin consists of two compartments: an epidermal component composed largely (>90%) of keratinocytes, and an underlying dermis composed of extracellular matrix proteins embedded with fibroblasts (Fig. 10-1). Fibroblasts and keratinocytes can both be used as targets of therapeutic gene transfer, depending on the nature of the disease.

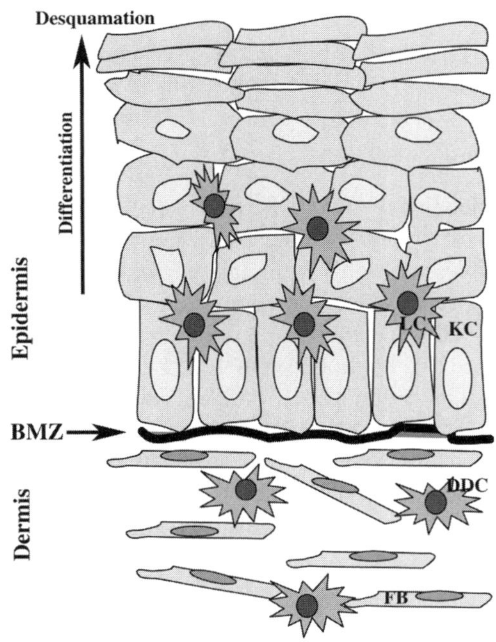

Figure 10-1 Major cellular components of skin targeted by gene transfer. Skin is composed of two distinct epidermal and dermal compartments separated by basement membrane (BMZ). Epidermis is a continuously renewing tissue, which is maintained by a population of stem cells in the basal layer of epidermis. Both epidermal keratinocytes (KCs) and dermal fibroblasts (FBs) are targets of gene transfer. Antigen-presenting cells residing in normal skin include Langerhans cells (LCs) and dermal dendritic cells (DDCs).

10.4.1 Epidermal Gene Transfer

For inherited skin disorders that involve the epidermis, keratinocytes are obvious targets of therapeutic gene transfer. There are well-characterized culture conditions to support keratinocyte proliferation, highly efficient methods of gene transfer to cultured keratinocytes, and advanced methods of tissue engineering and permanent skin regeneration in the clinic [Carretero et al. 2006; Mavilio et al. 2006]. However, because epidermis is a continuously renewing tissue, long-term epidermal gene therapy requires delivery of the therapeutic gene to keratinocyte stem cells located in the basal layer. Stem cell progeny either remain as stem cells or give rise to transit-amplifying cells, which after a few rounds of replication withdraw from the cell cycle, undergo terminal differentiation, and desquamate. Gene transfer to non-stem cells will result in transient transgene expression due to desquamation of the cells carrying the transgene. A major effort of cutaneous gene therapy has been directed at optimizing gene transfer to keratinocyte stem cells and achieving persistent transgene expression [Ghazizadeh and Taichman 2000].

10.4.2 Dermal Gene Transfer

Fibroblasts are easily propagated in culture, are much less susceptible to growth arrest and differentiation than keratinocytes, and are transduced efficiently by viral vectors. Cultured fibroblasts were widely used for proof-of-concept assessments in initial gene transfer studies to supply gene products to circulation. However, rapid transgene silencing in genetically modified fibroblasts in in vivo settings diminished enthusiasm for their use in clinical trials [Krueger 2000]. These problems have, however, been overcome by advances in vector design and cell transplantation. Fibroblasts are major recipients of gene transfer following direct intradermal injection of skin. A single intradermal injection of lentiviral vectors encoding an erythropoietin gene into human skin xenografts on immunodeficient mice resulted in sustained serum erythropoietin levels [Baek et al. 2001]. More recently, fibroblasts have proven to be the preferred therapeutic target over keratinocytes for genetic correction of type VII collagen deficiency in dystrophic EB [Goto et al. 2006]. Intradermal injection of collagen VII–expressing human fibroblasts has been shown to restore collagen VII expression in the basement membrane of regenerated human skin in vivo [Woodley et al. 2003]. More importantly, genetically modified fibroblasts injected into the mouse circulation home to the skin wounds allow treatment of widespread wounds that are often associated with blistering disorders of skin [Woodley et al. 2007].

10.5 METHODS OF GENE TRANSFER TO SKIN

A major factor in determining immune responses in gene therapy is the method of gene delivery. Skin is amenable to both ex vivo and in vivo approaches to gene transfer. Ex vivo transfer entails gene delivery to cells cultured outside the body and has several attractive features, including the ability to reduce or eliminate exposure of the host to vector as well as the possibility of verifying expression prior to engraftment back to the host. Both keratinocytes and fibroblasts are easily propagated in culture, are transduced efficiently by viral vectors, and can regenerate skin when grafted as a bilayer construct in vivo [Ghazizadeh and Taichman 2000].

The in vivo approach involves direct introduction of genetic material to skin using either viral (e.g., retroviral, lentiviral, or adenoviral vector transduction) or nonviral vectors (e.g., plasmid DNA delivered by particle bombardment, injection, or liposomes). The unique properties of each vector and the delivery method affect the efficiency of gene transfer, the longevity of transgene expression, and the type and intensity of immune responses to transgene expression (Table 10-1). For applications that require transient expression of a transgene (e.g., a growth factor during wound healing or an antigen for DNA vaccination), nonviral methods and in vivo gene transfer are most suitable. However, for long-term gene therapy, integrating vectors are required. To date recombinant retroviral and lentiviral vectors have proven to be the most suitable for long-term cutaneous gene therapy targeted to either keratinocytes or fibroblasts

TABLE 10-1 Comparison of Ex Vivo and In Vivo Cutaneous Gene Therapy

	In Vivo	Ex Vivo
Method of gene transfer	Direct transfer to tissue	Gene transfer in cultured cells followed by transplantation
Efficiency of gene transfer	Low efficiency and localized to the injection site	High efficiency of gene transfer
Type of vector	Integrating and nonintegrating vectors	Integrating vectors
Period of transgene expression	Transient or long-term	Long-term
Major applications	DNA vaccination, cancer gene therapy, and wound healing	Treatment of genetic disorders
Potential antigens	Viral protein and transgene products	Transgene products
Danger signals	Viral particles, inflammation	Inflammation

[Ghazizadeh and Taichman 2000]. Direct administration of these vectors to skin results in long-term transgene expression in both keratinocytes and fibroblasts at the site of injection [Woodley et al. 2004; Ghazizadeh and Taichman 2005]. More recently, novel strategies have been developed to address safety issues of viral vector systems, including gene transfer based on Sleeping Beauty transposons or ϕC31 bacteriophage integrase methodologies. Stable integration of large transgenes into primary cultures of human keratinocytes has been achieved using these technologies, although with lower efficiency than for viral vectors [Ortiz-Urda et al. 2003].

The backbones of integrating vectors are devoid of viral coding sequences and do not appear to induce adaptive host immune responses, although direct injection of defective viruses can induce innate immunity (e.g., by double-stranded RNA) and can potentiate transgene-specific responses. The activating signals provided to the immune system following in vivo administration of viral particles are avoided in ex vivo gene transfer, in which viral transduction takes place in culture. Therefore, a decreased risk of immune activation is expected in ex vivo gene therapy.

10.6 FEATURES OF CUTANEOUS IMMUNOLOGY RELEVANT TO GENE THERAPY

The type of cell and tissue producing a gene product is a major factor affecting the nature of host responses in gene therapy. For example, retrovirus-mediated gene transfer of *lacZ* or factor IX into the liver of immunocompetent dogs and rats resulted in long-term expression of the transgene [Ferry et al. 1991; Kay et al. 1993a,b], whereas expression of *lacZ* in skin keratinocytes leads to expression lasting only 2 to 3 weeks [Stockschlader et al. 1994; Ghazizadeh et al. 1999]. The differences in duration of transgene expression mirror the susceptibility of organs and tissue allografts to rejection following transplantation. For example, skin grafts are most susceptible to rejection; heart, kidney, and liver are progressively more readily accepted [Jones et al. 2001]. These differences point out the important role of the tissue microenvironment in the host response in gene therapy.

Skin covers most of the body's surface and provides the first line of defense against microorganisms. As an important immunological organ, it can initiate and direct an inflammatory response. Skin contains a large number of antigen-presenting cells (APCs), including epidermal Langerhans cells (LCs) and dermal dendritic cells (DCs), which are specialized in the initiation and regulation of immune responses, and a population of resident memory T cells that provide immune surveillance [Streilein 1990; Clark et al., 2006]. Dermal mast cells have an important role in both initiation and modulation of innate and adaptive immune responses, and in regulation of tolerance (see Table 10-2) [Waldmann 2006]. Keratinocytes also express or can be induced to express a number of immunologically important surface antigens, including the major histocompatibility complex (MHC) class II molecules, intercellular adhesion molecule 1 (ICAM-1), and the co-stimulatory molecule B7-H1, suggesting that these molecules have a potential role in the regulation of immune responses [Chu and Morris 2005]. Furthermore, keratinocytes produce a wide variety of soluble peptide mediators of inflammation, including interleukins, chemokines, growth factors, and angiogenic factors. When secreted they may act in an autocrine or paracrine fashion to influence multiple resident cell types within the skin, including endothelial cells, macrophages/dendritic cells, neutrophils, lymphocytes, fibroblasts, Langerhans cells, and keratinocytes [Kupper and Fuhlbrigge 2004].

Activation of keratinocytes by various stimuli, including injury, environmental stimuli, and microbial or viral pathogens, induces an inflammatory cascade with numerous effects on the modulation of leukocyte accumulation, antigen presentation, induction of innate immunity, promotion of vascular infiltration,

TABLE 10-2 Immune Response Elements Residing in Skin

	Cell Type	Major Function
Epidermis	Keratinocytes	Initiation of inflammatory response
	Langerhans cells	Antigen-presenting function
	Intraepithelial lymphocytes	Immune surveillance
Dermis	Dermal dendritic cells	Antigen-presenting function
	Mast cells	Immune regulation/immediate response
	Macrophages	Immune regulation
	CLA^+ memory T cells	Immune surveillance
	Endothelial cells	Leukocyte homing

and modulation of keratinocyte growth. Although these unique immunological features of skin have been utilized for the development of effective DNA immunization strategies, they are a major impediment for therapeutic gene transfer.

10.7 CUTANEOUS GENE TRANSFER FOR DNA VACCINATION

Delivery of plasmid DNA by a variety of methods, including direct intradermal injection, gene gun, hydrodynamic, electric pulse, or topical spray of liposomal DNA, results in the uptake of the DNA by skin cells. Although protein expression following transfer of plasmid DNA is often either transient or cannot be verified, gene transfer to skin has been shown to induce a long-lasting humoral and cellular immunity. Immunogenicity of DNA appears to depend on the presence of immunostimulatory CpG motifs within the bacteria-derived plasmid construct rather than the levels of antigenic protein expression [Sato et al. 1996; Hengge 2006]. In addition, there are quantitative differences in the type of immune responses induced by the various DNA delivery methods [Vogel 2000]. For example, responses to intradermal injection of plasmid DNA are dominated by Th1 cytokine production, while topical or gene gun DNA delivery methods may induce a Th2-type immune response [Feltquate et al. 1997]. These differences depend on several factors, including subcellular localization of antigen, type of cells targeted by gene transfer, and the pathway of antigen presentation [Boyle et al. 1997; Lauterbach et al. 2006]. Despite promising data obtained in experimental murine models, most preclinical studies in large animal models and clinical trials have been disappointing. Additional strategies to improve immunogenicity in large animal models include improved gene delivery, inclusion of various immunostimulatory compounds, and receptor-mediated targeting of plasmid DNA to LCs [Lisziewicz et al., 2005; Cristillo et al. 2007; Du et al. 2007].

10.8 SUITABLE ANIMAL MODELS FOR THE STUDY OF HOST RESPONSES IN CUTANEOUS GENE THERAPY

The role of immunological responses in the durability of transgene expression was ignored initially, as most of the initial gene transfer studies were focused on achieving sustained and targeted transgene expression in human keratinocytes and were carried out in immune-deficient mice. When transduced cultured keratinocytes or fibroblasts were grafted to immunocompetent animals, infection, poor engraftment, graft contracture, and host reepithelialization, as well as transcriptional gene silencing, often complicated the assessment of transgene-specific immune responses.

To explore host responses to neoantigen expression in skin, an in vivo transduction model in immunocompetent mice was developed (Fig. 10-2). Successful in vivo transduction of skin required the use of viral titers greater than 10^9 transducing units per milliliter and dermabrasion of the epidermis to induce stem cell

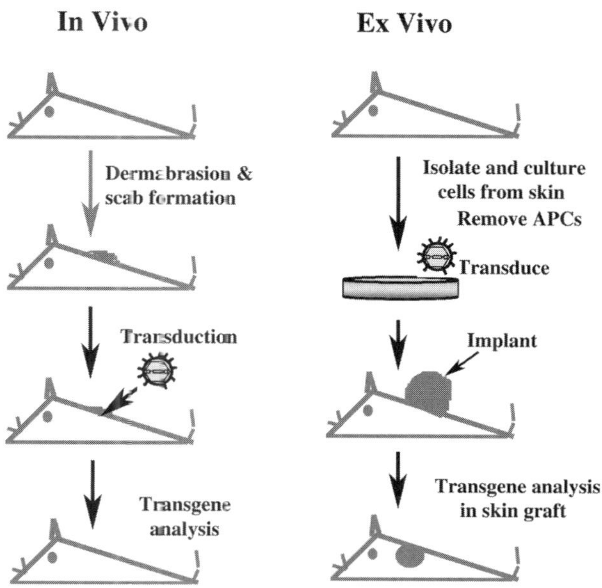

Figure 10-2 Two animal models developed to study transgene-specific immune responses in cutaneous gene therapy. In the case of in vivo gene transfer, the skin is dermabraded to induce proliferation of keratinocyte stem cell. Recombinant retroviruses are injected directly into the healing epidermis. In an ex vivo approach, target cells are removed from the skin and propagated in culture before being genetically modified by retroviral transduction. Transgenic skin is regenerated by implanting a mixture of genetically modified keratinocytes and fibroblasts as cell slurry on the fascia but under a transplantation chamber that is removed after one week.

replication and to allow access to these cells. Transduction of the hyperplastic epidermis with concentrated retroviral vectors encoding a neoantigen (e.g., lacZ or EGFP) results in stable gene transfer and expression of transgene in cutaneous epithelium. In mice that are tolerant to the neoantigen, prolonged expression is noted, but in nontolerant animals, expression is lost in 2 to 3 weeks [Ghazizadeh et al. 1999]. Analysis of humoral and cell-mediated responses indicate a direct correlation between induction of immune response and duration of transgene expression. Studies in transgene-tolerant mice that are immunocompetent suggest no significant role for integrated viral elements in the induction of immune responses mediating loss of transgene expression. Analysis of transgene expression in mice deficient in specific subsets of T cells indicates that $CD4^+$ and $CD8^+$ T cells have overlapping roles, and that either population can effectively eliminate transduced cells (Table 10-3) [Ghazizadeh et al. 2003]. Moreover, tissue-specific expression of the transgene by utilizing a retroviral vector with targeted expression to keratinocytes does not limit transgene-specific immune responses [Ghazizadeh et al. 2002; Lu and Ghazizadeh 2007].

TABLE 10-3 Analysis of Transgene Expression in the Epidermis of In Vivo–Transduced Mice with Defined Immune Deficiencies

Transgene Expression	C57Bl/6	$IgGh^{-/-}$	$\beta 2m^{-/-}$ (Class $I^{-/-}$)	$A\beta^{b-/-}$ (Class $II^{-/-}$)	$MHC^{-/-}$	Transgene Tolerant
1 week post-transduction	+(8/8)	+(6/6)	+(6/6)	+(4/4)	+(4/4)	+(8/8)
>3 weeks post-transduction	– (0/8)	– (0/6)	– (0/6)	– (0/6)	+ (4/4)	+ (8/8)

To evaluate immune responses in an ex vivo gene transfer approach, stable skin grafts are required. To achieve this, an all-murine model was adapted in which murine primary epidermal cells depleted of APCs are transduced in culture, mixed with syngeneic fibroblasts, and implanted orthotopically as cell slurry onto immunocompetent isogenic mice. Implantation of transgenenic keratinocytes on the back of transgene-tolerant mice results in establishment of stable skin grafts and long-term transgene expression. In nontolerant mice, however, transgene-specific immune responses reject the implanted genetically modified keratinocytes, identifying the transgene product as the dominant antigen responsible for rejection of transduced cells (Fig. 10-2) [Lu and Ghazizadeh 2005].

Animal models have been used to predict responses in human trials. In a clinical trial for treatment of epidermolysis bullosa, a patient with compound LAMB3 mutations allowing residual synthesis of laminin 5 was selected to ensure tolerance to transgene product [Mavilio et al. 2006]. The lack of laminin-specific antibodies or cell-mediated immunity throughout the follow-up and long-term retroviral-mediated transgene expression was predicted from earlier studies of murine models of cutaneous gene therapy. Large spontaneous immunocompetent animal models of some inherited skin disorders are now available and will be critical for accurate analysis of host responses for future cutaneous gene therapy trials.

10.9 PRESENTATION OF SKIN-DERIVED TRANSGENE PRODUCTS

Two predominant populations of DCs reside in the skin: dermal DCs and epidermal LCs. Skin-residing DCs can capture antigen in the epidermis or dermis, depending on the location of transgene, and migrate to the skin draining LNs, where they initiate and regulate T-cell responses [Richters et al. 2005]. Given the close proximity of LCs to keratinocytes that express a transgene, they are likely to play a predominant role in antigen presentation from epidermal keratinocytes and activation of naive T cells in the lymph nodes, although after activation of a small number of antigen-specific T cells, these cells can be amplified in skin itself. Expression of T-cell adhesion molecules in skin allows more efficient homing of activated T cells to skin [Kupper and Fuhlbrigge 2004]. Moreover, keratinocytes possess the ability to secrete an array of inflammatory cytokines and may act as antigen-presenting cells following up-regulation of MHC class II molecules [Albanesi et al. 1998].

Subsequent to the inoculation of vectors into skin, DCs may acquire transgene product either through direct transduction, or through uptake of viral particles containing some transgene product captured as the virus is budded off from the producer cell [Varmus 1988]. These antigen-contaminated viral particles could provide an exogenous source of antigen for presentation to MHC class II–restricted helper T cells. An endogenous source of antigens for presentation to MHC class I–restricted CTLs is provided either by direct transduction of DCs or via cross-presentation of internalized antigens [Heath and Carbone 2001a]. Cross-presentation requires transfer of antigenic transgene product to a specific subset of DCs ($CD8^+$ $CD205^+$ DCs) and processing of antigen into the MHC class I pathway for stimulation of cellular immunity [Heath et al. 2004; Dudziak et al. 2007]. The relative contribution of direct presentation versus cross-presentation in determining the nature and duration of immune responses to keratinocyte-derived antigens is not clear.

The nature of immune responses may also be affected by subcellular localization of transgene products. Bombardment of skin with DNA plasmids encoding secreted, cytoplasmic, or membrane-bound forms of ovalbumin (OVA) as a model antigen was shown to generate different type of immune responses. Gene transfer of cytoplasmic or transmembrane forms of OVA leads to strong OVA-specific CTL responses, but the secreted form of OVA failed to stimulate CTL responses, although antibody responses are generated [Morel et al. 2004]. The lack of CTL responses in the latter argues against a dominant role for cross-presentation of exogenous antigens, suggesting that soluble proteins are presented primarily by the exogenous antigen presentation route.

10.10 DANGER SIGNALS IN CUTANEOUS GENE THERAPY

Regulation of primary T-cell activation by DCs depends on at least two independent signals: an antigen-specific receptor (TCR) and co-stimulatory receptors, including CD28, CD40L, and inducible co-stimulator (ICOS) as well as on the induction of programmed death 1(PD-1) [Greenwald et al. 2005]. Co-stimulatory receptors are critical for regulation of T-cell activation and induction of proliferation and differentiation to effector, memory, or regulatory status. In the absence of co-stimulatory signals, the engagement of TCR results in anergy or hyporesponsiveness [Heath and Carbone 2001b; Mellman and Steinman 2001; Frauwirth and Thompson 2002]. Up-regulation of co-stimulatory molecules occurs during DC maturation and is triggered by exposure of DCs to a number of danger signals, including pathogen-associated molecular patterns (PAMPs) such as CpG DNA, dsRNA, and LPS, as well as various pro-inflammatory cytokines and tissue factors [Janeway 1992; McLellan et al. 1997; Chain, 2003]. In general, one may consider T-cell activation as a summation of positive and negative signals specified by expression of receptors and ligands on T cells and DCs. A negative signal in the absence of a positive signal can be tolerogenic. Conversely, positive signals could override negative signals.

Both models of in vivo and ex vivo cutaneous gene therapy are accompanied by initial inflammatory responses. The recombinant virus infection itself (e.g., double-stranded RNA) could induce innate immunity via interaction with Toll-like receptors and result in release of pro-inflammatory signals [Tan et al. 2005]. Tissue damage induced by needle injection, particle bombardment, abrasion-induced hyperplasia, or transplantation can induce a cascade of pro-inflammatory cytokine release by skin cells, including keratinocytes. Moreover, the remodeling that occurs during the initial stages of keratinocyte transplantation results in the release of apoptotic and necrotic cellular material along with transgene product and could be seen as danger signals by the immune system [Matzinger 1994].

10.11 EFFECTOR MECHANISMS MEDIATING TRANSGENE LOSS IN CUTANEOUS GENE TRANSFER

Although genetically modified epidermis expressing a neoantigen is rejected regardless of method of gene delivery, the mechanism of immune rejection appears to differ depending on whether an ex vivo or in vivo method of gene transfer is used. Effector mechanisms involved in the rejection of antigen-bearing cells are influenced by the microenvironment in which DCs encounter the antigen, the pathway of antigen presentation, and functional polarization of T cells [Rocha et al. 2003].

The loss of transgene expression following in vivo gene transfer to mouse skin was shown to be associated with Th1-type responses, as characterized by a prevalence of transgene-specific IgG2a in sera, secretion of high levels of gamma interferon by lymphocytes, intense tissue infiltration of CD4 and CD8 cells, and transgene-specific CTL activity and memory (Table 10-4). The fact that transient transgene expression is seen in mice deficient in either major histocompatibility complex (MHC) class I or class II molecules but long-term expression is seen in

TABLE 10-4 Transgene-Specific Responses in Murine Models of Retrovirus-Mediated Ex Vivo and In Vivo Epidermal Gene Transfer

	In Vivo	Ex Vivo
Type of tissue infiltrates	Lymphocytic	Atopic/eosinophils
Serum IgG isotype	IgG2a	IgG1
Cytokine profile	IFN-γ	IL4/IL-5
In vitro CTL activity	Yes	No
CTL memory	Yes	No
T-helper responses	Th1	Th2

$MHC^{-/-}$ mice lacking expression of both class I and class II MHC molecules suggests that inhibition of both $CD4^+$ or $CD8^+$ T cell-mediated responses are necessary for long-term skin-directed transgene expression (Table 10-3) [Ghazizadeh et al. 2003].

Nonviral cutaneous gene transfer with plasmid DNA delivered by intradermal injection where activation of immune responses is mediated in part by immunostimulatory CpG motifs within the bacterial DNA has also been shown to be dominated by Th1 cytokine production and to include antigen-specific $CD8^+$ CTLs and $CD4^+$ T helper cells [Larregina and Falo 2000]. Similar responses were induced when the cell-specific promoter K14 was used to target transgene expression to basal keratinocytes, suggesting that cross-priming mechanisms is sufficient to induce strong CTL responses in this model [Cho et al. 2001].

Contrary to Th1-type responses induced by in vivo gene transfer, implantation of keratinocytes expressing an intracellular antigen (ex vivo gene therapy) has been shown to induce a Th2-biased response, highlighted by increased secretion of IL-4 and IL-5 by T lymphocytes, elevated levels of anti-GFP IgG1 and IgE in sera, infiltration of numerous eosinophils and mast cells into the transduced skin, and lack of in vitro and in vivo CTL activity (Table 10-4). Intense eosinophilic infiltrates, significant tissue destruction in ex vivo–transduced skin, and a delayed rejection of genetically modified keratinocytes following suppression of eosinophil infiltration by IL-5 blockade suggest that eosinophils are the dominant effector cells mediating rejection of transgenic keratinocytes [Lu and Ghazizadeh 2007]. Eosinophils are recruited to the graft and exert cytotoxic activity through the release of several molecules, such as leukotriene, superoxides, major basic protein, and eosinophil cationic protein [Rocha et al. 2003]. It is worth noting, however, that although suppression of eosinophilia by IL-5 blockade is sufficient to prevent acute rejection of transduced cells, the gradual loss of transduced keratinocytes indicates that other effector pathways can mediate rejection of transduced cells in the absence of eosinophils [Lu and Ghazizadeh 2007].

The significant differences in the type of immune responses induced by two methods of gene transfer suggests that different strategies for suppression of destructive immune responses must be developed for ex vivo and in vivo gene therapy. Recent observations indicate that Th2 cells are more susceptible than Th1 cells to tolerance induction through the blockade of co-stimulatory signals [Kishimoto et al. 2000], making ex vivo methods of cutaneous gene transfer more amenable to immune modulation.

10.12 ALTERING TRANSGENE-SPECIFIC IMMUNE RESPONSES IN CUTANEOUS GENE THERAPY

Immunosuppressive strategies are likely required to control undesired transgene-specific immune responses in situations where the transgene product is an immunogen. These strategies may range from transient immunosuppressive therapy around the time of gene delivery to induction of long-term

TABLE 10-5 Potential Strategies for Local or Transient Modulation of Immune Responses in Cutaneous Gene Therapy

Immunosuppressive Strategy	Immune Alteration
Anti-inflammatory drugs	To suppress inflammation at the time of gene transfer
Transient anti-CD40L antibody and/or CTLA4-Ig treatment	To block co-stimulatory signals and T-cell activation around the time of gene delivery
Overexpression of PD-L1 in target cells	Local down-regulation of T cells to evade immune rejection
IDO expression in target cells	Local T-cell suppression

transgene-specific tolerance. Because DCs have a central role in controlling immune responses to cell-derived antigens, any bias in signals introduced by DCs has the potential to creat a long-term effect on the host's immune responses. In this way, it may be possible to direct DCs in the direction of peripheral tolerance rather than immunity [Heath and Carbone 2001b; Lechler et al. 2001]. As DCs provide a number of sequential signals to responding T cells, various strategies could be developed to manipulate DCs or their microenvironment to subvert destructive transgene-specific immune responses. Although the requirements for controlling immune responsiveness and generating peripheral tolerance in cutaneous gene therapy have not been defined, the strategies for inducting transgene-specific tolerance are likely to be similar to those being tested to control skin immune reaction to haptens or alloantigens. Some of these strategies are discussed below (see Table 10-5).

10.12.1 Dissociation of Danger Signal from Transgene Expression

An important aim of emerging immunosuppressive strategies is to ensure that antigen is perceived in a noninflammatory or tolerogenic context. In the absence of inflammatory stimuli, immature DCs are relatively poor inducers of the proliferation of naive T cells and induce regulatory T cells rather than effector T cells [Steinman et al. 2003]. According to this hypothesis, elimination of inflammation as a contributing factor (danger signal) may result in T cell ignorance or even tolerance of the transgene product. Studies of transgenic mice with targeted expression of OVA to various tissues, including epidermis, have shown that most interstitial DCs induce tolerance to tissue antigens as they traffic to lymph nodes in the steady state [Chen et al. 2004]. However, LCs residing in the epidermis seems to be an exception, as they present antigen to T cells in an immunogenic rather than a tolerogenic fashion as they traffic to lymph nodes in the steady state [Mayerova et al. 2004; Shibaki et al. 2004]. In both studies, adoptive transfer of naive TCR transgenic $CD8^+$ T cells into transgenic mice expressing the transgene in keratinocytes resulted in autoimmune skin disease, which was very different from the tolerogenic responses presented by APCs from other tissues expressing the same transgene. These studies suggest that suppression of inflammation at the time of gene transfer or cell transplantationis is not an effective strategy for avoiding or redirecting transgene-specific immune responses in epidermal gene therapy but will possibly be effective in dermal gene therapy.

10.12.2 Transient Blockade of Co-stimulatory Pathways

Since T-cell co-stimulatory pathways regulate T-cell activation and tolerance, numerous studies have evaluated the success of co-stimulation blockade in suppressing immune responses in autoimmunity, transplantation, and various inflammatory skin diseases [Chen 2004; Keir and Sharpe 2005]. One of the first pathways to be targeted in an attempt to modify allograft rejection was the CD28/B7 pathway by using a CTLA4Ig (a soluble form of the high-affinity inhibitory receptor to B7 molecule) [Lenschow et al. 1992; Linsley et al. 1992]. Blocking the CD28/B7 interaction was shown to suppress both $CD4^+$ T cells and alloantigen-specific $CD8^+$ T cells. Experimental applications of CTLA4Ig in mice have included prolongation of allogenic cardiac and pancreatic transplant survival and reduction of skin inflammatory diseases, including psoriasis [Baliga et al. 1994; Abrams et al. 2000; Yamashita et al. 2003]. The clinical use of CTLA4Ig, however, is aimed at achieving immunosuppression rather than tolerance, since combination therapies targeting multiple co-stimulatory pathways is probably required for a robust tolerogenic effect [Bluestone et al. 2006]. Other means of disrupting T-cell activation have been through blockade of the CD40/CD154 (also known as CD40L) pathway by an anti-CD154 antibody or CD40Ig [Quezada et al. 2004]. Administration of anti-CD154 antibody has been shown to suppress antigen-specific humoral responses following nonviral delivery of desmoglein 3 gene into skin of desmoglein 3-deficient mice [Ohyama et al. 2003]. Our own data demonstrate that transient blockade of CD40/CD154 interaction with anti-CD154 antibody at the time of cell transplantation in an ex vivo model of cutaneous gene therapy results in suppression of transgene-specific immune responses and long-term (>20 weeks) engraftment of genetically modified keratinocytes in the majority of mice, although transgene-specific tolerance is not achieved [Ghazizadeh 2007]. The lack of tolerance induction may be attributed to the mechanism of anti-CD154-induced immunosuppression, which has been shown to be mediated through selective depletion of activated T cells through FC-dependent mechanisms rather than blockade of the co-stimulatory signaling pathway [Monk et al. 2003]. The immunosuppressive effects of anti-CD154 treatment are limited to the ex vivo model of cutaneous gene transfer, which may be explained by the increased susceptibility of Th2 responses to co-stimulatory blockade, as has been shown in models of allogeneic transplantation [Kishimoto et al. 2000]. These data indicate that although targeting multiple co-stimulatory pathways may be required to induce a robust transgene-specific tolerogenic effect, it may not be necessary for achieving long-term transgene expression.

10.12.3 Evading Immune Rejection by Local Expression of Immunosuppressive Molecules

Microbes and tumor cells appear to exploit immune regulatory mechanisms to evade detection by the immune system. Similar strategies may be utilized to protect genetically modified cells. One such mechanism involves an inhibitory signal to T cells delivered by the PD-1/PD-L pathway, a newer member of the B7/CD28 family [Keir et al. 2007]. Contrary to the restricted expression of other CD28 family members, PD-1 is expressed broadly on activated T cells, NKT cells, B cells, and monocytes, and is involved in regulating T-cell activation and tolerance. One of the PD-1 ligands, PD-L1, is expressed on a wide variety of hematopoietic and nonhematopoietic cell types [Keir et al. 2007]. Recent evidence indicates that interactions between parenchymal cells and lymphocytes utilize PD-1/PD-L1 signaling to maintain tissue tolerance as well as controlling the intensity of T-cell effector responses, although the mechanism remains unclear [Keir et al. 2006]. In autoimmune diabetes in NOD mice and in autoimmune encephalitis model, tissue expression of the PD-L has been shown to have an important role in protecting tissues against immune attack [Hirata et al. 2005; Keir et al. 2006]. Therefore, overexpression of PD-L1 by genetically modified skin cells may protect them from immune attack, resulting in long-term transgene expression.

Another potential target of localized immunomodulatory strategies in cutaneous gene therapy is indolamine 2,3-dioxygenase (IDO), a tryptophan-catabolizing enzyme. IDO initiates the degradation of tryptophan along the kynurenine pathway, producing a series of immunosuppressive tryptophan metabolites that suppress T-cell proliferation and induce apoptosis. In addition, the cellular stress imposed by the depletion of tryptophan seems to mediate some of the immunosuppressive effects of IDO [Munn and Mellor 2007]. Ectopic overexpression of IDO in cells (including dermal fibroblasts) has been shown to render transduced cells capable of inhibiting T-cell proliferation in vitro and suppressing T-cell responses to cell and tissue xenografts in vivo [Li et al. 2004]. Interestingly, IDO has been implicated as a potential effector mechanism of regulatory T-cell-mediated immunosuppression through the CTLA4/B7 signaling pathway [Finger and Bluestone 2002; Grohmann et al. 2002; Mellor and Munn 2003]. Whether transgene-specific immune responses can be controlled by co-expression of IDO with an antigenic transgene product in genetically modified keratinocytes or by expression of IDO in fibroblasts implanted along with genetically modified keratinocyte awaits further investigation.

10.13 CONCLUSIONS

Cutaneous gene therapy brings a new dimension to the treatment of cutaneous as well as systemic disorders, where skin can act as a bioreactor to deliver a therapeutic protein to the systemic circulation. The successful transplantation of ex vivo–transduced keratinocytes to treat a rare form of junctional epidermolysis bullosa demonstrates the feasibility of cutaneous gene therapy. However, preclinical studies suggest that in patients carrying null mutations in the affected alleles, immune responses against the transgene product will limit the therapeutic effects of gene transfer. Therefore, controlling transgene-specific responses will be required to achieve effective therapy in these patients. Short courses of antibody treatment aimed at blocking the coreceptors CD4 and CD8 and/or co-stimulatory molecules such as CD40L or depleting activated T cells at the time of gene transfer may be required to protect genetically modified keratinocytes or fibroblasts from immune rejection. Moreover, modulation of the skin microenvironment by local expression of immunomodulatory molecules may protect genetically modified cells from chronic rejection. Preclinical studies in immunocompetent animal models may make it possible to define more precisely the requirements necessary to avoid the destructive immune responses to skin-derived transgene products.

REFERENCES

Abrams JR, Kelley SL, Hayes E, et al. 2000. Blockade of T lymphocyte costimulation with cytotoxic T lymphocyte-associated antigen 4-immunoglobulin (CTLA4Ig) reverses the cellular pathology of psoriatic plaques, including the activation of keratinocytes, dendritic cells, and endothelial cells. *J Exp Med* 192:681–694.

Albanesi C, Cavani A, and Girolomoni G. 1998. Interferon-gamma-stimulated human keratinocytes express the genes necessary for the production of peptide-loaded MHC class II molecules. *J Invest Dermatol* 110:138–142.

Baek SC, Lin Q, Robbins PB, Fan H, and Khavari PA. 2001. Sustainable systemic delivery via a single injection of lentivirus into human skin tissue. *Hum Gene Ther* 12:1551–1558.

Baliga P, Chavin KD, Qin L, et al. 1994. CTLA4Ig prolongs allograft survival while suppressing cell-mediated immunity. *Transplant* 58:1082–1090.

Bessis N, GarciaCozar FJ, and Boissier MC. 2004. Immune responses to gene therapy vectors: influence on vector function and effector mechanisms. *Gene Ther* 11(Suppl 1):S10–S17.

Bluestone JA, St Clair EW, and Turka LA. 2006. CTLA4Ig: bridging the basic immunology with clinical application. *Immunity* 24:233–238.

Boyle JS, Koniaras C, and Lew AM. 1997. Influence of cellular location of expressed antigen on the efficacy of DNA vaccination: cytotoxic T lymphocyte and antibody responses are suboptimal when antigen is cytoplasmic after intramuscular DNA immunization. *Int Immunol* 9:1897–1906.

Carretero M, Escamez MJ, Prada F, et al. 2006. Skin gene therapy for acquired and inherited disorders. *Histol Histopathol* 21:1233–1247.

Chain BM. 2003. Current issues in antigen presentation: focus on the dendritic cell. *Immunol Lett* 89:237–241.

Chen L. 2004. Co-inhibitory molecules of the B7-CD28 family in the control of T-cell immunity. *Nat Rev Immunol* 4:336–347.

Chen TC, Cobbold SP, Fairchild PJ, and Waldmann H. 2004. Generation of anergic and regulatory T cells following prolonged exposure to a harmless antigen. *J Immunol* 172:5900–5907.

Cho JH, Youn JW, and Sung YC. 2001. Cross-priming as a predominant mechanism for inducing CD8(+) T cell responses in gene gun DNA immunization. *J Immunol* 167:5549–5557.

Choate KA, Medalie DA, Morgan JR, and Khavari PA. 1996. Corrective gene transfer in the human skin disorder lamellar ichthyosis. *Nat (Med)* 2:1263–1267.

Chu AC and Morris JF. 2005. The keratinocyte. In *Skin Immune System: Cutaneous Immunology and Clinical Immunodermatology*, JD Bos, Ed. CRC Press, Boca Raton, FL, pp. 77–99.

Clark RA, Chong B, Mirchandani N, et al. 2006. The vast majority of CLA^+ T cells are resident in normal skin. *J Immunol* 176:4431–4439.

Cristillo AD, Lisziewicz J, He L, et al. 2007. HIV-1 prophylactic vaccine comprised of topical DermaVir prime and protein boost elicits cellular immune responses and controls pathogenic R5 SHIV162P3. *Virology* 366:197–211.

Del Rio M, Gache Y, Jorcano JL, Meneguzzi G, and Larcher F. 2004. Current approaches and perspectives in human keratinocyte-based gene therapies. *Gene Ther* 11(Suppl 1):S57–S63.

Du X, Zheng G, Jin H, et al. 2007. The adjuvant effects of co-stimulatory molecules on cellular and memory responses to HBsAg DNA vaccination. *J Gene Med* 9:136–146.

Dudziak D, Kamphorst AO, Heidkamp GF, et al. 2007. Differential antigen processing by dendritic cell subsets in vivo. *Science* 315:107–111.

Feltquate DM, Heaney S, Webster RG, and Robinson HL. 1997. Different T helper cell types and antibody isotypes generated by saline and gene gun DNA immunization. *J Immunol* 158:2278–2284.

Fenjves ES, Gordon DA, Pershing LK, Williams DL, and Taichman LB. 1989. Systemic distribution of apolipoprotein E secreted by grafts of epidermal keratinocytes: Implications for epidermal function and gene therapy. *Proc Natl Acad Sci U S A* 86:8803–8807.

Ferrari S, Pellegrini G, Mavilio F, and De Luca M. 2005. Gene therapy approaches for epidermolysis bullosa. *Clin Dermatol* 23:430–436.

Ferry N, Duplessis O, Houssin D, Danos O, and Heard JM. 1991. Retroviral-mediated gene transfer into hepatocytes in vivo. *Proc Natl Acad Sci U S A* 88:8377–8381.

Finger EB and Bluestone JA. 2002. When ligand becomes receptor: tolerance via B7 signaling on DCs. *Nat Immunol* 3:1056–1057.

Frauwirth KA and Thompson CB. 2002. Activation and inhibition of lymphocytes by costimulation. *J Clin Invest* 109:295–299.

Ghazizadeh S. 2007. Controlling transgene-specific immune responses in cutaneous gene therapy. *J Invest Dermatol* 127:S92.

Ghazizadeh S and Taichman LB. 2000. Virus-mediated gene transfer for cutaneous gene therapy. *Hum Gene Ther* 11:2247–2251.

Ghazizadeh S and Taichman LB. 2005. Organization of stem cells and their progeny in human epidermis. *J Invest Dermatol* 124:367–372.

Ghazizadeh S, Harrington R, and Taichman LB. 1999. In vivo transduction of mouse epidermis with recombinant retroviral vectors: implications for cutaneous gene therapy. *Gene Ther* 6:1267–1275.

Ghazizadeh S, Doumeng C, and Taichman LB. 2002. Durable and stratum-specific gene expression in epidermis. *Gene Ther* 9:1278–1285.

Ghazizadeh S, Kalish RS, and Taichman LB. 2003. Immune-mediated loss of transgene expression in skin: implications for cutaneous gene therapy. *Mol Ther* 7:296–303.

Goto M, Sawamura D, Ito K, et al. 2006. Fibroblasts show more potential as target cells than keratinocytes in COL7A1 gene therapy of dystrophic epidermolysis bullosa. *J Invest Dermatol* 126:766–772.

Greenwald RJ, Freeman GJ, and Sharpe AH. 2005. The B7 family revisited. *Annu Rev Immunol* 23:515–548.

Grohmann U, Orabona C, Fallarino F, et al. 2002. CTLA-4-Ig regulates tryptophan catabolism in vivo. *Nat Immunol* 3:1097–1101.

He Y and Falo LD. 2006. Induction of T cell immunity by cutaneous genetic immunization with recombinant lentivector. *Immunol Res* 36:101–117.

Heath WR and Carbone FR. 2001a. Cross-presentation in viral immunity and self-tolerance. *Nat Rev Immunol* 1:126–134.

Heath WR and Carbone FR. 2001b. Cross-presentation, dendritic cells, tolerance and immunity. *Annu Rev Immunol* 19:47–64.

Heath WR, Belz GT, Behrens GM, et al. 2004. Cross-presentation, dendritic cell subsets, and the generation of immunity to cellular antigens. *Immunol Rev* 199:9–26.

Hengge UR. 2006. Gene therapy progress and prospects: the skin: easily accessible, but still far away. *Gene Ther* 13:1555–1563.

Hirata S, Senju S, Matsuyoshi H, Fukuma D, Uemura Y, and Nishimura Y. 2005. Prevention of experimental autoimmune encephalomyelitis by transfer of embryonic stem cell–derived dendritic cells expressing myelin oligodendrocyte glycoprotein peptide along with TRAIL or programmed death-1 ligand. *J Immunol* 174:1888–1897.

Janeway CA Jr. 1992. The immune system evolved to discriminate infectious nonself from noninfectious self. *Immunol Today* 13:11–16.

Jones ND, Turvey SE, Van Maurik A, et al. 2001. Differential susceptibility of heart, skin, and islet allografts to T cell–mediated rejection. *J Immunol* 166:2824–2830.

Kay M, Rothenberg S, Landen CN, et al. 1993a. In vivo gene therapy of hemophilia B: sustained partial correction in factor IX–deficient dogs. *Science* 262:117–119.

Kay MA, Rothenberg S, Landen CN, et al. 1993b. In vivo gene therapy of hemophilia B: sustained partial correction in factor IX–deficient dogs. *Science* 262:117–119.

Keir ME and Sharpe AH. 2005. The B7/CD28 costimulatory family in autoimmunity. *Immunol Rev* 204:128–143.

Keir ME, Liang SC, Guleria I, et al. 2006. Tissue expression of PD-L1 mediates peripheral T cell tolerance. *J Exp Med* 203:883–895.

Keir ME, Francisco LM, and Sharpe AH. 2007. PD-1 and its ligands in T-cell immunity. *Curr Opin Immunol* 19:309–314.

Kishimoto K, Dong VM, Issazadeh S, et al. 2000. The role of CD154-CD40 versus CD28-B7 costimulatory pathways in regulating allogeneic Th1 and Th2 responses in vivo. *J Clin Invest* 106:63–72.

Krueger GG. 2000. Fibroblasts and dermal gene therapy: a minireview. *Hum Gene Ther* 11:2289–2296.

Kupper TS and Fuhlbrigge RC. 2004. Immune surveillance in the skin: mechanism and clinical consequences. *Nat Rev Immunol* 4:211–222.

Larregina AT and Falo LDJ. 2000. Generating and regulating immune responses through cutaneous gene delivery. *Hum Gene Ther* 11:2301–2305.

Lauterbach H, Gruber A, Ried C, Cheminay C, and Brocker T. 2006. Insufficient APC capacities of dendritic cells in gene gun-mediated DNA vaccination. *J Immunol* 176:4600–4607.

Lechler R, Ng WF, and Steinman RM. 2001. Dendritic cells in transplantation: friend or foe? *Immunity* 14:357–368.

Lenschow DJ, Zeng Y, Thistlethwaite JR, et al. 1992. Long-term survival of xenogeneic pancreatic islet grafts induced by CTLA4lg. *Science* 257:789–792.

Li Y, Tredget EE, Kilani RT, et al. 2004. Expression of indoleamine 2,3-dioxygenase in dermal fibroblasts functions as a local immunosuppressive factor. *J Invest Dermatol* 122:953–964.

Linsley PS, Wallace PM, Johnson J, et al. 1992. Immunosuppression in vivo by a soluble form of the CTLA-4 T cell activation molecule. *Science* 257:792–795.

Lisziewicz J, Trocio J, Whitman L, et al. 2005. DermaVir: a novel topical vaccine for HIV/AIDS. *J Invest Dermatol* 124:160–169.

Lu Z and Ghazizadeh S. 2005. Host immune responses in ex vivo approaches to cutaneous gene therapy targeted to keratinocytes. *Exp Dermatol* 14:727–735.

Lu Z and Ghazizadeh S. 2007. Loss of transgene following ex vivo gene transfer is associated with a dominant Th2 response: implications for cutaneous gene therapy. *Mol Ther* 15:954–961.

Marchetto MC, Muotri AR, Burns DK, Friedberg EC, and Menck CFM. 2004. Gene transduction in skin cells: preventing cancer in xeroderma pigmentosum mice. *Proc Natl Acad Sci U S A* 101:17759–17764.

Matzinger P. 1994. Tolerance, danger, and the extended family. *Annu Rev Immunol* 12:991–1045.

Mavilio F, Pellegrini G, Ferrari S, et al. 2006. Correction of junctional epidermolysis bullosa by transplantation of genetically modified epidermal stem cells. *Nat Med* 12:1397–1402.

Mayerova D, Parke EA, Bursch LS, Odumade OA, and Hogquist KA. 2004. Langerhans cells activate naive self-antigen-specific CD8T cells in the steady state. *Immunity* 21:391–400.

McLellan AD, Sorg RV, Fearnley DB, et al. 1997. T lymphocyte mediated regulation of costimulator molecule expression on human dendritic cells. *Adv Exp Med Biol* 417:203–206.

Mellman I and Steinman RM. 2001. Dendritic cells: specialized and regulated antigen processing machines. *Cell* 106:255–258.

Mellor AL and Munn DH. 2003. Tryptophan catabolism and regulation of adaptive immunity. *J Immunol* 170:5809.

Monk NJ, Hargreaves REG, Marsh JE, et al. 2003. Fc-dependent depletion of activated T cells occurs through CD40L-specific antibody rather than costimulation blockade. *Nat Med* 9:1275–1280.

Morel PA, Falkner D, Plowey J, Larregina AT, and Falo J. 2004. DNA immunisation: altering the cellular localisation of expressed protein and the immunisation route allows manipulation of the immune response. *Vaccine* 22:447–456.

Munn DH and Mellor AL. 2007. Indoleamine 2,3-dioxygenase and tumor-induced tolerance. *J Clin Invest* 117:1147–1154.

Ohyama M, Ota T, Aoki M, et al. 2003. Suppression of the immune response against exogenous desmoglein 3 in desmoglein 3 knockout mice: an implication for gene therapy. *J Invest Dermatol* 120:610–615.

Ortiz-Urda S, Thyagarajan B, Keene DR, Lin Q, Calos MP, and Khavari PA. 2003. C31 Integrase-mediated nonviral genetic correction of junctional epidermolysis bullosa. *Hum Gene Ther* 14:923–928.

Quezada SA, Jarvinen LZ, Lind EF, and Noelle RJ. 2004. CD40/CD154 interactions at the interface of tolerance and immunity. *Annu Rev Immunol* 22:307–328.

Richters CD, Hoekstra MJ, du Pont JS, Kreis RW, and Kamperdijk EWA. 2005. Immunology of skin transplantation. *Clin Dermatol* 23:338–342.

Rocha PN, Plumb TJ, Crowley SD, and Coffman TM. 2003. Effector mechanisms in transplant rejection. *Immunol Rev* 196:51–64.

Sato Y, Roman M, Tighe H, et al. 1996. Immunostimulatory DNA sequences necessary for effective intradermal gene immunization. *Science* 273:352–354.

Shibaki A, Sato A, Vogel JC, Miyagawa F, and Katz SI. 2004. Induction of GVHD-like skin disease by passively transferred $CD8^+$ T cell receptor transgenic T cells into keratin 14-ovalbumin transgenic mice. *J Invest Dermatol* 123:109–115.

Steinman RM, Hawiger D, and Nussenzweig MC. 2003. Tolerogenic dendritic cells. *Annu Rev Immunol* 21:685–711.

Stockschlader MA, Schuening FG, Graham TC, and Storb R. 1994. Transplantation of retrovirus-transduced canine keratinocytes expressing the β-galactosidase gene. *Gene Ther* 1:317–322.

Streilein JW. 1990. Skin-associated lymphoid tissues (SALT): the next generation. In *Skin Immune System*, JD Bos, Ed. CRC Press, Boca Raton, FL, pp. 25–48.

Taichman LB. 1999. Systemic replacement therapy from genetically modified epidermal keratinocytes. *Proc Assoc Am Physicians* 111:206–210.

Tan PH, Beutelspacher SC, Xue SA, et al. 2005. Modulation of human dendritic-cell function following transduction with viral vectors: implications for gene therapy. *Blood* 105:3824–3832.

Uitto J and Pulkkinen L. 2000. The genodermatoses: candidate diseases for gene therapy. *Hum Gene Ther* 11:2267–2275.

Varmus H. 1988. Retroviruses. *Science* 240:1427–1435.

Vogel JC. 2000. Nonviral skin gene therapy. *Hum Gene Ther* 11:2253–2259.

Waldmann H. 2006. Immunology: protection and privilege. *Nature* 442:987–988.

Woodley DT, Krueger GG, Jorgensen CM, et al. 2003. Normal and gene-corrected dystrophic epidermolysis bullosa fibroblasts alone can produce type VII collagen at the basement membrane zone. *J Invest Dermatol* 121:1021–1028.

Woodley DT, Keene DR, Atha T, et al. 2004. Intradermal injection of lentiviral vectors corrects regenerated human dystrophic epidermolysis bullosa skin tissue in vivo. *Mol Ther* 10:318–326.

Woodley DT, Remington J, Huang Y, et al. 2007. Intravenously injected human fibroblasts home to skin wounds, deliver type VII collagen, and promote wound healing. *Mol Ther* 15:628–635.

Yamashita K, Masunaga T, Yanagida N, et al. 2003. Long-term acceptance of rat cardiac allografts on the basis of adenovirus mediated CD40Ig plus CTLA4Ig gene therapies. *Transplant* 76:1089–1096.

11

IMMUNE RESPONSES TO PULMONARY GENE THERAPY

CHRISTIAN MÜLLER, PH.D., AND TERENCE R. FLOTTE, M.D.

Department of Pediatrics, University of Massachusetts Medical School, Worcester, Massachusetts

11.1 INTRODUCTION

The lung is a crucial target organ for gene therapy since this organ is associated with the pathophysiology of monogenetic disorders such as cystic fibrosis, α1-antitrypsin deficiency, and polygenic disorders such as acute respiratory

Gene Therapy Immunology, Edited by Roland Herzog

distress syndrome (ARDS), asthma, and chronic obstructive pulmonary disease (COPD), among others. The latter chronic inflammatory diseases result from an imbalance in immune responses of the lung. Immunomodulatory gene therapy could potentially help to attenuate these imbalances and reestablish a homeostatic immune environment. Similarly, gene therapy can be suited to target lung cancers by using a tumor-associated antigen to target a specific cell population where gene therapy vectors target the cancerous cells with suicide genes or transgenes that promote an immune response. The accessibility of the lungs to gene transfer vectors through the airways and vasculature makes it potentially attractive for gene therapy. However, there is one aspect of this accessibility that has made pulmonary gene therapy more challenging than originally anticipated. The lung's defense mechanisms allow it to "manage" and effectively neutralize potential harmful particles from its day-to-day contact with the environment. Once delivered to the lung, gene therapy vectors encounter highly evolved defenses that continually clear allergens, viruses, bacteria, and other foreign particles. Despite the many studies that have demonstrated the feasibility of gene transfer to the lung, the therapeutic potential in humans has failed to meet the expectations of clinicians and patients. Although many advances have been made in delivery methods and overall vector design, significant limitations are imposed by the lung's natural defenses. The purpose of this chapter is to review the current understanding of the immune mechanisms in play during pulmonary gene therapy and to summarize the different immune responses elicited by various gene transfer agents tested in the lung.

11.2 THE LUNG

The lung is a complex organ that forms a substantial boundary between the external environment and the blood. The surface area of this interface in adults is estimated to be between 70 and 90 m^2, roughly the size of a tennis court [Effros et al. 1997]. The large surface area is needed to enable the alveolar membrane of the lung to take up oxygen efficiently and eliminate carbon dioxide. As a result of this immense interface with the environment, the lung has evolved various mechanisms to deal with the burden of foreign particles inspired on a daily basis. These range from mechanical barriers to innate and adaptive immune systems. The most basic of these mechanisms are anatomical barriers. These include the production of mucus, the beating of cilia on the respiratory epithelial cells, and the cough reflex, which all combine to create the highly effective mucociliary escalator. The nasopharyngeal barriers prevent the penetration into the lower airways of particles larger than 2 to 3 μm. These particles are trapped in the mucus and are then processed by the host's immune defense mechanisms.

11.3 INNATE IMMUNE RESPONSES AND THE MUCOCILIARY APPARATUS

The innate system is an older immune system, which is always active and is able to mount immediate responses by recognizing microbial and viral products entering the lung in a non-antigen-specific manner. This system is composed of mucins, humoral response elements such as soluble factors that include surfactant proteins, lectin-binding protein, C3b, and cellular responses orchestrated by macrophages and neutrophils.

Particles that are carried into the conducting airways get trapped onto the mucociliary surface of the airways. This is one of the first barriers encountered by inhaled pathogens. The extracellular mucus coats the ciliated epithelium of the lung. The upward beat of the cilia assists the mucociliary escalator to transport particles from the terminal bronchioles to the trachea at speeds varying between 100 and 30 $\mu m\ s^{-1}$, where the particles eventually exit the lungs by coughing or swallowing [Sleigh 1983; Sleigh et al. 1988]. This mucociliary apparatus in the airway surface liquid (ASL) consists of the low-viscosity sol phase, also known as the periciliary liquid, which is about 5 to 10 μm thick. This phase allows the cilia to beat and the high-viscosity gel phase (2 to 20 μm) to flow on top of it to create the transport mechanism (Fig. 11-1). The major components of the mucus are mucoglycoproteins and proteoglycans that are produced and secreted from surface goblet cells and submucosal glands. The high carbohydrate content and intrinsic hydrophilic and negatively charged nature of these proteins provide the physical viscosity of mucus and its ability to bind inspired particles. The dense mucuslike mixture of carbohydrates, glycoproteins, and polysaccharides has also been termed the glycocalyx (Fig. 11-1).

Of the nine mucins identified to date, MUC1 is of special interest to gene therapy researchers. Unlike other mucins, this extensively sialylated transmembrane protein is anchored to airway epithelial cells by a hydrophobic domain linked to a bound 69-amino acid cytoplasmic tail. This mucin extends far out above the apical membrane, where it is thought to interfere with cell-to-cell contact by hindering integrin binding. Such properties help the lung restrict the binding of potential pathogens, such as bacteria and viruses, which require binding to the airway surface before they are able to penetrate the epithelium. Adenoviral vectors enter epithelial cells with the help of integrins after their initial binding to the coxsackievirus and adenovirus receptor and thus are susceptible to steric inhibition by MUC1. Arcasoy et al. [1997] have shown that MUC1 had inhibitory effects on the binding of adenovirus to primary bronchial epithelia cells. This inhibitory effect was reversed upon the addition of neuroaminidase to remove the sialic residues from the MUC1-expressing epithelial cells. In other studies, Pickles et al. [2000] have determined that the glycocalyx and mucociliary clearance are two significant innate barriers limiting vector exposure to the epithelial

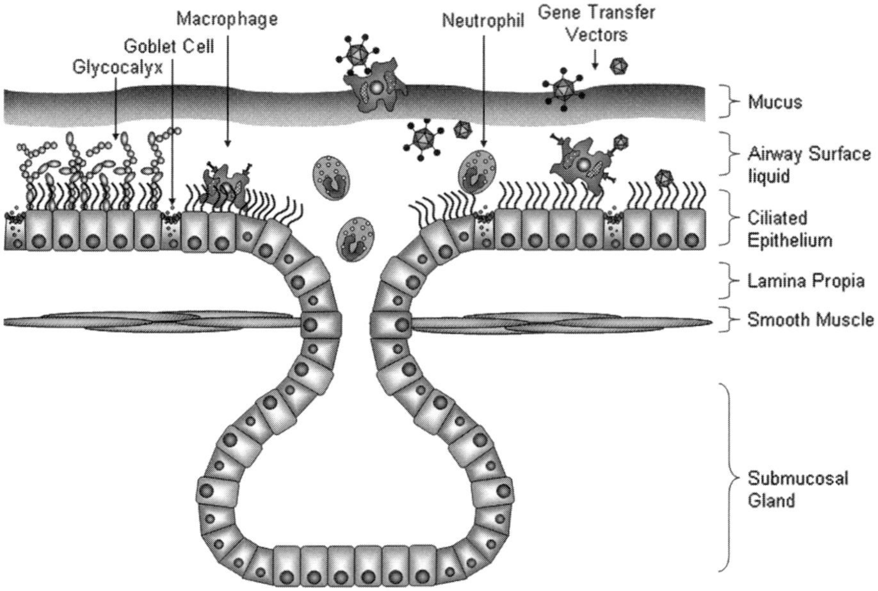

Figure 11-1 In the large conducting airways the pseudostratified epithelial cells are covered by a thick layer of mucus that rides on the airway surface liquid (ASL) layer. The ASL normally exists in two phases: a low-viscosity sol phase, which occupies the periciliary space, and a high-viscosity gel phase, which contains the mucins. A mucociliary escalator is created when cilia on the surface of the epithelial cells beat upward within the sol phase, allowing the gel phase and mucus to ride on top. The ASL is made up of antimicrobial proteins and defensins such as lysozyme and lactoferrin. Resident neutrophils and macrophages are also found in this layer, along with the carbohydrate-rich glycocalyx.

surface. By holding the viral vectors at a distance from the epithelium, the glycocalyx offers the alveolar macrophages the opportunity to ingest and destroy the virus. More recent studies highlight the fact that hypoosmotic permeabilization of the glycocalyx allows viral vectors increased access to the tight junctions and epithelium, thereby increasing their uptake [Rudolph et al. 2005].

11.3.1 Soluble Proteins and Pattern Recognition Receptors

Important soluble proteins contributing to lung defenses are carried within the mucus. Among these constituents in the conducting airways are lysozyme, a muramidase that degrades glycosidic linkage of bacterial membranes, and lactoferrin, which sequesters iron, limiting its availability for bacterial metabolism. Other important proteins include IgA, IgG, and defensins, which are antimicrobial peptides released by leukocytes and respiratory epithelial cells [Becker et al. 2000; Lehrer 2004]. Bronchoalveolar lavage (BAL) fluids of human patients also contain high levels of LPS-binding protein (LBP) and soluble CD14 [Dubin et al. 1996; Lin et al. 2004]. These are key molecules for the recognition of bacterial LPS by alveolar macrophages. LBP is produced by type II pneumocytes, while soluble CD14 is released from the surface of alveolar macrophages after protease digestion [Dentener et al. 2000].

An additional group of soluble proteins that are important in promoting phagocytosis of foreign particles by alveolar macrophages are the collectin family. Collectins (short for "collagen-binding lectins") are members of the C-type lectin superfamily. Collectins share a carbohydrate recognition domain that helps them recognize and bind to microorganisms. This interaction facilitates the adhesion and subsequent phagocytosis into alveolar macrophages after agglutination and opsonization [Hickling et al. 2004]. Each collectin can differ on the specificity of the microbial sugars they bind. The main members of this family involved in innate lung defense are surfactant protein A (SP-A), surfactant protein D (SP-D), and the mannose-binding lectin (MBL). SP-A and SP-D are produced by alveolar type II cells and Clara cells In addition to SP-A's and SP-D's surfactant properties, which lower the surface tension in the lung, they bind to organisms entering the pulmonary tree. This facilitates uptake of the organisms by alveolar macrophages. SP-A is composed of six trimeric units, resembling the structure of the complement component C1q, the trimeric units from homotrimers that oligomerize to form highly ordered structures. SP-A has been shown to bind gram-positive and gram-negative bacteria, yeasts, and viruses [Lawson and Reid 2000]. Specifically, it binds rough LPS, the glycoprotein of *Pneumocystis jiroveci*, and the outer membrane protein of *Haemophilus influenzae* as well as lipoarabinomanna from mycobacteria [Sano and Kuroki 2005]. Much of our understanding of SP-A was elucidated by a series of experiments conducted by Levine et al. in SP-A-knockout mice. In these experiments Levine showed that SP-A-knockout mice had decreased clearance of *H. influenzae* and *Pseudomonae aeruginosa*. The decreased clearance was tied to a reduction in bacterial uptake by alveolar macrophages. Reduced clearance of viral pathogens such as respiratory syncytial virus (RSV), influenza virus, and adenovirus has also been observed in these mice [Benne et al. 1997; Harrod et al. 1999]. The adenovirus is of considerable interest to the field of gene therapy since it is a commonly used viral vector for lung gene therapy. In addition to binding microbial antigens, SP-A can function to increase the production of reactive oxygen species in macrophages and alternatively, to attenuate the inflammatory process [Sano and Kuroki 2005]. Crouch et al. demonstrated that SP-A-knockout mice have higher inflammatory cytokine responses to infectious challenges compared to wild-type mice [Crouch and Wright 2001]. Additional roles for SP-A include reducing the inflammatory process by enhancing the phagocytosis of apoptotic neutrophils and increasing the secretion of the anti-inflammatory cytokine TGF-β [Reidy and Wright 2003].

SP-D has a different structure than SP-A, as it is composed of four trimers and more closely resembles bovine conglutinin. SP-D is also a pattern recognition receptor; however, less is known about this surfactant protein. It has been shown to bind mycobacterial lipoarabinomannan and *Mycoplasma pneumoniae*

[Sano and Kuroki 2005]. SP-D-knockout mice were found to have normal clearance rates for bacteria, but there was an increased severity of *Pneumocystis carinii* infection, leading to higher inflammatory responses and decreased survival [Atochina et al. 2004a–c]. Similarly, the clearance of RSV was shown to be reduced in SP-D knockouts by Levine et al. [2004]. This relationship with RSV is actually seen in humans, as certain SP-D polymorphsims have been associated with increased neonatal RSV infection in the clinic [Lahti et al. 2002].

A third member of the collectin family is the mannose-binding lectin (MBL). In addition to binding the clareticulin receptor to increase monocyte activity, MBL acts as a direct opsonin by binding carbohydrate residues on microorganisms and has also been implicated in binding bacterial DNA [Palaniyar et al. 2003; Hickling et al. 2004]. MBL-deficient mice have increased susceptibility to fungal asthma [Hogaboam et al. 2004]. MBL polymorphisms act as modifier genes in cystic fibrosis and are associated with worsening of pulmonary disease [Gabolde et al. 1999].

As described above, the innate system relies heavily on soluble proteins being able to recognize pathogen-associated molecular patterns (PAMPs). An additional line of defense is provided by pattern recognition receptors (PRRs). These receptors allow a host to mount a quick immune response to specific patterns on foreign particles entering the lung. The most common of these receptors are the Toll-like receptors (TLRs), a highly conserved family of type 1 transmembrane domains. Their structure is characterized by an NH_2-terminal extracellular leucine-rich domain with a COOH–intracellular tail [Basu and Fenton 2004]. Their specificity is a function of the variability in the leucine-rich domain, while the signaling in the 10 mammalian TLRs discovered to date is mediated by a conserved intracellular domain and the MyD88 adaptor protein [Takeuchi et al. 2000; Takeda and Akira 2001]. The best characterized TLRs are TLR2 and TLR4, where lung inflammation in response to LPS on gram-negative bacteria is regulated by TLR4 and responses to lipotechoic acid on gram-positive bacteria are orchestrated by TLR2. For a comprehensive review of TLR function, the reader is referred to the review by Basu and Fenton [2004].

One important TLR to consider when using gene transfer agents is TLR9; this receptor is responsible for the recognition of unmethylated cytosine–pyrimidine–guanine (CpG) island motifs on DNA from a bacterial origin. Bacterial-derived plasmid DNA is something that all gene therapy approaches have in common. Plasmid DNA used for gene transfer is usually derived from bacterial plasmid production systems, which will certainly contain unmethylated CpG dinucleotide sequences. On the other hand, eukaryotic DNA tends to have methylated cytosines and far fewer CpG dinucleotide repeats. Recognition by TLR9 of bacterially derived plasmid DNA is particularly an issue for nonviral gene transfer, where the DNA is not encapsulated. Early indications of inflammatory reactions mediated by TLR9 were observed in CF clinical trials using aerosolized liposomes and cationic lipids containing bacterially derived plasmid DNA [Chadwick et al. 1997; Alton et al. 1999; Krieg 2002]. Clearly, the innate immune system may be encountered by both viral and nonviral gene transfer agents. The presence of carbohydrate motifs on viral vectors and the exposed bacterially derived DNA on nonviral delivery agents would be recognized and targeted by collectins and TLRs for opsonization or macrophage uptake.

11.3.2 Alveolar Macrophages

Alveolar macrophages make up about 85% of the cell populations recovered from BALs. These bone marrow–derived cells are the immune sentinels of the lung. Blood monocytes entering the lung compartment differentiate into mature macrophages and take residence in alveoli and alveolar ducts, where they accumulate in concentrations of 50 to 100 cells per alveolus. Their location and overwhelming presence make them most likely to be the first cells encountered by particles entering the lung. These cells are usually the only phagocytic cells present in the lower airways, which is why the alveolar macrophage plays a crucial role in innate lung defense. They avidly phagocytose inspired particles and bacteria. As mentioned above, their ability to interact with microbes is mediated by surface receptors that recognize lipopolysaccharides, polysaccharides, complement proteins, and pathogens tagged with collectins, such as MBL, LBP, SP-A, and SP-D. Once ingested the microbes are targeted to the phagolysosomal compartment for digestion. The bactericidal properties of alveolar macrophages are a result of lysozyme, reactive oxygen intermediates such as superoxide anions, hydrogen peroxide, and hydroxyl radicals. In addition to their scavenging properties, macrophages can initiate local immune responses. They initiate inflammation through the release of IL-1α, IL-β, and TNF-α, which in turn leads to a release of IL-8 and GM-CSF and up-regulation of adhesion molecules on epithelial cells [Nicod 1999]. Just as efficiently, they are also responsible for maintaining lung homeostasis by actively suppressing T-cell proliferation [Holt 1993a,b; Thepen et al. 1994]. They accomplish this by releasing TNF-soluble receptors, IL-1 receptor antagonists, prostaglandins, nitric oxide, and IL-10, thereby inhibiting the development of acquired immune response to innocuous inspired antigens [Nicod et al. 1995]. For example, the ability of macrophages to suppress T-cell proliferation is crucial in the prevention of sensitization to allergens that would lead to asthma. Ultimately, macrophages are also responsible for lung remodeling and repair. Through cytokine regulation macrophages can express metalloelasteases, metalloproteases, and collagenase and can then remodel the matrix by fibrin deposition and release of fibroblast growth factors [Lacraz et al. 1994a,b].

Due to the avid scavenging nature and wide distribution of alveolar macrophages, it is not surprising that they may ultimately be responsible for the uptake and destruction of many gene transfer agents entering the lung. Kuzmin et al. [1997] demonstrated this elegantly when examining adenoviral gene transfer to the lung. They depleted macrophages from the lung by delivering dichloromethylene diphosphate to the lung, where it accumulates inside alveolar macrophages, eventually leading them to undergo apoptosis. In doing so, Kuzmin et al. were able to increase the persistence of adenovirus vector genomes and transgene expression in lung epithelial cells. These results help highlight the fact that alveolar macrophages represent an important barrier to gene transfer in the lung. Lung gene therapy would be greatly served by transient macrophage suppression or gene transfer agents that can bypass macrophage uptake and degradation.

11.4 ADAPTIVE IMMUNE RESPONSES

Whereas innate immune responses are immediate and may be responsible for effectively blocking and preventing transduction of lung tissue by gene transfer agents, acquired immune responses are responsible for clearing transduced cells and preventing readministration of gene transfer agents. These effects fall along the lines of the cell-mediated immune responses, specifically those directed at cells expressing viral or transgene proteins, eventually clearing transduced cells. At the other end of the adaptive response spectrum are humoral immune responses directed at viral vector capsid proteins or ligands and peptides on molecular conjugates, effectively neutralizing the repeated administration of gene therapy transfer agents.

11.4.1 Cellular Immune Responses

About 10% of the cells in the normal alveolus are lymphocytes, of which 50% are CD4, 30% CD8, 15% killer and natural killer (NK) cells, and 5% B cells. Cell-mediated responses are carried out by $CD8^+$ cells and are crucial for the lung's defense against pulmonary viral infections. These responses are initiated by dendritic cells that have either been infected or become associated with viral-infected cells and have been activated with the help of TLR stimulation or pro-inflammatory cytokines. These cells then home to the draining lymph nodes or locally to bronchus-associated lymphoid tissues (BALTs), where they increase the expression of co-stimulatory molecules and process the viral proteins in peptide fragments for presentation via the MHC molecules [Sallusto et al. 2000]. Importantly for lung host responses, this activation of dendritic cells (DCs) is divided into two phenotypes. Myeloid DCs express TLR4, TLR1, TLR2, and TLR3, which endow them with the ability to respond to LPS, mycopeptides, and viral RNA by producing IL-12. On the other hand, plasmacytoid DCs express TLR9 and TLR7, which permit them to respond to bacterial DNA and viruses by producing IFN-α [Ardavin 2003; Leon et al. 2004; Liu 2005]. Equally important is the context of the MHC molecule presentation. Peptide fragments presented in the draining lymph nodes on MHC class I are recognized by $CD8^+$ cytotoxic lymphocytes (CTL). $CD8^+$ cytotoxic lymphocytes are effectively activated if the MHC class I presentation is accompanied by a second signal, usually provided by co-stimulatory molecules. Once activated, $CD8^+$ cells migrate back to the lung, where they target infected cells presenting specific pathogen peptides on their cell surface. Antigen-specific CD8 CTLs appear in the lung parenchyma within a week after viral infection [Wyde and Cate 1978].

It is this antigen-specific lysis that presents a challenge for gene therapy, because if viral vectors induce such a response, all the therapeutically transduced cells are quickly eradicated. This is especially true in replication-competent vectors, where the antigenic peptide is continually produced. It is important to note that not only can viral antigens elicit such responses, but as is the case in many gene therapy approaches, the transgenes themselves can be immunogenic. This is particularly true in diseases involving the absence of protein translation or premature stop codons, where T cells directed against these novel antigens were not deleted during thymic development.

11.4.2 Humoral Immune Responses

Much in the same way in which CD8 CTL responses are initiated, humoral CD4 T-cell responses originate in the draining lymph nodes or BALTs with an activated DC. The difference is the context of the peptide presentation. Pathogen-associated peptides that are proteolyticaly processed and presented on MHC class II peptides are recognized by CD4 T helper cells. These cells can mount dichotomous mutually inhibitory types of responses. They have been termed T helper 1 (Th1) and T helper 2 (Th2) responses based mostly on their cytokine-secreting profiles. Type 1 responses have a cytokine profile that includes IFN-γ, IL-2, TNF-α, and GM-CSF and are responsible for activating macrophages to kill intracellular pathogens such as *Mycobacterium tuberculosis*. In addition, Th1 responses also promote the production of IgG2a. Alveolar macrophages depend on CD4 Th1 T cells in order to activate their STAT1-dependent effector mechanism [Punturieri et al. 2004]. Individual microbial antigens may favor the development of either Th1 or Th2 responses. For example, IL-12 secreted by infected macrophages helps create an environment that favors the development of Th1 responses [Hsieh et al. 1993; Ferrick et al. 1995]. On the other hand, Th2 CD4 T cells secrete IL-4, IL-13, IL-5, IL-9, and IL-10. These responses serve to down-regulate type 1–associated inflammation but can also lead to fibrosis [Jakubzick et al. 2004; Kaufman et al. 2004]. More important, Th2 responses favor B-cell antibody class isotype switching from IgM to IgE, IgA, IgG1, and IgG4 and the growth and maturation of eosinophils and basophils. It is this arm of the $CD4^{+}$T-cell responses that directs the production of neutralizing antibodies (NABs) against viral vectors or peptide molecular conjugates used for gene therapy. This effectively prevents the administration of gene transfer agents that have elicited NAB formation. This barrier to gene therapy is not only observed upon readministration of gene transfer agents but also the patients will often have naturally occurring NABs to the viral vectors, due to prior exposure to the wild-type viruses from which the vectors are derived, effectively rendering the first administration inefficient.

11.5 PULMONARY VIRAL GENE TRANSFER

11.5.1 Adenovirus

Adenovirus is a nonenveloped DNA virus with a genome between 36 and 40 kb. Most of the adenovirus that has been used for recombinant gene therapy vectors is based on serotypes 2 and 5. It is known that the viral capsid interacts with the coxsackievirus adenovirus receptor (CAR) as an initial binding step followed by secondary engagement of the integrin co-receptors $\alpha5\beta1$, $\alpha\nu\beta3$, $\alpha\nu\beta5$, and $\alpha M\beta2$. It then enters the cells and escapes the endosome, after which it enters the nucleus via microtubules using nuclear pore complexes to inject its genome. Adenovirus is naturally associated with infectious diseases such as upper respiratory infections and conjunctivitis and can cause liver, kidney, and urinary tract infections. Thus, it is not surprising that adenovirus can infect successfully a wide variety of cells, including respiratory epithelial cells, myoblasts, macrophages, hepatocytes, and glial cells [Engelhardt et al. 1994; Horellou et al. 1994; Ghadge et al. 1995]. Serological testing revealed that 55% of North Americans have NABs to adenovirus type 5 [Chirmule et al. 1999]. Adenovirus vectors are known to elicit Th1 and Th2 immunogenic responses and to cause inflammation as well as cytotoxicity [Brody et al. 1994; Yang et al. 1995]. More specifically, mice studies have shown that adenovirus-mediated gene transfer to the lung elicited both Th1 and Th2 responses, characterized by the enhanced production of IgG1, IgG2a, and IgA antibodies [van Ginkel et al. 1995, 1997].

Although adenoviral vector–mediated transfer to the lung epithelium is moderately efficient, gene expression is only transient [Zabner et al. 1994]. In an effort to reduce immunogenicity, the viral gene products E1A and E1B were deleted from the first-generation adenoviral vectors, thus creating replication-deficient vectors. The idea was to limit the amount of viral proteins being produced after vector delivery and to expand the packaging capacity of the vector. Yang et al. [1994a,b] reported that this second generation still elicited cellular immunity, so they were modified further to delete the E2A, E3, and E4 genes. Clinical trials conducted with these adenoviral vectors delivering the CFTR gene to six CF patients achieved a dose-dependent, although transient (30 days) CFTR expression [Crystal et al. 1994]. Moreover, readministration of the vector did not achieve the original CFTR expression levels, and no expression was observed with the third administration. The transient nature of expression and the decrease in expression with successive administrations indicate both cellular and humoral adaptive immune responses to the adenoviral vector. Similar findings were seen in a study involving 11 CF patients using adenoviral vectors devoid of the E1 and E4 genes. The expression after delivery was low and sustained only for 42 days. In this study, adenovirus-specific CD8 T cells were recorded in the majority of the subjects [Zuckerman et al. 1999]. Further modifications of the adenoviral vectors with the deletion of all viral gene products termed helper-dependent adenoviral vectors have been generated, although there are difficulties in large-scale production and helper virus contamination [Morsy et al. 1998; Amalfitano and

Parks 2002; Koehler et al. 2005, 2006; Palmer and Ng 2005; Brunetti-Pierri et al. 2006; Flotte et al. 2007].

"Stealth" adenoviral vectors were created by steric coating of adenovirus with polyethylene glycol, and intratracheal delivery of these vectors had markedly reduced NAB and T-cell responses [Croyle et al. 2001]. Other strategies being used to reduce the immonogenicity of the vectors are the use of serotypes not prevalent in the human population, as well as transient immunosupression at the time of administration. Blocking of co-stimulation has been shown to inhibit the activation of T cells in various animal models of gene therapy. In this respect, CTLA4-Ig and anti-CD40 ligand, which block the interactions of B7-CD80/86 and CD40-CD40L, have demonstrated the ability to reduce the adenovirus-specific T-cell and humoral responses in the lung and liver of mice, and even permitting readministration of viral vectors [Yang et al. 1996a,b; Kay et al. 1997; Jooss et al. 1998].

11.5.2 Adeno-associated Virus

Adeno-associated virus (AAV) is a member of the Dependovirus family and the Parvovirinae subfamily. This helper-dependent parvovirus has a single-stranded DNA genome of 4.7 kb that is flanked by 145-nt palindromic GC-rich inverted terminal repeats (ITRs) [Berns and Giraud 1996]. Wild-type AAV2 can uniquely integrate into a site termed AAVS1 on the q arm of human chromosome 19 [Kotin et al. 1990]. The virion is a naked nonenveloped icosahedron, approximately 25 nm in size consisting of three capsid proteins co-linearly encoded but with alternate translational starting sites (VP1,VP2, and VP3). The use of overlapping reading frames to encode its capsid proteins maximizes the relatively limited packaging space of the virion but also creates a smaller number of epitopes that immune cells can target. Unfortunately, this also allows for varying degrees of cross-neutralization among different serotypes [Gao et al. 2002]. Recombinant AAV (rAAV) vectors are manufactured by removing all of the viral ORFs and replacing them with the transgene of interest flanked only by the ITRs. This leaves the expressed transgene and the input capsid as the only potential immunogenic antigens. In comparison with other viral vectors, these features allow rAAV vectors to have a low immunogenic profile. One additional feature that makes this vector suitable for lung gene therapy is the ability to transduce nondividing as well as dividing cell populations efficiently and has led to sustained expression of one or more years [Flotte et al. 1994; McCown et al. 1996; McKeon and Samulski 1996; Rubenstein et al. 1997].

A wide range of preclinical studies and a limited number of clinical trials all indicate that there is no detectable toxicity from administration of rAAV, even at the highest deliverable doses used to date. Expression profiling of infected cells with microarray analysis indicates that host cell gene expression is remarkably unperturbed after rAAV infection. While some humoral immune responses to the AAV capsid are observed, a series of studies indicate that cell-mediated immune responses to AAV are uncommon in the absence of adenovirus co-infection

[Hernandez et al. 1999]. Recombinant AAV–cystic fibrosis transmembrane conductance regulator (CFTR) vectors that have been developed for treatment of cystic fibrosis (CF) were tested in New Zealand white rabbits and in rhesus macaques by the endobronchial route [Flotte et al. 1993; Afione et al.1996; Conrad et al. 1996]. Vector DNA transfer and mRNA expression were detectable for more than six months in each instance without any indication of inflammation or any other toxicity. Studies in rhesus monkeys also indicated that the likelihood of rescue of rAAV by concomitant wild-type AAV and adenovirus infection was low [Afione et al. 1996]. In addition, delivery of rAAV2-CFTR to rhesus monkey lungs had no inflammatory effect on the lung, and CFTR mRNA was detected 180 days post-administration [Conrad et al. 1996]. These studies provided the preclinical data necessary for initiation of phase I clinical trials of rAAV in CF patients. AAV vectors have been demonstrated to be safe and effective in transferring CFTR cDNA to the respiratory and nasal epithelium of human patients [Wagner et al. 1998; Wang et al. 1999]. However, two studies of repeated aerosol dosing of rAAV encoding the complete human CFTR (tgAAVCF) showed clearly that neutralizing antibodies were raised, rendering subsequent doses ineffective for DNA transfer. In the larger study, 33% of the patients in the tgAAVCF and 31% of the placebo groups were positive for AAV2 NABs at baseline, after the first dose 59% in the tgAAV2CF group had a fourfold or greater rise in NAB compared with 2% in the placebo group. Even more after the second aerosolized dose 100% of the patients in the tgAAV2CF had serum AAV2 NAB levels rise fourfold or more compared with only 2% in the placebo group [Moss et al. 2004, 2007].

Although CTL responses have not been recorded for rAAV gene therapy targeting the lung, there is evidence that NABs to the viral capsid can limit rAAV transduction. In humans the presence of serum antibodies directed against AAV1, 2, 3, and 5 are common. For AAV1, 2, and 3, seroepidimiological studies determined that by age 10 they are present in about 60% of the population [Blacklow et al. 1971]. The dynamics of AAV5 are slightly different, with a peak of 50% of the population having antibodies by age 20 [Georg-Fries et al. 1984]. Importantly, not all the antibodies detected are NAB and there are still conflicting data from studies performed with AAV2-specific antibodies. In one of these studies, 96% of 74 human samples tested positive for AAV2 antibodies, but of these only 32% were effective at neutralizing AAV2 [Chirmule et al. 1999]. In a separate study, 80% of 32 samples were positive for AAV2 antibodies, of which 67% were NABs [Erles et al. 1999]. A third study by Moskalenko et al. found that 80% of 50 human samples were positive for AAV2 antibodies by ELISA, but only 18% were NABs [Moskalenko et al. 2000].

The effects that serum antibodies have specifically on lung delivery are equally conflicting. Studies performed on rAAV readministration in rabbits where NABs were formed after primary administration yielded no positively stained cells in the lung upon second administrations [Halbert et al. 1997]. On the contrary, a study using rAAV delivered GFP to rabbit lungs could detect expression following subsequent administration in the presence of circulating NABs [Beck et al. 1999].

11.6 PULMONARY NONVIRAL GENE TRANSFER

Although traditionally less efficient, nonviral gene transfer has been considered safer, noninfectious, and less immunogenic and thus a real alternative to viral gene transfer. Nonviral gene transfer can be as basic as naked DNA or employ the use of cationic polymers or cationic liposomes. The latter two offer significant advantages over naked DNA, which is inefficient in the lung and is rapidly degraded by the endonucleases found in the lung. To prevent the endonuclease degradation of naked DNA, plasmids have been complexed with either cationic liposomes or cationic polymers. These molecular complexes have resulted in more efficient gene transfer in the lung; however, they have proven to be less efficient and more transient than most viral vectors [Ziady et al. 2003a]. Moreover, in some cases these molecular complexes have unmasked host innate immune responses associated with the unmethylated cytosine–pyrimidine–guanine (CpG) repeats found in bacterially derived plasmid DNA. Thus, although a feasible alternative to viral vectors, these gene transfer agents are faced with unique obstacles.

11.6.1 Cationic Liposomes

Cationic liposomes have been studied in the lung as a nonviral gene transfer vector for treating cystic fibrosis. These delivery systems compromise cationic lipids that are usually mixed with cholesterol and dioleoylphophatidyl ethanolamine (DOPE). When mixed with DNA, they bind via electrostatic interaction and complex to form positively charged particles ranging from 100 to 500 nm in diameter, which can fuse with cell membranes and enter cells. The DNA–lipid complexes are then resistant to nuclease degradation and unlike viral vectors, offer no limit to the size of DNA that can be delivered. This makes liposomes attractive since tissue-specific promoters and locus control regions can be delivered along with the gene of interest, making gene expression of the therapeutic protein more biologically accurate. A number of studies have shown that cationic liposomes can mediate the transfection of epithelial cells in the lung. Cationic lipids include the formulation from Genzyme termed GL-67, which was shown to have 100-fold greater expression over other liposomes in the mouse lung [Lee et al. 1996]. Early studies by Scheule et al. [1997] in BALB/c mice revealed that GL-67 had in vivo toxicity associated with lung infiltration of neutrophils and to a lesser extent, macrophages and lymphocytes as well as elevated lung levels of the pro-inflammatory cytokines IL-6, TNF-α, and IFN-γ. Subsequent studies with GL-67 on humans have focused on CF patients. In one of the more successful studies, conducted by Alton et al. [1999], cationic liposomes containing the CFTR gene were delivered to CF patients by nasal perfusion. The study resulted in partial correction of nasal potential differences, a common measure associated with functional chloride secretion. However, CFTR expression could not be directly verified by the detection of CFTR mRNA. Unfortunately, patients in this study developed fever and increased levels of IL-6 after GL-67 administration. These side effects were attributed to innate inflammatory responses orchestrated by TLR 9 in response to the recognition of bacterially derived unmethylated CpG repeats. The immune response to GL-67 was further characterized in another study by Ruiz et al. [2001] in which he performed a dose escalation with aerosolized delivery. Patients in this study also responded with fever and increased serum levels of IL-6 as quickly as 1 hour after gene administration. They went on to determine that peripheral blood mononuclear cells taken from patients responded to plasmid DNA, and a more robust synergistic response was observed when plasmid DNA was complexed to GL-67. Interestingly, they also observed a milder response to GL-67 conjugated with eukaryotic DNA, suggesting that at least in part the immune response is independent of the unmethylated CpG repeats. Clearly, cationic liposomes need to be developed further to be considered workable in the clinical setting. Strategies that have been employed to reduce inflammatory outcomes include the reduction of nonessential CpG sequences or the use of chloroquine as an inhibitor of the CpG signaling pathway [Yew et al. 2000; Zhao et al. 2000].Alternatively, methylation of the CpG motifs, although successful at reducing inflammation, was also associated with a severe reduction in transgene expression [Yew et al. 1999].

11.6.2 Cationic Polymers

Another class of nonviral vectors used for gene therapy are cationic polymers such as poly-L-lysine (polyK), polyethyleneimine (PEI), and polyamidoamine dedrimers. In a fashion similar to cationic liposomes, polymers are able to condense DNA into small nuclease-resistant particles. Due to their net positive charge, the polymers can bind to cells via electrostatic interactions with the negatively charged membrane. In addition, PEI's endosomal release is facilitated because in branched form their amines act as proton sinks that cause endosomes to swell and burst [Boussif et al. 1995]. In mouse studies PEI vectors have been shown to localize to the lung preferentially after intravenous delivery. Transfection efficiency was 1 to 5% and restricted to the distal and branched airways close to the alveoli, including pneumocytes, endothelial cells, but few epithelial cells [Zou et al. 2000]. In contrast, aerosol delivery to mice lungs localized primarily to the epithelial cells [Gautam et al. 2001a,b]. Unfortunately, high-molecular-mass PEI complexes are not biodegradable; additionally, PEI's efficiency is tied to its ability to rupture endosomes, which has been shown to cause toxicity both in vitro and in vivo [Gebhart and Kabanov 2001; Chollet et al. 2002]. For these reasons, cationic polymer delivery has recently focused more on the use of polymers of L-amino acids such as polyK. An additional advantage is that these polymers can easily be conjugated with targeting peptides for cell-specific and enhanced uptake. Although manufacturing large quantities of peptides for large animals may be cost prohibitive, this approach has been used in mice. Specifically, the human CFTR gene was delivered to mouse lungs using polyK conjugated with a ligand to the serpin–enzyme complex receptor (SecR). This is a receptor found on hepatocytes, macrophages, and the apical surface of airway epithelia, which is responsible for binding and internalizing protease inhibitors once they have bound and inactivated their ligands. In these studies, although vector expression was transient (~12 days), Ziady et al. [2002] observed a partial correction in chloride secretion. Although immune responses to polyK were not observed, an antibody response to the SecR ligand was observed, hindering the possibility of readministration. Similar to the strategy used to create stealth adenoviral vectors, polyethylene glycol (PEG) has been used to modify the side chains of polyK. The results of this were twofold: The polyK complexes were stabilized in physiological saline instead of the usual 1 M NaCl solution, and additionally, PEG–polyK complexes were further protected from CpG-mediated immune responses and showed no toxicity in vivo (Ziady et al. 2003a;b]. These PEGylated polyK CFTR complexes were then delivered to the lower nasal airways of 12 CF patients in three escalating doses. Importantly, nasal potential difference correction was observed in eight of the 12 patients for up to six days, and no adverse events were associated with the treatment [Konstan et al. 2004].

11.7 CONCLUSIONS

The studies reviewed in this chapter highlight the significant immunological hurdles that have been met in the field of pulmonary gene therapy. Clearly, both physical and immunological defense mechanisms have to be resolved adequately before successful pulmonary gene therapy becomes a reality. The major challenges for viral gene therapy include viral pathogenicity and CTL clearance in the case of adenoviral vectors. Repeated administrations are crucial for diseases such as cystic fibrosis and α1-antitrypsin, and they are currently being hindered by NABs in most viral delivery methods. For nonviral gene transfer, issues with cell toxicity and CpG-mediated inflammation pose a significant barrier. Importantly, for all gene transfer agents the role of innate and adaptive immune responses in the airways need ongoing research to better define mechanisms at play and to develop methods to overcome them. Strategies to modulate and suppress the host immune responses transiently need to be investigated further to determine if they will eventually be clinically applicable.

REFERENCES

Afione SA, Conrad CK, et al. 1996. In vivo model of adeno-associated virus vector persistence and rescue. *J Virol* 70:3235–3241.

Alton EW, Stern M, et al. 1999. Cationic lipid-mediated CFTR gene transfer to the lungs and nose of patients with cystic fibrosis: a double-blind placebo-controlled trial. *Lancet* 353:947–954.

Amalfitano A and Parks RJ. 2002. Separating fact from fiction: assessing the potential of modified adenovirus vectors for use in human gene therapy. *Curr Gene Ther* 2:111–133.

Arcasoy SM, Latoche J, et al. 1997. MUC1 and other sialoglycoconjugates inhibit adenovirus-mediated gene transfer to epithelial cells. *Am J Respir Cell Mol Biol* 17:422–435.

Ardavin C. 2003. Origin, precursors and differentiation of mouse dendritic cells. *Nat Rev Immunol* 3:582–590.

Atochina EN, Beck JM, et al. 2004a. Enhanced lung injury and delayed clearance of *Pneumocystis carinii* in surfactant protein A-deficient mice: attenuation of cytokine responses and reactive oxygen–nitrogen species. *Infect Immun* 72:6002–6011.

Atochina EN, Beers MF, et al. 2004b. Surfactant protein-D, a mediator of innate lung immunity, alters the products of nitric oxide metabolism. *Am J Respir Cell Mol Biol* 30:271–279.

Atochina EN, Gow AJ, et al. 2004c. Delayed clearance of *Pneumocystis carinii* infection, increased inflammation, and altered nitric oxide metabolism in lungs of surfactant protein-D knockout mice. *J Infect Dis* 189:1528–1539.

Basu S and Fenton MJ. 2004. Toll-like receptors: function and roles in lung disease. *Am J Physiol Lung Cell Mol Physiol* 286:L887–L892.

Beck SE, Jones LA, et al. 1999. Repeated delivery of adeno-associated virus vectors to the rabbit airway. *J Virol* 73:9446–9455.

Becker MN, Diamond G, et al. 2000. CD14-dependent lipopolysaccharide-induced beta-defensin-2 expression in human tracheobronchial epithelium. *J Biol Chem* 275:29731–29736.

Benne CA, Benaissa-Trouw B, et al. 1997. Surfactant protein A, but not surfactant protein D, is an opsonin for influenza A virus phagocytosis by rat alveolar macrophages. *Eur J Immunol* 27:886–890.

Berns KI and Giraud C. 1996. Biology of adeno-associated virus. *Curr Top Microbiol Immunol* 218:1–23.

Blacklow NR, Hoggan MD, et al. 1971. A seroepidemiologic study of adenovirus-associated virus infection in infants and children. *Am J Epidemiol* 94:359–366.

Boussif O, Lezoualc'h F, et al. 1995. A versatile vector for gene and oligonucleotide transfer into cells in culture and in vivo: polyethylenimine. *Proc Natl Acad Sci U S A* 92:7297–7301.

Brody SL, Metzger M, et al. 1994. Acute responses of non-human primates to airway delivery of an adenovirus vector containing the human cystic fibrosis transmembrane conductance regulator cDNA. *Hum Gene Ther* 5:821–836.

Brunetti-Pierri N, Ng T, et al. 2006. Improved hepatic transduction, reduced systemic vector dissemination, and long-term transgene expression by delivering helper-dependent adenoviral vectors into the surgically isolated liver of nonhuman primates. *Hum Gene Ther* 17:391–404.

Chadwick SL, Kingston HD, et al. 1997. Safety of a single aerosol administration of escalating doses of the cationic lipid GL-67/DOPE/DMPE-PEG5000 formulation to the lungs of normal volunteers. *Gene Ther* 4:937–942.

Chirmule N, Propert K, et al. 1999. Immune responses to adenovirus and adeno-associated virus in humans. *Gene Ther* 6:1574–1583.

Chollet P, Favrot MC, et al. 2002. Side-effects of a systemic injection of linear polyethylenimine–DNA complexes. *J Gene Med* 4:84–91.

Conrad CK, Allen SS, et al. 1996. Safety of single-dose administration of an adeno-associated virus (AAV)-CFTR vector in the primate lung. *Gene Ther* 3:658–668.

Crouch E and Wright JR. 2001. Surfactant proteins a and d and pulmonary host defense. *Annu Rev Physiol* 63:521–554.

Croyle MA, Chirmule N, et al. 2001. "Stealth" adenoviruses blunt cell-mediated and humoral immune responses against the virus and allow for significant gene expression upon readministration in the lung. *J Virol* 75:4792–4801.

Crystal RG, McElvaney NG, et al. 1994. Administration of an adenovirus containing the human CFTR cDNA to the respiratory tract of individuals with cystic fibrosis. *Nat Genet* 8:42–51.

Dentener MA, Vreugdenhil AC, et al. 2000. Production of the acute-phase protein lipopolysaccharide–binding protein by respiratory type II epithelial cells: implications for local defense to bacterial endotoxins. *Am J Respir Cell Mol Biol* 23:146–153.

Dubin W, Martin TR, et al. 1996. Asthma and endotoxin: lipopolysaccharide-binding protein and soluble CD14 in bronchoalveolar compartment. *Am J Physiol* 270:L736–744.

Effros RM, Darin C, et al. 1997. Water transport and the distribution of aquaporin-1 in pulmonary air spaces. *J Appl Physiol* 83:1002–1016.

Engelhardt JF, Litzky L, et al. 1994. Prolonged transgene expression in cotton rat lung with recombinant adenoviruses defective in E2a. *Hum Gene Ther* 5:1217–1229.

Erles K, Sebokova P, et al. 1999. Update on the prevalence of serum antibodies (IgG and IgM) to adeno-associated virus (AAV). *J Med Virol* 59:406–411.

Ferrick DA, Schrenzel MD, et al. 1995. Differential production of interferon-gamma and interleukin-4 in response to Th1- and Th2-stimulating pathogens by gamma delta T cells in vivo. *Nature* 373:255–257.

Flotte TR, Afione SA, et al. 1993. Stable in vivo expression of the cystic fibrosis transmembrane conductance regulator with an adeno-associated virus vector. *Proc Natl Acad Sci U S A* 90(22):10613–10617.

Flotte TR, Afione SA, et al. 1994. Adeno-associated virus vector gene expression occurs in nondividing cells in the absence of vector DNA integration. *Am J Respir Cell Mol Biol* 11:517–521.

Flotte TR, Ng P, et al. 2007. Viral vector-mediated and cell-based therapies for treatment of cystic fibrosis. *Mol Ther* 15:229–241.

Gabolde M, Muralitharan S, et al. 1999. Genotyping of the three major allelic variants of the human mannose-binding lectin gene by denaturing gradient gel electrophoresis. *Hum Mutat* 14:80–83.

Gao GP, Alvira MR, et al. 2002. Novel adeno-associated viruses from rhesus monkeys as vectors for human gene therapy. *Proc Natl Acad Sci U S A* 99:11854–11859.

Gautam A, Densmore CL, et al. 2001a. Transgene expression in mouse airway epithelium by aerosol gene therapy with PEI–DNA complexes. *Mol Ther* 3:551–556.

Gautam A, Densmore CL, et al. 2001b. Pulmonary cytokine responses associated with PEI–DNA aerosol gene therapy. *Gene Ther* 8:254–257.

Gebhart CL and Kabanov AV. 2001. Evaluation of polyplexes as gene transfer agents. *J Control Release* 73:401–416.

Georg-Fries B, Biederlack S, et al. 1984. Analysis of proteins, helper dependence, and seroepidemiology of a new human parvovirus. *Virology* 134:64–71.

Ghadge GD, Roos RP, et al. 1995. CNS gene delivery by retrograde transport of recombinant replication-defective adenoviruses. *Gene Ther* 2:132–137.

Halbert CL, Standaert TA, et al. 1997. Transduction by adeno-associated virus vectors in the rabbit airway: efficiency, persistence, and readministration. *J Virol* 71:5932–5941.

Harrod KS, Trapnell BC, et al. 1999. SP-A enhances viral clearance and inhibits inflammation after pulmonary adenoviral infection. *Am J Physiol* 277:L580–L588.

Hernandez YJ, Wang J, et al. 1999. Latent adeno-associated virus infection elicits humoral but not cell-mediated immune responses in a nonhuman primate model. *J Virol* 73:8549–8558.

Hickling TP, Clark H, et al. 2004. Collectins and their role in lung immunity. *J Leukoc Biol* 75:27–33.

Hogaboam CM, Takahashi K, et al. 2004. Mannose-binding lectin deficiency alters the development of fungal asthma: effects on airway response, inflammation, and cytokine profile. *J Leukoc Biol* 75:805–814.

Holt PG. 1993a. Macrophage: dendritic cell interaction in regulation of the IgE response in asthma. *Clin Exp Allergy* 23:4–6.

Holt PG. 1993b. Pulmonary dendritic cell populations. *Adv Exp Med Biol* 329:557–562.

Horellou P, Vigne E, et al. 1994. Direct intracerebral gene transfer of an adenoviral vector expressing tyrosine hydroxylase in a rat model of Parkinson's disease. *Neuroreport* 6:49–53.

Hsieh CS, Macatonia SE, et al. 1993. Pathogen-induced Th1 phenotype development in $CD4^+$ alpha beta-TCR transgenic T cells is macrophage dependent. *Int Immunol* 5:371–382.

Jakubzick C, Kunkel SL, et al. 2004. Therapeutic targeting of IL-4- and IL-13-responsive cells in pulmonary fibrosis. *Immunol Res* 30:339–349.

Jooss K, Turka LA, et al. 1998. Blunting of immune responses to adenoviral vectors in mouse liver and lung with CTLA4Ig. *Gene Ther* 5:309–319.

Kaufman J, Sime PJ, et al. 2004. Expression of CD154 (CD40 ligand) by human lung fibroblasts: differential regulation by IFN-gamma and IL-13, and implications for fibrosis. *J Immunol* 172:1862–1871.

Kay MA, Meuse L, et al. 1997. Transient immunomodulation with anti-CD40 ligand antibody and CTLA4Ig enhances persistence and secondary adenovirus-mediated gene transfer into mouse liver. *Proc Natl Acad Sci U S A* 94:4686–4691.

Koehler DR, Frndova H, et al. 2005. Aerosol delivery of an enhanced helper-dependent adenovirus formulation to rabbit lung using an intratracheal catheter. *J Gene Med* 7:1409–1420.

Koehler DR, Martin B, et al. 2006. Readministration of helper-dependent adenovirus to mouse lung. *Gene Ther* 13:773–780.

Konstan MW, Davis PB, et al. 2004. Compacted DNA nanoparticles administered to the nasal mucosa of cystic fibrosis subjects are safe and demonstrate partial to complete cystic fibrosis transmembrane regulator reconstitution. *Hum Gene Ther* 15:1255–1269.

Kotin RM, Siniscalco M, et al. 1990. Site-specific integration by adeno-associated virus. *Proc Natl Acad Sci U S A* 87:2211–2215.

Krieg AM. 2002. CpG motifs in bacterial DNA and their immune effects. *Annu Rev Immunol* 20:709–760.

Kuzmin AI, Finegold MJ, et al. 1997. Macrophage depletion increases the safety, efficacy and persistence of adenovirus-mediated gene transfer in vivo. *Gene Ther* 4:309–316.

Lacraz S, Dayer JM, et al 1994a. 1,25-Dihydroxyvitamin D3 dissociates production of interstitial collagenase and 92-kDa gelatinase in human mononuclear phagocytes. *J Biol Chem* 269:6485–6490.

Lacraz S, Isler P, et al. 1994b. Direct contact between T lymphocytes and monocytes is a major pathway for induction of metalloproteinase expression. *J Biol Chem* 269:22027–22033.

Lahti M, Lofgren J, et al. 2002. Surfactant protein D gene polymorphism associated with severe respiratory syncytial virus infection. *Pediatr Res* 51:696–699.

Lawson PR and Reid KB. 2000. The roles of surfactant proteins A and D in innate immunity. *Immunol Rev* 173:66–78.

Lee ER, Marshall J, et al. 1996. Detailed analysis of structures and formulations of cationic lipids for efficient gene transfer to the lung. *Hum Gene Ther* 7:1701–1717.

Lehrer RI. 2004. Primate defensins. *Nat Rev Microbiol* 2:727–738.

Leon B, Martinez del Hoyo G, et al. 2004. Dendritic cell differentiation potential of mouse monocytes: monocytes represent immediate precursors of $CD8^-$ and $CD8^+$ splenic dendritic cells. *Blood* 103 2668–2676.

LeVine AM, Elliott J, et al. 2004. Surfactant protein-d enhances phagocytosis and pulmonary clearance of respiratory syncytial virus. *Am J Respir Cell Mol Biol* 31(2):193–199.

Lin SM, Frevert CW, et al. 2004. Differential regulation of membrane CD14 expression and endotoxin-tolerance in alveolar macrophages. *Am J Respir Cell Mol Biol* 31:162–170.

Liu YJ. 2005. IPC: professional type 1 interferon-producing cells and plasmacytoid dendritic cell precursors. *Annu Rev Immunol* 23:275–306.

McCown TJ, Xiao X, et al. 1996. Differential and persistent expression patterns of CNS gene transfer by an adeno-associated virus (AAV) vector. *Brain Res* 713:99–107.

McKeon C and Samulski RJ. 1996. NIDDK Workshop on AAV Vectors: Gene Transfer into Quiescent Cells. *Hum Gene Ther* 7:1615–1619.

Morsy MA, Gu M, et al. 1998. An adenoviral vector deleted for all viral coding sequences results in enhanced safety and extended expression of a leptin transgene. *Proc Natl Acad Sci U S A* 95:7866–7871.

Moskalenko M, Chen L, et al. 2000. Epitope mapping of human anti-adeno-associated virus type 2 neutralizing antibodies: implications for gene therapy and virus structure. *J Virol* 74:1761–1766.

Moss RB, Rodman D, et al. 2004. Repeated adeno-associated virus serotype 2 aerosol-mediated cystic fibrosis transmembrane regulator gene transfer to the lungs of patients with cystic fibrosis: a multicenter, double-blind, placebo-controlled trial. *Chest* 125:509–521.

Moss RB, Milla C, et al. 2007. Repeated aerosolized AAV-CFTR for treatment of cystic fibrosis: a randomized placebo-controlled phase 2B trial. *Hum Gene Ther* 18:726–732.

Nicod LP. 1999. Pulmonary defence mechanisms. *Respiration* 66:2–11.

Nicod LP, el Habre F, et al. 1995. Interleukin-10 decreases tumor necrosis factor alpha and beta in alloreactions induced by human lung dendritic cells and macrophages. *Am J Respir Cell Mol Biol* 13:83–90.

Palaniyar N, Nadesalingam J, et al. 2003. Innate immune collectins bind nucleic acids and enhance DNA clearance in vitro. *Ann N Y Acad Sci* 1010:467–470.

Palmer DJ and Ng P. 2005. Helper-dependent adenoviral vectors for gene therapy. *Hum Gene Ther* 16:1–16.

Pickles RJ, Fahrner JA, et al. 2000. Retargeting the coxsackievirus and adenovirus receptor to the apical surface of polarized epithelial cells reveals the glycocalyx as a barrier to adenovirus-mediated gene transfer. *J Virol* 74:6050–6057.

Punturieri A, Alviani RS, et al. 2004. Specific engagement of TLR4 or TLR3 does not lead to IFN-beta-mediated innate signal amplification and STAT1 phosphorylation in resident murine alveolar macrophages. *J Immunol* 173:1033–1042.

Reidy MF and Wright JR. 2003. Surfactant protein A enhances apoptotic cell uptake and TGF-beta1 release by inflammatory alveolar macrophages. *Am J Physiol Lung Cell Mol Physiol* 285:L854–L861.

Rubenstein RC, McVeigh U, et al. 1997. CFTR gene transduction in neonatal rabbits using an adeno-associated virus (AAV) vector. *Gene Ther* 4:384–392.

Rudolph C, Schillinger U, et al. 2005. Aerosolized nanogram quantities of plasmid DNA mediate highly efficient gene delivery to mouse airway epithelium. *Mol Ther* 12:493–501.

Ruiz FE, Clancy JP, et al. 2001. A clinical inflammatory syndrome attributable to aerosolized lipid–DNA administration in cystic fibrosis. *Hum Gene Ther* 12:751–761.

Sallusto F, Mackay CR, et al. 2000. The role of chemokine receptors in primary, effector, and memory immune responses. *Annu Rev Immunol* 18:593–620.

Sano H and Kuroki Y. 2005. The lung collectins, SP-A and SP-D, modulate pulmonary innate immunity. *Mol Immunol* 42:279–287.

Scheule RK, St George JA, et al. 1997. Basis of pulmonary toxicity associated with cationic lipid–mediated gene transfer to the mammalian lung. *Hum Gene Ther* 8:689–707.

Sleigh MA. 1983. Ciliary function in transport of mucus. *Eur J Respir Dis* (Suppl 128, Pt 1):287–292.

Sleigh MA, Blake JR, et al. 1988. The propulsion of mucus by cilia. *Am Rev Respir Dis* 137:726–741.

Takeda K and Akira S. 2001. Regulation of innate immune responses by Toll-like receptors. *Jpn J Infect Dis* 54:209–219.

Takeuchi O, Hoshino K, et al. 2000. Cutting edge: TLR2-deficient and MyD88-deficient mice are highly susceptible to *Staphylococcus aureus* infection. *J Immunol* 165:5392–5396.

Thepen T, Kraal G, et al. 1994. The role of alveolar macrophages in regulation of lung inflammation. *Ann N Y Acad Sci* 725:200–206.

van Ginkel FW, Liu C, et al. 1995. Intratracheal gene delivery with adenoviral vector induces elevated systemic IgG and mucosal IgA antibodies to adenovirus and beta-galactosidase. *Hum Gene Ther* 6:895–903.

van Ginkel FW, McGhee JR, et al. 1997. Adenoviral gene delivery elicits distinct pulmonary-associated T helper cell responses to the vector and to its transgene. *J Immunol* 159:685–693.

Wagner JA, Reynolds T, et al. 1998. Efficient and persistent gene transfer of AAV–CFTR in maxillary sinus. *Lancet* 351:1702–1703.

Wang D, Fischer H, et al. 1999. Efficient CFTR expression from AAV vectors packaged with promoters: the second generation. *Gene Ther* 6:667–675.

Wyde PR and Cate TR. 1978. Cellular changes in lungs of mice infected with influenza virus: characterization of the cytotoxic responses. *Infect Immun* 22:423–429.

Yang Q, Chen F, et al. 1995. Inhibition of cellular and SV40 DNA replication by the adeno-associated virus Rep proteins. *Virology* 207:246–250.

Yang Y, Nunes FA, et al. 1994a. Cellular immunity to viral antigens limits E1-deleted adenoviruses for gene therapy. *Proc Natl Acad Sci U S A* 91:4407–4411.

Yang Y, Nunes FA, et al. 1994b. Inactivation of E2a in recombinant adenoviruses improves the prospect for gene therapy in cystic fibrosis. *Nat Genet* 7:362–369.

Yang Y, Greenough K, et al. 1996a. Transient immune blockade prevents formation of neutralizing antibody to recombinant adenovirus and allows repeated gene transfer to mouse liver. *Gene Ther* 3:412–420.

Yang Y, Su Q, et al. 1996b. Transient subversion of CD40 ligand function diminishes immune responses to adenovirus vectors in mouse liver and lung tissues. *J Virol* 70:6370–6377.

Yew NS, Wang KX, et al. 1999. Contribution of plasmid DNA to inflammation in the lung after administration of cationic lipid:pDNA complexes. *Hum Gene Ther* 10:223–234.

Yew NS, Zhao H, et al. 2000. Reduced inflammatory response to plasmid DNA vectors by elimination and inhibition of immunostimulatory CpG motifs. *Mol Ther* 1:255–262.

Zabner J, Petersen DM, et al. 1994. Safety and efficacy of repetitive adenovirus-mediated transfer of CFTR cDNA to airway epithelia of primates and cotton rats. *Nat Genet* 6:75–83.

Zhao H, Cheng SH, et al. 2000. Requirements for effective inhibition of immunostimulatory CpG motifs by neutralizing motifs. *Antisense Nucleic Acid Drug Dev* 10:381–389.

Ziady AG, Kelley TJ, et al. 2002. Functional evidence of CFTR gene transfer in nasal epithelium of cystic fibrosis mice in vivo following luminal application of DNA complexes targeted to the serpin–enzyme complex receptor. *Mol Ther* 5:413–419.

Ziady AG, Gedeon CR, et al. 2003a. Transfection of airway epithelium by stable PEGylated poly-L-lysine DNA nanoparticles in vivo. *Mol Ther* 8:936–947.

Ziady AG, Gedeon CR, et al. 2003b. Minimal toxicity of stabilized compacted DNA nanoparticles in the murine lung. *Mol Ther* 8:948–956.

Zou SM, Erbacher P, et al. 2000. Systemic linear polyethylenimine (L-PEI)-mediated gene delivery in the mouse. *J Gene Med* 2:128–134.

Zuckerman JB, Robinson CB, et al. 1999. A phase I study of adenovirus-mediated transfer of the human cystic fibrosis transmembrane conductance regulator gene to a lung segment of individuals with cystic fibrosis. *Hum Gene Ther* 10:2973–2985.

12

INDUCTION OF IMMUNE TOLERANCE THROUGH GENE TRANSFER TO HEMATOPOIETIC STEM CELLS

JESSAMYN BAGLEY, PH.D., CHAORUI TIAN, M.D., AND JOHN IACOMINI, PH.D.

Transplantation Research Center, Renal Division, Brigham and Women's Hospital, and Children's Hospital, Harvard Medical School, Boston, Massachusetts

Gene Therapy Immunology, Edited by Roland Herzog

12.1 INTRODUCTION

The primary function of the immune system is to protect organisms from disease by recognizing and destroying a diverse variety of pathogens, including viruses, parasites, and bacteria. The success of the normal immune system in rapidly eliminating foreign antigens and protecting from disease is potently demonstrated by the existence of immune defect diseases such as severe combined immunodeficiency syndrome (SCID) and acquired immune deficiency syndrome (AIDS), where in the absence of a functional immune system, the patient is rapidly overwhelmed with opportunistic infections (reviewed by Kumar et al. [2006]). These syndromes highlight the fact that the ability to recognize and respond to foreign antigens efficiently is critical for the survival of the organism. However, these powerful responses to foreign antigens can sometimes be deleterious. In organ transplantation, immune responses to the foreign organ lead to immunological rejection and graft failure. It would be of great clinical benefit to induce an inability of the immune system to respond to foreign antigens expressed on organ grafts. In many gene therapy applications the introduction of a therapeutic gene results in the elimination of encoded proteins by the immune response. The induction of specific tolerance to these proteins may greatly improve the efficacy of gene therapy approaches to the treatment of disease. Finally, autoimmunity is caused by aberrant responses of the immune system to self-proteins, and the ability to induce specific tolerance could result in the development of treatments for these diseases.

Because of the potential clinical applications, a great deal of research has been focused on strategies to induce specific tolerance. In this chapter we focus on the induction of molecular chimerism to establish tolerance. In this approach, bone marrow–derived hematopoietic stem cells are genetically engineered to express the protein of interest, usually through viral gene transfer. When these genetically engineered cells are transplanted into conditioned hosts, cells derived from the transduced progenitors repopulate the immune system. Thus, the immune system is functionally reconstituted in the presence of the introduced antigen, which is recognized as "self" (Fig. 12-1). This approach allows the fundamental reprogramming of the immune system and results in B- and T-cell tolerance to a wide variety of antigens introduced by genetic engineering of hematopoietic stem cells.

12.2 MECHANISMS OF SELF-TOLERANCE

The basis of immune system function is the ability of the immune system to distinguish between antigens that occur in the normal healthy organism (self) and those that are derived from foreign pathogens (nonself). The inability of the immune system to respond to self-antigens is the result of the development of tolerance during immune system maturation. An organism that is tolerant to an antigen is specifically and permanently unable to mount an immune response to

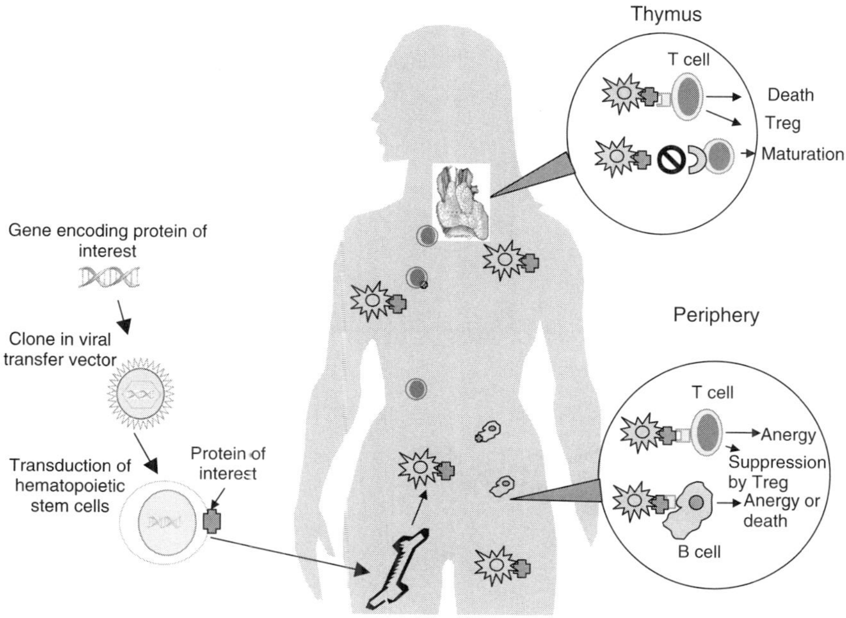

Figure 12-1 Tolerance induction through genetic engineering of hematopoietic progenitors.

that antigen while retaining the ability to respond to other, third-party antigens. The retention of the ability to respond to third-party antigen is a crucial distinction in the definition of immunologic tolerance. The term *tolerance* is often used loosely to refer to immune system hyporesponsiveness, in which responses to a specific antigen are temporarily decreased, or to a state of generalized immunosuppression, similar to that seen with the immunosuppressive drugs cyclosporine and rapamycin, in which responses to third-party antigens are also impaired. Although strategies that result in general immunosuppression or hyporesponsiveness to a particular antigen may be relevant in some clinical settings, they cannot be considered to result in tolerance. The induction of true immunologic tolerance to antigens without the need for immunosuppression would have a significant impact in the fields of transplantation, gene therapy, and autoimmune disease by ablating specific responses while leaving responses to pathogens intact.

12.2.1 T-Cell Tolerance

Intensive investigation into the mechanisms through which T cells are made tolerant to self-antigen has greatly increased our understanding of these events. Immature T-cell progenitors are generated from hematopoietic stem cells in the

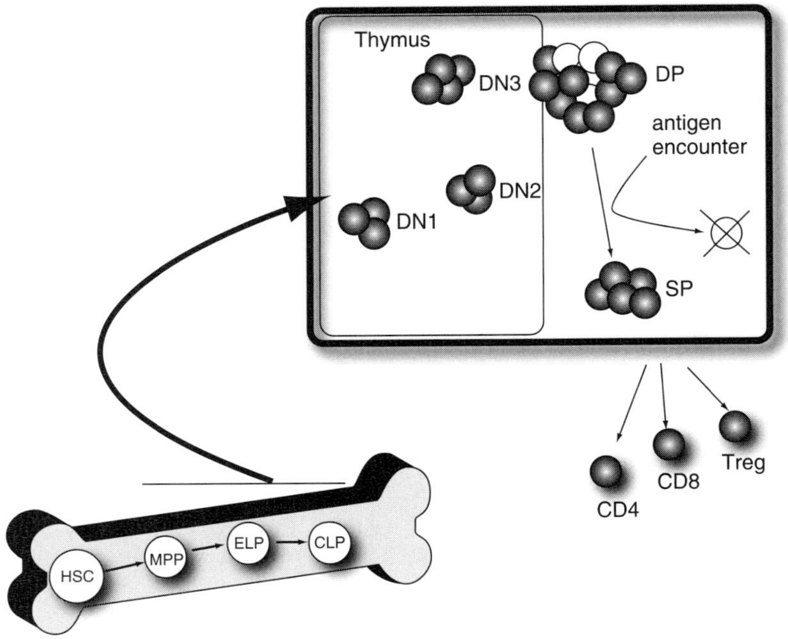

Figure 12-2 T-cell development. HSC, hematopoietic stem cell; MPP, multipotent progenitor; ELP, early lymphoid progenitor; CLP, common lymphoid progenitor; DN, double negative; DP, double positive; SP, single positive; CD4, $CD4^+$ T cells; CD8, $CD8^+$ T cells; Treg, regulatory T cell.

bone marrow and migrate to the thymus, where they complete their maturation (Fig. 12-2). Self-renewing multipotent hematopoietic stem cells (HSCs) in the bone marrow lack expression of lineage markers, are CD117 $(Kit)^+$ express Sca-1 and are $Flt3^-$ [Spangrude et al. 1988]. These cells give rise to nonrenewing multipotent progenitors that are $Lin^-Sca\text{-}1^+Kit^+Flt3^+$ and have a greatly decreased capacity to develop into myeloid cells [Adolfsson et al. 2001]. A subset of these cells also expresses *Rag* genes and have been termed early lymphoid progenitors [Igarashi et al. 2002]. These, in turn, give rise to common lymphoid progenitor cells (CLPs), which possess T- and B-cell lineage potential [Kondo et al. 1997]. While the stages of development of these progenitors in the bone marrow have been fairly well defined, it is not known which cell type migrates through the blood to the thymus. Although HSCs can develop into T cells when injected directly into the thymus, after intravenous injection HSCs do not home to the thymus, suggesting that other cell types move from bone marrow to thymus under physiologic conditions [Bhandoola et al. 2007].

Once reaching the thymus, double-negative 1 (DN1) progenitors, which are $CD3^-$ $CD8^-$ $CD44^+$ $CD25^-Kit^{hi}$, are found initially in the cortex immediately adjacent to the medulla [Shimonkevitz et al. 1987; Godfrey et al. 1993; Shortman and Wu 1996]. These cells differentiate into DN2 cells ($Lin^{lo}CD44^{+}Kit^{hi}CD25^{+}$) cells that migrate outward from sites of entry in the perimedullary cortex to the inner cortex [Shortman and Wu 1996; Lind et al. 2001]. Upon migrating to the outer cortex, they undergo further differentiation to become DN3 cells ($Lin^{lo}CD44^{lo}Kit^{lo}CD25^{+}$) that are committed to the T-cell lineage [Shortman and Wu 1996] and begin rearrangement of T-cell receptor (TCR) β genes. DN3 cells continue to proliferate [Penit et al. 1995; Petrie et al. 1995]; however, the factors that support DN3 growth remain undefined. Cells that rearrange the β-chain successfully move to the subcapsular zone [Dudley et al. 1994] and begin to express to pre-T complex [Saint-Ruf et al. 1994]. At this stage, cells become $CD4^{+}$ $CD8^{+}$ double-positive (DP) thymocytes, move out of the subcapsular zone, and stop proliferating. These DP thymocytes initiate rearrangement of the TCRα locus and develop unique TCRs that recognize major histocompatibility complex (MHC) proteins in complex with self-peptides.

Self-peptides are presented in the context of MHC molecules expressed by thymic epithelia, and T cells that are capable of binding these complexes receive signals which allow their survival and further development (reviewed by Alberola-Ila and Hernandez-Hoyos [2003]). This process of positive selection ensures that all T cells can recognize self-MHC molecules, but also enriches for self-reactive cells, making all T cells potentially self-reactive. These potentially autoreactive cells then migrate to the thymic medulla via CCR7-dependent signaling [Kurobe et al. 2006], where self-antigen/MHC peptides are again presented by medullary epithelial cells, and by bone marrow–derived antigen-presenting cells (reviewed by Takahama [2006]). Through the process of negative selection, potentially autoreactive T cells that recognize self-antigens with high avidity are eliminated by clonal deletion. Thus, antigens that are present in the thymus at the time of T-cell development eliminate T-cell clones that are capable of recognizing and responding to them (Kappler et al. 1987], reviewed by Siggs et al. [2006]).

The thymus is capable of presenting many self-antigens that are normally expressed outside the thymus in a tissue-specific fashion or during restricted developmental stages. The promiscuous expression of peripheral antigens in thymic epithelial cells is regulated by the autoimmune regulator (AIRE). AIRE has been shown to regulate the expression of insulin [Anderson et al. 2002], interphotoreceptor retinoid-binding protein [DeVoss et al. 2006], and α-fodrin [Kuroda et al. 2005] in the thymus, thus making peptides derived from these self-proteins available to developing T cells. The presence of these proteins during development allows for the elimination of most T cells bearing high-avidity receptors for self-MHC/peptide complexes and plays a major role in preventing autoimmunity in peripheral organs. AIRE is mutated in autoimmune polyendocrinopathy syndrome type 1, a recessive Mendelian disorder characterized by a spectrum of organ-specific autoimmune diseases that variably targets the parathyroid, adrenal glands, ovaries, and other tissues [Anderson et al. 2002]. The severity of this syndrome highlights the critical importance of central tolerance to immune system function [Liston et al. 2003].

The process of negative selection eliminates most, but not all, autoreactive T cells. Low-avidity autoreactive T cells are not all negatively selected in the thymus (reviewed by Gallegos and Bevan [2006]) and migrate to peripheral sites. In normal individuals these autoreactive T cells are controlled by peripheral mechanisms. One potential mechanism for the control of autoreactive T cells is the induction of anergy, in which T cells remain alive but are incapable of responses to antigen [Schwartz 2003]. This antigen nonresponsive state can be induced when the T-cell receptor is ligated in the absence of co-stimulation (reviewed by Abbas et al. [2004]). In vitro, T-cell clones that recognize antigen require a "second signal" delivered by one or more co-stimulatory molecules to be capable of productive immune response. T cells express a large number of surface molecules that can transmit either positive or negative co-stimulatory signals [Kroczek et al. 2004]. These co-stimulatory receptors are engaged by ligands expressed on the surface of antigen-presenting cells, which contribute to the immune response through their ability to present antigens and to promote an inflammatory environment through pathogen-specific receptors, such as Toll receptors, expressed on their surface [Lutz and Schuler 2002; Schwarz et al. 2003; Gwyer et al. 2006; Nocentini et al. 2007].

Autoreactive T cells are also controlled in the periphery through active suppression mediated by regulatory T cells (Tregs). Various types of T cells, including $CD8^+$ and $CD4^-$ $CD8^-$ cells, may have a regulatory function (reviewed by Jiang et al. [2006]); however, the most extensively studied Treg population in rodents is CD4 positive and expresses the IL-2 receptor CD25. The selective depletion of $CD4^+$ $CD25^+$ T cells from mice has been shown to result in the development of autoimmune disease [Taguchi and Takahashi 1996; McHugh and Shevach 2002]. In mice, Tregs are also predominantly FoxP3 positive, and the deletion of the gene encoding FoxP3 results in the "scurfy" phenotype, which is subject to overwhelming autoimmunity, indicating the importance of this gene in maintaining self-tolerance [Brunkow et al. 2001]. In humans, immune dysregulation, polyendocrinopathy, enteropathy, and X-linked syndrome (IPEX) is caused by mutations of FoxP3 [Bennett et al. 2001; Wildin et al. 2001]. FoxP3-positive regulatory T cells have been shown to develop both in the thymus during maturation [Bensinger et al. 2001; Jordan et al. 2001] and in the periphery in response to antigen [Kretschmer et al. 2005]. Thus, the evidence gathered from animal models appears to suggest that the maintenance of natural tolerance is dependent on both peripheral and central mechanisms, since when either of these mechanisms is impaired, autoimmunity results. The increased understanding of events involved in the induction of self-tolerance has led to attempts to manipulate the immune response to induce tolerance to foreign antigens, in the case of transplantation immunology and gene therapy, and to restore natural tolerance to self-antigens in autoimmunity.

12.2.2 B-Cell Tolerance

B-lymphocyte development occurs when immunoglobulin (Ig) genes are recombined to form a productive B-cell receptor. Heavy chain recombination occurs in early pro-B cells. Cells that undergo a productive heavy chain rearrangement expand at the late pro-B stage and then initiate further rearrangements at light chain loci during the pre-B stage. The successfully recombined B cell receptors transduce a signal that turns off *Rag1* and *Rag2*, which prevents further rearrangements at Ig loci. This results in allelic exclusion, whereby individual cells express only a single heavy chain and a single light chain. Signaling through this receptor in immature B cells results in positive selection which B cells gain the ability to leave the bone marrow. It has been estimated that up to half of these newly developed B cells are autoreactive [Rajewsky 1996]. Thus, mechanisms to prevent the further development of these autoreactive cells are critical for the prevention of autoimmunity and the induction of tolerance. Exposure of developing B cells to self-antigens results in editing of the specificity of the B-cell receptor, or if the receptor cannot be edited successfully, recognition of self-antigens leads to apoptosis [reviewed by Nemazee et al. 2006] or anergy [Goodnow et al. 1988]. Thus, the presence of antigen in the bone marrow during B-cell development leads to selection pressure that prevents the emergence of autoreactive B-cell specificities. Furthermore, the participation of T cells is required for optimal B-cell activation and antibody production in the periphery. Thus, the elimination of antigen-specific T cells can prevent the development of a B-cell response to that antigen.

12.3 INDUCED TOLERANCE

Increased understanding of the mechanisms that control self-tolerance in healthy individuals has led to interest in exploiting these mechanisms to induce therapeutic tolerance to antigens in organ transplantation, gene therapy, and autoimmunity.

12.3.1 Induction of Tolerance to Alloantigens: Major Histocompatibility Complex

The use of transplantation to treat end-stage organ failure of heart, kidney, liver, and lung has great potential in the treatment of a wide variety of otherwise fatal conditions, and the number of patients receiving an organ transplant reached an all-time high of 28,930 in 2006 (United Network on Organ Sharing). The discovery of powerful immunosuppressives such as cyclosporine and rapamycin has greatly decreased the incidence of acute organ graft rejection and has been critical to the success of organ transplantation as a therapy. However, use of these nonspecific immunosuppressive agents is associated with significant morbidity and mortality due both to the toxicity of these drugs and to increased incidence of infection and malignancy due to generalized suppression of the immune system [Ozduran et al. 2005; Singh 2005; Fishman 2007]. In addition, while the incidence of acute rejection immediately following organ transplantation has decreased greatly, the incidence of chronic rejection of organ allografts after months or years remains high. Indeed, the major cause of graft loss is currently chronic rejection [Meier-Kriesche et al. 2004; Vadivel et al. 2007]. Thus, the ability to generate specific unresponsiveness, or tolerance, to organ allografts without requiring generalized immunosuppression remains a top priority in transplantation research.

It has long been established in animal models that specific tolerance to transplantation antigens, the most important of which are the major histocompatibility (MHC) genes, can be achieved through transplantation of allogeneic hematopoietic stem cells [Billingham et al. 1953]. However, there are several barriers to the clinical effectiveness of such a strategy, including the proven difficulty of inducing such chimerism in humans [Fudaba et al. 2006], the extensive and undesirable conditioning regimens that would be required in patients already requiring an organ transplant, the risk of graft failure, and the potentially fatal consequences of graft versus host disease (GVHD), in which T cells from the bone marrow graft attack the host tissue. These factors combine to make it difficult for bone marrow chimerism for the induction of tolerance to attain wide clinical significance.

In principle, the induction of *molecular* rather than cellular chimerism through the use of genetic engineering to express alloantigens on recipient bone marrow cells can overcome some of the drawbacks associated with bone marrow transplantation. For example, because cells derived from the recipient are used as the target of gene transfer, GVHD cannot occur. Early studies indicated that gene transfer of MHC class I genes into bone marrow cells resulted in a prolongation of allogeneic skin grafts [Sykes et al. 1993; Wong et al. 1996], although neither expression of the gene nor graft survival was permanent. Although skin grafts were significantly prolonged, they were all eventually rejected. This phenomena was controlled through the helper pathway [Fraser et al. 1995; Mayfield et al. 1997], since additional helper determinants expressed by allogeneic grafts were capable of reversing immune hyporesponsiveness and accelerating skin graft rejection. Although these early experiments were not able to demonstrate acceptance of skin grafts, or tolerance, the hyporesponsiveness induced appeared to be sufficient to induce "operational" tolerance to heart grafts [Wong et al. 1999; Fry et al. 2002]. However, the hyporesponsiveness was transient and is quite distinct from tolerance in which specific and durable unresponsiveness to an antigen is achieved in the presence of responses to third-party antigen. It was hypothesized that the failure to induce tolerance in these initial experiments may have been related to the low and transient levels of protein expression that were achieved following gene transfer. To test this hypothesis, improved retroviral vectors encoding the MHC class I gene H-2K^b were produced [Bagley et al. 2002]. These vectors were then used to transduce bone marrow stem cells from a mouse that encoded only the H-2K^k allele. Transduced bone marrow cells were transplanted into conditioned recipients, and the immune system was allowed to reconstitute, generating bone marrow–derived cells that expressed both H-2K^b and H-2K^k. Relatively high and durable levels of H-2K^b could be detected in all cell lineages following reconstitution, suggesting that hematopoietic stem cells had been targeted efficiently. After full reconstitution, animals were found to accept allogeneic skin grafts expressing H-2K^b indefinitely, while at the same time they were able rapidly to reject third-party grafts. This was therefore the first demonstration that molecular chimerism was able to induce T-cell tolerance to MHC class I antigens [Bagley et al. 2002].

To explore whether durable expression of the introduced gene was required, retroviral vectors encoding H-2K^b were used to transduce bone marrow cells from a H-2K^k mouse. Transduced bone marrow cells were transplanted into conditioned recipients, and the immune system was allowed to reconstitute. After reconstitution, animals were then treated with a H-2K^b-specific depleting antibody [Tian et al. 2006]. This created mice that had expressed H-2K^b during immune reconstitution, in which H-2K^b expression had subsequently been ablated. When allogeneic skin grafts expressing H-2K^b were placed on these animals, it was found that in the absence of expression of H-2K^b, tolerance was not maintained, and grafts were rejected [Tian et al. 2006]. Thus, the maintenance of antigen expression is required for tolerance after expression of MHC class I in hematopoietic stem cells. Therefore, the hypothesis that low and transient levels of gene expression following gene transfer into bone marrow cells results in transient hyporesponsiveness while higher and prolonged expression results in tolerance appears to have been confirmed.

Further investigation has served to elucidate the mechanisms whereby the introduced gene product expressed in hematopoietic stem cells induces tolerance. Central deletional mechanisms are detectable in animals that received bone marrow transduced with retrovirus encoding H-2K^b, as CD8 T-cell clones specific for H-2K^b were completely deleted in the thymus of these animals [Kang and Iacomini 2002]. However, this approach also appears to involve the development of regulatory tolerance mechanisms. When CD4 T-cell clones that were specific for peptides derived from H-2K^b were examined, it was apparent that while central deletion could be observed, not all H-2K^b reactive CD4 T cells were deleted [Forman et al. 2006]. H-2K^b reactive CD4 T cells could be detected in the periphery of mice that had received hematopoietic stem cells transduced with a retrovirus encoding H-2K^b, although these T cells remained unresponsive. Despite the fact that recipients contain alloreactive CD4 T cells, tolerance remains intact, and skin grafts survive indefinitely. The maintenance of tolerance in this model appears to depend on the action of Tregs in the periphery, and it was shown that the transfer of CD4$^+$CD25$^+$ Tregs from molecular chimeras could delay H-2K^b-expressing skin graft rejection in secondary recipients compared with graft rejection in mice that have received control T cells [Forman et al. 2006]. This stands in contrast to data reported from bone marrow chimeras, in which strong regulatory T-cell generation does not appear to occur [Adams et al. 2001; Kurtz et al. 2004a,b]. This raises the possibility that the induction of molecular chimerism may be a more powerful technique than the induction of cellular chimerism alone.

The finding that the introduction of MHC class I genes into hematopoietic stem cells followed by bone marrow transplantation resulted in T-cell tolerance was followed up by the observation that tolerance to MHC class II antigens could be induced in a similar way [Wong et al. 2003]. In large-animal models, transfer of MHC class I and II was found to have an effect on graft rejection in pigs [Sonntag et al. 2001]. However, it is unclear whether tolerance was induced, since gene expression was low and variable. Overall, these experiments confirm the potential for using gene-transduced hematopoietic cells to establish immunologic tolerance and prevent organ allograft rejection. In a baboon model of xenograft rejection, transfer of MHC class II genes may have some effect on the development of immune responses [Ierino et al. 1999]. But again, since expression of the transgene was neither pronounced nor prolonged, it seems unlikely that tolerance to the antigen was achieved. As in mouse studies, further work with improved viral vectors might serve to greatly improve results and induce tolerance rather than hyporesponsiveness.

12.3.2 Induction of Tolerance to a Carbohydrate Antigen

Although the principal determining factor in the rejection of organ allografts is the MHC, the transplantation of organ grafts between different species, xenografts, has additional immunological barriers. It has been observed that grafts from phylogenetically disparate species are rejected within minutes after transplantation. This process of hyperacute rejection is due to the presence of pre-formed natural antibodies in the host directed against epitopes on the donor. In the pig-to-primate transplantation model, the most heavily investigated to date, it has been shown that the pre-formed natural antibodies primarily recognize a single target, the Galα1-3Galβ1-4GlcNAc-R (αGal) carbohydrate antigen. All placental mammals with the exception of humans and Old World monkeys express the enzyme galactose:β-D-galactosyl-1,4-*N*-acetyl-D-glucosaminide α(1–3) galactosyltransferase (αGT). Because humans do not express a functional αGT gene, the carbohydrate antigen is not present in humans, and antibodies to this epitope form at high frequency (reviewed by Bracy et al. [1999]). Since the presence of these antibodies results in extremely rapid rejection of grafts from other species, attempts to use xenografts to address organ shortages have proven futile. It has been shown in a mouse model that the reconstitution of mice in which the αGT gene has been knocked out (and therefore produce αGal antibodies) with a mixture of wild-type and knockout bone marrow cells completely inhibits the production of αGal antibodies [Yang et al. 1998]. This indicates that expression of αGal epitopes on bone marrow–derived hematopoietic cells is sufficient to induce tolerance. However, for this approach to work in a pig-to-primate model, it would require that pig bone marrow engraft in primates, which is not feasible using current technology. It was therefore hypothesized that tolerance to αGal could be induced through molecular rather than cellular chimerism through gene transfer to hematopoietic stem cells. When mice were reconstituted with bone marrow transduced with a retrovirus encoding αGT, it was shown that the development of αGal antibodies was completely inhibited [Bracy et al. 1998]. Expression of αGT was multilineage, persisted for the lifetime of the animal, and could be transferred to secondary recipients. No αGal antibodies were observed in mice even after multiple immunizations with cells bearing the αGal epitope, indicating that B-cell tolerance was induced [Bracy and Iacomini 2000]. Further investigation showed that when wild-type heart grafts, which express αGal, were transplanted into αGT-knockout mice, grafts were acutely rejected in an αGal antibody-dependent fashion [Bracy and Iacomini 2002]. In contrast, when wild-type heart grafts were transplanted into αGT-knockout mice that had been reconstituted with hematopoietic stem cells transduced with virus encoding αGT, cardiac grafts were not rejected by αGal antibody mechanisms. However, recipients were eventually able to reject these grafts, due to minor antigen disparities between the donor and recipient strains, indicating that responses to third-party antigens were intact, and that true tolerance had been achieved in these animals. Similar results were later reported using lentiviral rather than retroviral vectors [Kearns-Jonker et al. 2004].

The induction of B-cell tolerance through molecular chimerism is extremely robust, showing the ability to fundamentally reshape the immune repertoire even in the face of pre-formed antibodies. Indeed, even when αGT-knockout mice were sensitized by extensive immunization with cells expressing the αGal epitope, reconstitution with bone marrow cells engineered to express αGT completely prevented the generation of αGal antibodies [Bracy and Iacomini 2002]. These data expand the potential clinical utility of molecular chimerism by indicating that this technique could be used in patients who have already developed deleterious B-cell responses, such as pre-sensitized patients who require organ transplants. In these patients, exposure to foreign MHC either through blood transfusion or childbirth has resulted in sensitization to MHC molecules, significantly decreasing their chance of receiving a suitable organ allograft and increasing the chances that any allograft received would be rapidly rejected. The potential clinical application of molecular chimerism is underscored by the observation that molecular chimerism can be obtained using clinically relevant nonmyeloablative conditioning regimens [Forman et al. 2005; Mitsuhashi et al. 2006]. Furthermore, preliminary experiments in large-animal models suggest that the goal of αGT expression following gene transfer into bone marrow cells may be attained [Fischer-Lougheed et al. 2007]. Unfortunately, despite success with HIV-based vectors in the mouse model, expression of αGT in rhesus following transplantation with bone marrow transduced with these vectors was extremely low, with αGal epitopes being undetectable on most lineages 50 days after transplant. In addition, it was found that reconstitution of these animals with bone marrow expressing αGal resulted in an increase in the production of anti-αGal IgG, indicating that tolerance was not achieved. Substantially better expression data were obtained with SIV-based vectors; however, anti-αGal IgG levels were not measured, making it difficult to determine if tolerance was achieved in this large-animal model [Fischer-Lougheed et al. 2007]. Recent reports using αGT-knockout pigs have indicated that the elimination of αGal reactivity is not sufficient to ablate antibody responses to xenografts [Chen et al. 2005], suggesting that this approach will not on its own overcome humoral immunity to pig organs. Therefore, the greater importance of this work is the proof that the expression of antigen in bone marrow–derived cells is sufficient to induce B-cell tolerance and to prevent humoral immune responses to antigen. This has potential applications both for blood group–incompatible organ transplantation, in which pre-formed antibodies to the A and B blood group antigens results in rapid rejection of mismatched grafts, and for gene therapy and autoimmune applications, in which it would be desirable to eliminate deleterious antibody responses.

12.3.3 Induction of Tolerance to Products of Gene Therapy

Green Fluorescent Protein To determine if the strategy of gene transfer into bone marrow–derived stem cells would be effective for inducing tolerance in a wider variety of applications, such as inducing tolerance to products of gene therapy, it first needed to be determined if this approach worked for secreted proteins, or proteins expressed in the cell cytoplasm as well as cell surface molecules such as MHC or αGal. Early experiments with secreted or cytoplasmic forms of MHC class I resulted in induction of hyporesponsiveness rather than tolerance, probably due to expression issues [Bagley et al. 2000]. Further experiments performed using improved retroviral vectors indicated that the expression of the cytoplasmic protein enhanced green fluorescent protein (EGFP) in hematopoietic stem cells eliminated the immune response to EGFP in recipients while leaving third-party responses intact [Tian et al. 2003]. This work had significant implications for gene therapy applications of tolerance induction through molecular chimerism since it suggested that the product of any gene introduced into bone marrow stem cells through genetic engineering was capable of inducing tolerance. Follow-up work confirmed that the induction of molecular chimerism under nonmyeloablative conditions was also sufficient to induce tolerance to EGFP and to prolong indefinitely skin grafts expressing EGFP [Andersson et al. 2003a,b]. Similarly, it has been shown that tolerance to β-galactosidase can be obtained through the induction of molecular chimerism [Pichard et al. 2006]. Together, these data suggest that molecular chimerism may be a useful strategy for many applications in which tolerance induction is desired.

In large-animal models, it has been shown that introduction of the neomycin resistance gene (neo) through retroviral-mediated transduction of rhesus macaque bone marrow cells and reconstitution results in long-term persistence of cells producing neo, and the absence of immune response to this protein [Heim et al. 2000]. Responses to GFP were ablated in primates receiving myeloablative conditioning, and bone marrow engineered to express GFP [Kung et al. 2003]. Rigorous immunization with purified GFP adjuvant failed to elicit anti-GFP responses, suggesting that tolerance was achieved. Significantly, no response to either neo or GFP was detected in a model in which nonmyeloablative conditioning was used to allow for the engraftment of retrovirally transduced bone marrow in macaques [Kang et al. 2001]. Together, these data suggest that genetic engineering of hematopoietic stem cells could be used to induce tolerance in a clinically relevant fashion.

Hemophilia One potential application would be in the treatment of hemophilia A and B. Hemophilia A is a congenital bleeding disorder caused by the functional inactivation of coagulation factor VIII (FVIII) through truncation or mis-sense mutations in the gene that encodes this protein [Oldenburg et al. 2004]. Because patients do not produce wild-type FVIII, they are able to generate immune responses to this protein, and 25 to 30% of patients who are exposed to repeated administration of FVIII develop antibodies that inhibit FVIII function [Ehrenforth et al. 1992]. The development of inhibitors renders the exogenous administration of FVIII ineffective and can pose serious risks for uncontrolled bleeding. The development of clinically relevant strategies to eliminate inhibitor development is therefore a major goal in the treatment of hemophilia A. Using an engineered variant of FVIII protein, it was shown that the transplantation of genetically engineered autologous bone marrow can be used successfully to treat hemophilia in mice, resulting in sustained production of FVIII and a decrease in production of antibodies to FVIII [Moayeri et al. 2004, 2005]. In hemophilia A patients in whom the FVIII protein is absent or mutated, the immune system does not recognize FVIII as a self-protein and therefore responds with vigorous T- and B-cell-mediated immunity. Whereas B-cell-mediated antibody responses are of the most concern when FVIII proteins are being infused, T-cell-mediated responses become important for gene therapy approaches in which autologous cells are induced to produce FVIII. These cells can be recognized by FVIII-specific T cells and eliminated, representing a significant risk when liver or muscle cells are targeted by gene therapy. It is therefore of great importance to gene therapy applications that tolerance to FVIII can be induced through the targeting of bone marrow–derived cells. Similarly, hemophilia B is caused by mutations in coagulation factor IX (FIX). Although inhibitor generation is less common in hemophilia B than in hemophilia A, it can still occur in 2 to 4% of patients. In addition, attempts to correct the hemophilia B phenotype by gene therapy are confounded by the generation of vigorous T- and B-cell responses, which are capable of eliminating the FIX transgene. The expression of human FIX in hematopoietic stem cells through gene transfer leads to the long-term correction of the hemophilia B phenotype in mice, suggesting that immune responses to FIX are eliminated. Furthermore, no antibody to FIX can be detected in animals reconstituted with stem cells expressing FIX, even after immunization with human FIX, further confirming that tolerance has been achieved [Bigger et al. 2006]. Thus, it is apparent that the induction of molecular chimerism has the ability to reshape the immune repertoire in hemophiliac mice and to prevent the development of immune responses to exogenously administrated coagulation factors.

12.3.4 Induction of Tolerance to Autoantigens

Type 1 Diabetes Another potential application of molecular chimerism is the restoration of self-tolerance in autoimmune disease models. One such model that has been studied extensively is autoimmune or type 1 diabetes. Type 1 diabetes is caused by T-cell-mediated autoimmune destruction of insulin-producing β cells in the pancreas. Although patients can be kept alive by the administration of exogenous insulin, there is presently no cure. Several genes contribute to the development of type 1 diabetes, but the principal determining genetic component in humans is the inheritance of mutant MHC alleles associated with susceptibility to disease (at-risk alleles) [Morel et al. 1988; Wicker et al. 1995; McDevitt 1998; Nepom and Kwok 1998]. These alleles are characterized by the lack of a charged amino acid at position 57 of the MHC class II β-chain [Davies et al. 1994; Mein et al. 1998]. Conversely, inheritance of MHC class II alleles containing a charged amino acid at position 57 of the β-chain is associated with protection from disease. In the NOD model of spontaneous type 1 diabetes, the MHC class II region encodes a single MHC class II molecule, I-A^{g7}, which contains polymorphisms that are strikingly similar to at-risk human alleles [Hattori et al. 1986]. Since at-risk alleles appear to have abnormalities in peptide presentation that may lead to abnormal T-cell selection in the thymus, and therefore autoimmunity, it was hypothesized that the introduction of a MHC class II I-Aβ-chain molecule that contains a charged amino acid at position 76 through genetic engineering of hematopoietic bone marrow stem cells might be sufficient to prevent the occurrence of spontaneous diabetes in NOD recipients. When pre-diabetic mice were tested, it was found that while animals reconstituted with bone marrow transduced with control virus developed spontaneous diabetes, mice that were reconstituted with bone marrow genetically engineered to express the I-$A\beta^{d}$ gene were completely protected from disease. This phenomenon was robust, since mice treated with the diabetes-precipitating compound cyclophosphamide were also protected completely. When islets from mice reconstituted with bone marrow genetically engineered to express the I-$A\beta^{d}$ gene were examined, no cellular infiltrate was observed, indicating a lack of immune response to islets, and insulin storage was normal. No T-cell responses to islet antigens could be detected in ELISPOT assays, which was interpreted as further evidence of restored self-tolerance. To elucidate the mechanism of tolerance in this model, a MHC tetramer staining reagent coupled to a peptide known to be recognized by diabetogenic T cells was used (BDC15). Populations of T cells that recognize the BDC15–tetramer complex develop in control NOD mice and in mice treated with bone marrow transduced with control virus. However, in mice that were reconstituted with bone marrow genetically engineered to express the I-$A\beta^{d}$ gene, T cells that recognized the BDC15–tetramer complex were present in the thymus only at developmental stages prior to negative selection. These data indicate that diabetogenic T cells can be eliminated by negative selection in pre-diabetic NOD mice expressing protective MHC class II genes on bone marrow–derived cells.

These data suggest that genetic engineering of autologous hematopoietic stem cells could be used to prevent diabetes occurrence in high-risk individuals who inherit diabetes-permissive MHC class II alleles. However, it would be more clinically relevant to be able to treat individuals in whom diabetes has already developed. It was recently shown that in addition to being able to prevent diabetes, the introduction of protective MHC class II genes through gene transfer into hematopoietic stem cells can also cure T1 diabetes. Spontaneously diabetic NOD mice were reconstituted with bone marrow transduced with retrovirus encoding either I-Aβ^d or control virus. Animals were maintained on insulin until reconstitution was complete. After confirming that the mice remained diabetic following bone marrow transplantation, each animal received an islet transplant. Mice that were reconstituted with bone marrow transduced with retrovirus encoding I-Aβ^d became normoglycemic within 24 hours and remained nondiabetic indefinitely, suggesting that autoimmunity was eliminated in these animals. In contrast, mice reconstituted with bone marrow transduced with control virus were transiently normoglycemic, indicating that the islet grafts were functional, and then became diabetic within three days following transplantation, presumably due to autoimmune destruction of the islets. These data suggest that tolerance induction through gene transfer into hematopoietic stem cells can act both to eliminate the development of diabetogenic T cells in pre-diabetic animals, and to control the function of autoimmune T cells already present in the periphery of diabetic mice. Interestingly, it was found that the administration of PDL1 antibody, which normally precipitates diabetes in NOD mice within 48 hours, was not able to induce diabetes in NOD mice treated with bone marrow transduced with virus encoding I-Aβ^d (Tian and Iacomini, personal communication). This suggests that the expression of I-Aβ^d fundamentally reshapes the immune repertoire of NOD mice.

Another approach to curing autoimmunity in T1D is to target the islet antigen recognized by diabetogenic T cells. This is complicated somewhat by the fact that the primary islet antigens responsible for eliciting an autoimmune response have not been clearly identified. However, there are some indications that T-cell responses to insulin are a major precipitating factor in the development of T1D. In diabetic humans, a high frequency of T cells isolated from the pancreatic lymph nodes are insulin reactive [Kent et al. 2005], and T-cell clones from diabetic NOD mice have been shown to be insulin reactive and initiate diabetes [Wegmann et al. 1994; Nakayama et al. 2005]. To determine if tolerance to insulin could be induced, bone marrow cells were transduced with virus encoding proinsulin or control virus, and transferred into pre-diabetic NOD mice [Chan et al. 2006]. Histological assessment of islets 8 weeks after transfer showed a substantial decrease in the incidence of insulitis in mice that expressed pro-insulin compared with controls. While the incidence of diabetes was not reported, previous studies using a similar strategy in which bone marrow cells expressing insulin were transferred into NOD recipients [Steptoe et al. 2003] suggests that diabetes incidence may also be reduced.

Depending on the nature of the underlying immune defect that has allowed autoimmunity to occur, it may not be possible for expression of antigen on bone marrow–derived cells to restore tolerance. We know that molecular chimerism appears to induce both central deletion and the generation of regulatory T cells (Tregs). One might expect that if self-tolerance to a particular antigen was controlled by peripheral mechanisms such as Tregs and that in an autoimmune person the ability to generate regulatory T cells was impaired, the introduction of antigen on autologous bone marrow–derived cells may not restore self-tolerance, since the ability to generate Tregs would remain impaired. On the other hand, it might be found that the induction of molecular chimerism would generate a central deletional response that would eliminate the requirement for Tregs, and autoimmunity would be eliminated. Further work determining if tolerance to insulin has in fact been induced in this model will be of particular interest since it would indicate that tolerance to individual autoantigens can be induced through molecular chimerism in autoimmune persons without repairing the underlying defect that resulted in a break of central tolerance.

Experimental Autoimmune Encephalitis Further exploration of the ability of molecular chimerism to induce tolerance in autoimmune persons has been performed using bone marrow cells expressing phospholipid protein (PLP) in a model for relapsing, remitting experimental autoimmune encephalomyelitis (EAE) [Xu et al. 2006], a mouse model of multiple sclerosis. Animals from susceptible strains can be injected with several different proteins or with peptides derived from proteins that make up the components of myelin, including myelin basic protein (MBP), myelin oligodendrocyte glycoprotein, and phospholipid protein, resulting in acute, or relapsing remitting demyelination of neurons. When susceptible mice were reconstituted with bone marrow cells transduced with full-length PLP, they were completely protected from the incidence of EAE for as long as 120 days following challenge with the PLP139-151 peptide. In contrast, mice reconstituted with bone marrow transduced with control virus developed relapsing remitting disease. A substantial decrease in proliferation in response to stimulation with PLP of T cells from mice reconstituted with bone marrow expressing PLP compared with controls further supports the suggestion that these mice are tolerant to PLP. These data indicate that the introduction of PLP on hematopoietic cells induces tolerance and prevents the occurrence of disease. However, it would be more clinically relevant to determine if the induction of molecular chimerism has an effect on animals that have already developed disease. Susceptible mice that had developed mild EAE were conditioned and reconstituted with bone marrow transduced with virus encoding PLP or control virus. After reconstitution, mice that received bone marrow expressing PLP experienced little further development of disease, suggesting that demyelination was no longer occurring, while controls went on to develop severe disease. Thus, as observed in the diabetes model, the expression of antigen on hematopoietic cells by gene transfer appears to have the ability to both prevent the development of autoimmune T cells and to functionally inactivate existing autoimmune cells.

Contrasting data have been generated in the same model system using MBP [Peters et al. 2000]. In this system, cDNA-encoding mouse MBP was introduced into the hematopoietic stem cells of B10.PL, SJL, and B10 mice by retrovirus-mediated gene transfer. Modest expression of MBP was detected in the peripheral blood and thymus after bone marrow transplantation. However, the expression did not result in deletion of MBP-specific T cells or tolerance to MBP in the susceptible strains B10.PL and SJL. However, gene transfer did result in resistant B10 mice developing mild EAE. The reasons for this surprising finding are not clear. They may be due to technical issues of expression level or to the use of guinea pig MBP for EAE induction. However, they may also indicate that tolerance cannot be induced to all antigens in autoreactive mice.

12.4 OVERCOMING THE NEED FOR BONE MARROW TRANSPLANTATION

The induction of molecular chimerism through the genetic engineering of hematopoietic stem cells has proven to be a powerful technique for the induction of tolerance. However, several obstacles need to be overcome before this technique becomes clinically relevant. The major drawback to this approach is the requirement for bone marrow transplantation, which exposes patients to significant risks, including the risk of graft failure and complications due to conditioning regimens. While the development of non-myeloablative conditioning regimens that allow for the induction of molecular chimerism does decrease the drawbacks associated with bone marrow transplants, significant risks do exist. The identification of mature cell lineages derived from hematopoietic progenitors that are responsible for the induction of tolerance would raise the possibility of induction tolerance without the requirement for bone marrow transplantation.

12.4.1 Induction of Tolerance Through Genetic Engineering of Mature B Cells

The use of gene therapy to transfer genes encoding the protein of interest in frame at the N-terminus of an IgG heavy chain into B cells has been studied for many years. B cells possess several advantages for the induction of tolerance: They are relatively long-lived, can be transplanted into immunocompetent recipients, and can be tolerogenic under some conditions. This approach has been shown to induce nonresponsiveness to the antigen presented in the context of the Ig carrier protein in autoimmune models of experimental uveitis, lupus, multiple sclerosis, and diabetes. In the latter model a single injection of B cells encoding GAD 65 Ig fusion protein or insulin Ig fusion protein were sufficient to reduce the incidence of diabetes significantly. Although not all animals were protected from disease, this may reflect the diversity of islet antigens to which diabetogenic T cells can respond, rather than a failure to induce hyporesponsiveness to Gad65 and insulin. In a mouse model of hemophilia A, mice injected with B cells transduced with virus encoding a FVIII-Ig fusion protein did not respond to FVIII even after immune challenge, indicating that tolerance to FVIII was achieved using only mature B cells. The mechanism of tolerance induction in this system is not well understood; however, MHC class II expression on presenting B cells is important, and Fc receptors are not required. In addition, in the diabetes model, protection from disease was partially abrogated by the depletion of $CD25^+$ cells, suggesting that regulatory T cells play a role in the maintenance of tolerance.

12.4.2 Induction of Tolerance Through Genetic Engineering of Mature T Cells

In attempting to identify the mature bone marrow–derived cells that are responsible for tolerance induction, it was found that Rag-deficient hematopoietic progenitors, which are not capable of developing into T or B cells, were not able to induce tolerance following transplantation. These data suggest that the expression of antigen by either T or B cells is required for tolerance induction. Although the induction of tolerance through the genetic engineering of B cells is effective in many model systems, the expression of allogeneic MHC on B cells is not sufficient to induce transplantation tolerance [Tian et al. 2002]. Whether this failure on the part of B cells to induce tolerance in a transplantation model is due to the higher precursor frequency of T cells that are alloreactive compared with the frequency that responds to other protein antigens is not clear. However, when antigen was expressed on mature T cells, tolerance to MHC antigens was induced [Tian et al. 2004]. These data indicate that expression of antigen on mature T cells may be sufficient to induce tolerance without the need for bone marrow transplantation.

REFERENCES

Abbas AK, Lohr J, et al. 2004. T cell tolerance and autoimmunity. *Autoimmun Rev* 3:471–475.

Adams AB, Durham MM, et al. 2001. Costimulation blockade, busulfan, and bone marrow promote titratable macrochimerism, induce transplantation tolerance, and correct genetic hemoglobinopathies with minimal myelosuppression. *J Immunol* 167:1103–1111.

Adolfsson J, Borge OJ, et al. 2001. Upregulation of Flt3 expression within the bone marrow Lin(-)Sca1(+)c-Kit(+) stem cell compartment is accompanied by loss of self-renewal capacity. *Immunity* 15:659–669.

Alberola-Ila J and Hernandez-Hoyos G. 2003. The Ras/MAPK cascade and the control of positive selection. *Immunol Rev* 191:79–96.

Anderson MS, Venanzi ES, et al. 2002. Projection of an immunological self shadow within the thymus by the aire protein. *Science* 298:1395–1401.

Andersson G, Denaro M, et al. 2003a. Engraftment of retroviral EGFP-transduced bone marrow in mice prevents rejection of EGFP–transgenic skin grafts. *Mol Ther* 8:385–391.

Andersson G, Illigens BM, et al. 2003b. Nonmyeloablative conditioning is sufficient to allow engraftment of EGFP-expressing bone marrow and subsequent acceptance of EGFP-transgenic skin grafts in mice. *Blood* 101:4305–4312.

Bagley J, Wu Y, et al. 2000. Defining the requirements for peptide recognition in gene therapy-induced T cell tolerance. *J Immunol* 165:4842–4847.

Bagley J, Tian C, et al. 2002. Induction of T-cell tolerance to an MHC class I alloantigen by gene therapy. *Blood* 99:4394–4399.

Bennett CL, Christie J, et al. 2001. The immune dysregulation, polyendocrinopathy, enteropathy, X-linked syndrome (IPEX) is caused by mutations of FOXP3. *Nat Genet* 27:20–21.

Bensinger SJ, Bandeira A, et al. 2001. Major histocompatibility complex class II-positive cortical epithelium mediates the selection of CD4(+)25(+) immunoregulatory T cells. *J Exp Med* 194:427–438.

Bhandoola A, von Boehmer H, et al. 2007. Commitment and developmental potential of extrathymic and intrathymic T cell precursors: plenty to choose from. *Immunity* 26:678–689.

Bigger BW, Siapati EK, et al. 2006. Permanent partial phenotypic correction and tolerance in a mouse model of hemophilia B by stem cell gene delivery of human factor IX. *Gene Ther* 13:117–126.

Billingham RE, Brent L, et al. 1953. Actively acquired tolerance of foreign cells. *Nature* 172:603–606.

Bracy JL and Iacomini J. 2000. Induction of B-cell tolerance by retroviral gene therapy. *Blood* 96:3008–3015.

Bracy J and Iacomini J. 2002. Engraftment of genetically modified bone marrow cells in sensitized hosts. *Mol Ther* 6:252–257.

Bracy JL, Sachs DH, et al. 1998. Inhibition of xenoreactive natural antibody production by retroviral gene therapy. *Science* 281:1845–1847.

Bracy JL, Cretin N, et al. 1999. Xenoreactive natural antibodies. *Cell Mol Life Sci* 56:1001–1007.

Brunkow ME, Jeffery EW, et al. 2001. Disruption of a new forkhead/winged-helix protein, scurfin, results in the fatal lymphoproliferative disorder of the scurfy mouse. *Nat Genet* 27:68–73.

Chan J, Clements W, et al. 2006. Transplantation of bone marrow genetically engineered to express proinsulin II protects against autoimmune insulitis in NOD mice. *J Gene Med* 8:1281–1290.

Chen G, Qian H, et al. 2005. Acute rejection is associated with antibodies to non-Gal antigens in baboons using Gal-knockout pig kidneys. *Nat Med* 11:1295–1298.

Davies JL, Kawaguchi Y, et al. 1994. A genome-wide search for human type 1 diabetes susceptibility genes. *Nature* 371:130–136.

DeVoss J, Hou Y, et al. 2006. Spontaneous autoimmunity prevented by thymic expression of a single self-antigen. *J Exp Med* 203:2727–2735.

Dudley EC, Petrie HT, et al. 1994. T cell receptor beta chain gene rearrangement and selection during thymocyte development in adult mice. *Immunity* 1:83–93.

Ehrenforth S, Kreuz W, et al. 1992. Factor VIII inhibitors in haemophiliacs. *Lancet* 340:253.

Fischer-Lougheed JY, Tarantal AF, et al. 2007. Gene therapy to inhibit xenoantibody production using lentiviral vectors in non-human primates. *Gene Ther* 14:49–57.

Fishman JA. 2007. Infection in renal transplant recipients. *Semin Nephrol* 27:445–461.

Forman D, Kang ES, et al. 2006. Induction of alloreactive CD4T cell tolerance in molecular chimeras: a possible role for regulatory T cells. *J Immunol* 176:3410–3416.

Forman D, Tian C, et al. 2005. Induction of donor-specific tolerance in sublethally irradiated recipients by gene therapy. *Mol Ther* 12:353–359.

Fraser CC, Sykes M, et al. 1995. Specific unresponsiveness to a retrovirally-transferred class I antigen is controlled through the helper pathway. *J Immunol* 154:1587–1595.

Fry JW, Morris PJ, et al. 2002. Adenoviral transfer of a single donor-specific MHC class I gene to recipient bone marrow cells can induce specific immunological unresponsiveness in vivo. *Gene Ther* 9:220–226.

Fudaba Y, Spitzer TR, et al. 2006. Myeloma responses and tolerance following combined kidney and nonmyeloablative marrow transplantation: in vivo and in vitro analyses. *Am J Transplant* 6:2121–2133.

Gallegos AM and Bevan MJ. 2006. Central tolerance: good but imperfect. *Immunol Rev* 209:290–296.

Godfrey DI, Kennedy J, et al. 1993. A developmental pathway involving four phenotypically and functionally distinct subsets of $CD3^-CD4^-CD8^-$ triple-negative adult mouse thymocytes defined by CD44 and CD25 expression. *J Immunol* 150:4244–4252.

Goodnow CC, Crosbie J, et al. 1988. Altered immunoglobulin expression and functional silencing of self-reactive B lymphocytes in transgenic mice. *Nature* 334:676–682.

Gwyer E, Snelgrove R, et al. 2006. The therapeutic potential of positive and negative immune cell co-stimulation during inflammation. *Biochem Soc Trans* 34:1032–1036.

Hattori M, Buse JB, et al. 1986. The NOD mouse: recessive diabetogenic gene in the major histocompatibility complex. *Science* 231:733–735.

Heim DA, Hanazono Y, et al. 2000. Introduction of a xenogeneic gene via hematopoietic stem cells leads to specific tolerance in a rhesus monkey model. *Mol Ther* 1:533–544.

Ierino FL, Gojo S, et al. 1999. Transfer of swine major histocompatibility complex class II genes into autologous bone marrow cells of baboons for the induction of tolerance across xenogeneic barriers. *Transplantation* 67:1119–1128.

Igarashi H, Gregory SC, et al. 2002. Transcription from the RAG1 locus marks the earliest lymphocyte progenitors in bone marrow. *Immunity* 17:117–130.

Jiang S, Lechler RI, et al. 2006. Regulatory T cells and transplantation tolerance. *Hum Immunol* 67:765–776.

Jordan MS, Boesteanu A, et al. 2001. Thymic selection of $CD4^+CD25^+$ regulatory T cells induced by an agonist self-peptide. *Nat Immunol* 2:301–306.

Kang E, Giri N, et al. 2001. In vivo persistence of retrovirally transduced murine long-term repopulating cells is not limited by expression of foreign gene products in the fully or minimally myeloablated setting. *Hum Gene Ther* 12:1663–1672.

Kang ES and Iacomini J. 2002. Induction of central deletional T cell tolerance by gene therapy. *J Immunol* 169:1930–1935.

Kappler JW, Roehm N, et al. 1987. T cell tolerance by clonal elimination in the thymus. *Cell* 49:273–280.

Kearns-Jonker M, Fischer-Lougheed J, et al. 2004. Use of lentiviral vectors to induce long-term tolerance to gal(+) heart grafts. *Transplantation* 77:1748–1754.

Kent SC, Chen Y, et al. 2005. Expanded T cells from pancreatic lymph nodes of type 1 diabetic subjects recognize an insulin epitope. *Nature* 435:224–228.

Kondo M, Weissman IL, et al. 1997. Identification of clonogenic common lymphoid progenitors in mouse bone marrow. *Cell* 91:661–672.

Kretschmer K, Apostolou I, et al. 2005. Inducing and expanding regulatory T cell populations by foreign antigen. *Nat Immunol* 6:1219–1227.

Kroczek RA, Mages HW, et al. 2004. Emerging paradigms of T-cell co-stimulation. *Curr Opin Immunol* 16:321–327.

Kumar A, Teuber SS, et al. 2006. Current perspectives on primary immunodeficiency diseases. *Clin Dev Immunol* 13:223–259.

Kung SK, An DS, et al. 2003. Induction of transgene-specific immunological tolerance in myeloablated nonhuman primates using lentivirally transduced $CD34^+$ progenitor cells. *Mol Ther* 8:981–991.

Kurobe H, Liu C, et al. 2006. CCR7-dependent cortex-to-medulla migration of positively selected thymocytes is essential for establishing central tolerance. *Immunity* 24:165–177.

Kuroda N, Mitani T, et al. 2005. Development of autoimmunity against transcriptionally unrepressed target antigen in the thymus of Aire-deficient mice. *J Immunol* 174:1862–1870.

Kurtz J, Shaffer J, et al. 2004a. Mechanisms of early peripheral CD4T-cell tolerance induction by anti-CD154 monoclonal antibody and allogeneic bone marrow transplantation: evidence for anergy and deletion but not regulatory cells. *Blood* 103:4336–4343.

Kurtz J, Wekerle T, et al. 2004b. Tolerance in mixed chimerism: a role for regulatory cells? *Trends Immunol* 25:518–523.

Lind EF, Prockop SE, et al. 2001. Mapping precursor movement through the postnatal thymus reveals specific microenvironments supporting defined stages of early lymphoid development. *J Exp Med* 194:127–134.

Liston A, Lesage S, et al. 2003. Aire regulates negative selection of organ-specific T cells. *Nat Immunol* 4:350–354.

Lutz MB and Schuler G. 2002. Immature, semi-mature and fully mature dendritic cells: which signals induce tolerance or immunity? *Trends Immunol* 23:445–449.

Mayfield RS, Hayashi H, et al. 1997. The mechanism of specific prolongation of class I–mismatched skin grafts induced by retroviral gene therapy. *Eur J Immunol* 27:1177–1181.

McDevitt HO. 1998. The role of MHC class II molecules in susceptibility and resistance to autoimmunity. *Curr Opin Immunol* 10:677–681.

McHugh RS and Shevach EM. 2002. Cutting edge: depletion of $CD4^+CD25^+$ regulatory T cells is necessary, but not sufficient, for induction of organ-specific autoimmune disease. *J Immunol* 168:5979–5983.

Meier-Kriesche HU, Schold JD, et al. 2004. Lack of improvement in renal allograft survival despite a marked decrease in acute rejection rates over the most recent era. *Am J Transplant* 4:378–383.

Mein CA, Esposito L, et al. 1998. A search for type 1 diabetes susceptibility genes in families from the United Kingdom. *Nat Genet* 19:297–300.

Mitsuhashi N, Fischer-Lougheed J, et al. 2006. Tolerance induction by lentiviral gene therapy with a nonmyeloablative regimen. *Blood* 107:2286–2293.

Moayeri M, Hawley TS, et al. 2005. Correction of murine hemophilia A by hematopoietic stem cell gene therapy. *Mol Ther* 12:1034–1042.

Moayeri M, Ramezani A, et al. 2004. Sustained phenotypic correction of hemophilia A mice following oncoretroviral-mediated expression of a bioengineered human factor VIII gene in long-term hematopoietic repopulating cells. *Mol Ther* 10:892–902.

Morel PA, Dorman JS, et al. 1988. Aspartic acid at position 57 of the HLA-DQ beta chain protects against type I diabetes: a family study. *Proc Natl Acad Sci U S A* 85:8111–8115.

Nakayama M, Abiru N, et al. 2005. Prime role for an insulin epitope in the development of type 1 diabetes in NOD mice. *Nature* 435:220–223.

Nemazee D, Gavin A, et al. 2006. Immunology: Toll-like receptors and antibody responses. *Nature* 441:E4; discussion E4.

Nepom GT and Kwok WW. 1998. Molecular basis for HLA-DQ associations with IDDM. *Diabetes* 47:1177–1184.

Nocentini G, Ronchetti S, et al. 2007. GITR/GITRL: more than an effector T cell co-stimulatory system. *Eur J Immunol* 37:1165–1169.

Oldenburg J, Ananyeva NM, et al. 2004. Molecular basis of haemophilia A. *Haemophilia* 10 (Suppl 4):133–139.

Ozduran V, Yamani MH, et al. 2005. Survival beyond 10 years following heart transplantation: The Cleveland Clinic Foundation experience. *Transplant Proc* 37:4509–4512.

Penit C, Lucas B, et al. 1995. Cell expansion and growth arrest phases during the transition from precursor ($CD4^-8^-$) to immature ($CD4^+8^+$) thymocytes in normal and genetically modified mice. *J Immunol* 154:5103–5113.

Peters TR, Bodine DM, et al. 2000. Retrovirus mediated gene transfer of the self antigen MBP into the bone marrow of mice alters resistance to experimental autoimmune encephalomyelitis. *J Neuroimmunol* 103:51–62.

Petrie HT, Livak F, et al. 1995. T cell receptor gene recombination patterns and mechanisms: cell death, rescue, and T cell production. *J Exp Med* 182:121–127.

Pichard V, Bellodi-Privato M, et al. 2006. Mixed hematopoietic molecular chimerism results in permanent transgene expression from retrovirally transduced hepatocytes in mice. *J Gene Med* 8:425–432.

Rajewsky K. 1996. Clonal selection and learning in the antibody system. *Nature* 381:751–758.

Saint-Ruf C, Ungewiss K, et al. 1994. Analysis and expression of a cloned pre-T cell receptor gene. *Science* 266:1208–1212.

Schwartz RH. 2003. T cell anergy. *Annu Rev Immunol* 21:305–334.

Schwarz K, Storni T, et al. 2003. Role of Toll-like receptors in costimulating cytotoxic T cell responses. *Eur J Immunol* 33:1465–1470.

Shimonkevitz RP, Husmann LA, et al. 1987. Transient expression of IL-2 receptor precedes the differentiation of immature thymocytes. *Nature* 329:157–159.

Shortman K and Wu L. 1996. Early T lymphocyte progenitors. *Annu Rev Immunol* 14:29–47.

Siggs OM, Makaroff LE, et al. 2006. The why and how of thymocyte negative selection. *Curr Opin Immunol* 18:175–183.

Singh N. 2005. Infectious complications in organ transplant recipients with the use of calcineurin-inhibitor agent-based immunosuppressive regimens. *Curr Opin Infect Dis* 18:342–345.

Sonntag KC, Emery DW, et al. 2001. Tolerance to solid organ transplants through transfer of MHC class II genes. *J Clin Invest* 107:65–71.

Spangrude GJ, Heimfeld S, et al. 1988. Purification and characterization of mouse hematopoietic stem cells. *Science* 241:58–62.

Steptoe RJ, Ritchie JM, et al. 2003. Transfer of hematopoietic stem cells encoding autoantigen prevents autoimmune diabetes. *J Clin Invest* 111:1357–1363.

Sykes M, Sachs DH, et al. 1993. Specific prolongation of skin graft survival following retroviral transduction of bone marrow with an allogeneic major histocompatibility complex gene. *Transplantation* 55:197–202.

Taguchi O and Takahashi T. 1996. Administration of anti-interleukin-2 receptor alpha antibody in vivo induces localized autoimmune disease. *Eur J Immunol* 26:1608–1612.

Takahama Y. 2006. Journey through the thymus: stromal guides for T-cell development and selection. *Nat Rev Immunol* 6:127–135.

Tian C, Bagley J, et al. 2004. Induction of central tolerance by mature T cells. *J Immunol* 173:7217–7222.

Tian C, Bagley J, et al. 2002. Expression of antigen on mature lymphocytes is required to induce T cell tolerance by gene therapy. *J Immunol* 169:3771–3776.

Tian C, Bagley J, et al. 2005. Persistence of antigen is required to maintain transplantation tolerance induced by genetic modification of bone marrow stem cells. *Am J Transplant* 6:2202–2207.

Tian C, Bagley J, et al. 2003. Induction of T cell tolerance to a protein expressed in the cytoplasm through retroviral-mediated gene transfer. *J Gene Med* 5:359–365.

Vadivel N, Tullius SG, et al. 2007. Chronic allograft nephropathy. *Semin Nephrol* 27:414–429.

Wegmann DR, Norbury-Glaser M, et al. 1994. Insulin-specific T cells are a predominant component of islet infiltrates in pre-diabetic NOD mice. *Eur J Immunol* 24:1853–1857.

Wicker LS, Todd JA, et al. 1995. Genetic control of autoimmune diabetes in the NOD mouse. *Annu Rev Immunol* 13:179–200.

Wildin RS, Ramsdell F, et al. 2001. X-linked neonatal diabetes mellitus, enteropathy and endocrinopathy syndrome is the human equivalent of mouse scurfy. *Nat Genet* 27:18–20.

Wong W, Billing JS, et al. 2003. Retroviral transfer of donor MHC class I or MHC class II genes into recipient bone marrow cells can induce operational tolerance to alloantigens in vivo. *Hum Gene Ther* 14:577–590.

Wong W, Fry J, et al. 1999. Haematopoietic stem cells transduced with a single donor class I major histocompatibility complex gene can induce operational tolerance to fully allogeneic cardiac allografts. *Transplant Proc* 31:886.

Wong W, Morris PJ, et al. 1996. Syngeneic bone marrow expressing a single donor class I MHC molecule permits acceptance of a fully allogeneic cardiac allograft. *Transplantation* 62:1462–1468.

Xu B, Haviernik P, et al. 2006. Bone marrow transplantation combined with gene therapy to induce antigen-specific tolerance and ameliorate EAE. *Mol Ther* 13:42–48.

Yang YG, deGoma E, et al. 1998. Tolerization of anti-Galalpha1-3Gal natural antibody-forming B cells by induction of mixed chimerism. *J Exp Med* 187:1335–1342.

13

RECONSTITUTION OF THE IMMUNE SYSTEM BY GENE THERAPY

WASEEM QASIM, M.D., PH.D., AND ADRIAN THRASHER, M.D., PH.D.
Centre for Immunodeficiency, Institute of Child Health, and Great Ormond Street Hospital NHS Trust, London, UK

13.1 INTRODUCTION

Allogeneic haematopoietic stem cell transplantation (HSCT) has been used to treat primary immunodeficiencies for almost 30 years [Buckley et al. 1999; Antoine et al. 2003], and these disorders are now highly attractive targets for correction by gene therapy. The most serious conditions, severe combined immune deficiencies (SCIDs), were the first to benefit from strategies using retroviral vectors for the addition of corrected gene copies to host cells [Cavazzana-Calvo

Gene Therapy Immunology, Edited by Roland Herzog

et al. 2000; Aiuti et al. 2002a]. This in turn allowed reconstitution of functional immunity in otherwise profoundly immunodeficient hosts. In this chapter we review ways in which gene-based strategies can be used to correct autologous hematopoietic stem cells (HSCs) and reconstitute lifesaving immunity in primary immune disorders. We also discuss how gene-modified allogeneic T cells have been used to support cellular immunity in the wider HSCT setting.

SCID disorders have a heterogeneous molecular basis (Table 13-1) but share a common pattern of clinical presentation, usually in the first few months of life. Poor growth and recurrent or opportunistic infections are characteristic [Fischer 2001; Buckley 2004]. The commonest form of SCID is X-linked and is caused by defects in the common cytokine gamma chain (γc). This molecule combines with an additional receptor chain (α-chain) or chains (α and β) to form interleukin receptors essential for T-cell and natural killer cell development and function (Fig. 13-1). B cells are produced in normal numbers but are dysfunctional, and in the absence of helper T-cell function, immunoglobulin production is defective, and profound T- and B-cell immune deficiency results. A second, less common disorder, adenosine deaminase deficiency (ADA) SCID,

TABLE 13-1 Molecular Basis of Severe Combined Immune Deficiency Disorders[a]

Disorder	Mutated Gene	Molecular Defect
SCID-X1	Common γ-chain	Absence of receptors for IL-2, -4, -7, -9, -15, and -21
JAK3 deficiency	JAK3	Defect of signalling via IL-2, -4, -7, -9, -15, and -21
IL-7 receptor deficiency	IL-7 receptor α	Absence of IL-7 receptor α
RAG-1, -2 deficiency	RAG-1 and RAG-2	Defective VDJ recombination
Artermis deficiency	Artermis	Defective VDJ recombination; radiation sensitivity
Ligase IV deficiency	Ligase IV	Defective VDJ recombination; radiation sensitivity
Cernunnos	Cernunnos	Defective VDJ recombination; radiation sensitivity
Adenosine deaminase deficiency	ADA	Block in purine salvage metabolism
Purine nucleoside phosphorylase deficiency	PNP	Block in purine salvage metabolism
T-cell receptor deficiencies	CD3 γ/δ/ε	Defective T-cell signaling
ZAP70 deficiency	ZAP70	Defective T-cell signaling
ORAI-1	ORAI-1	Defective T-cell signaling
CD45 deficiency	CD45	Defective T- and B-cell signaling

[a]A molecular basis can be established for over 80% of cases. The SCID-X1 and ADA deficiencies have been treated successfully using retroviral gene therapy.

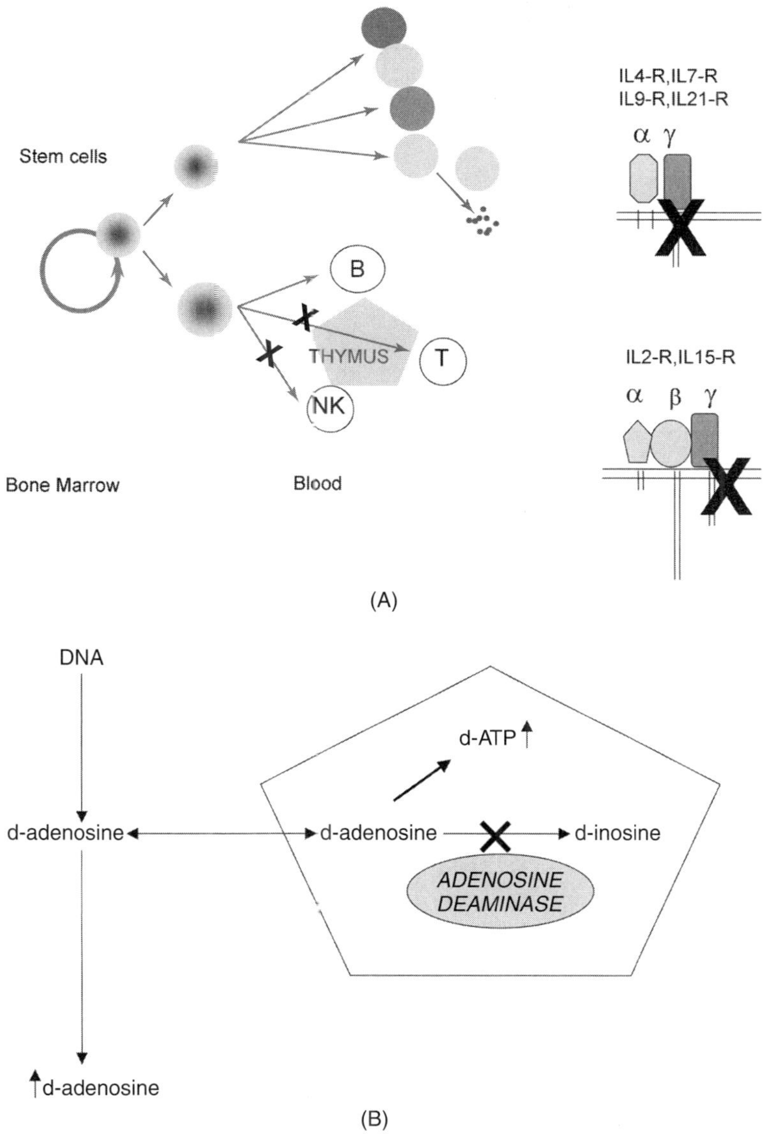

Figure 13-1 (A) SCID-X1 is caused by defective expression of the common cytokine γ-chain, which leads to failed T- and NK-cell production. B cells do develop but are functionally incompetent. (B) In adenosine deaminase (ADA) deficiency, accumulation of the purine metabolites 2′-deoxyadenosine and deoxyadenosinetrisphosphate (d-ATP) leads to inhibition of DNA synthesis, impaired cell division, and apoptosis of lymphocytes.

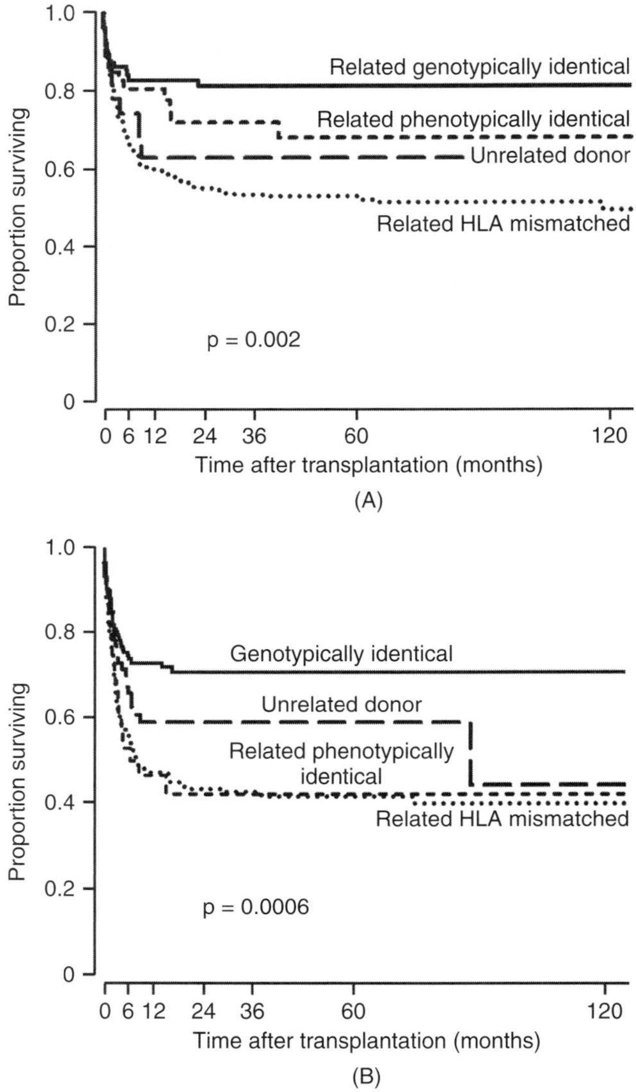

Figure 13-2 Survival following allogeneic HSCT for SCID (A) and non-SCID (B) disorders based on the level of HLA matching. (From Antoine et al. 2003.)

has a recessive inheritance. The ADA enzyme is ubiquitous, with particularly high levels of activity in the thymus and lymphoid tissues. ADA deficiency results in an accumulation of 2′-deoxyadenosine and deoxyadenosinetrisphosphate (d-ATP), leading to inhibition of DNA synthesis, impaired cell division, and apoptosis. Polyethylene-glycolated bovine enzyme (PEG-ADA) can mediate systemic detoxification and thereby permits a degree of immune reconstitution. This is now first-line therapy in patients awaiting stem cell transplantation and can provide satisfactory protection if combined with immunoglobulin replacement therapy, although there are concerns about the durability of its effects in the longer term [Husain et al. 2007]. In the majority of SCID disorders, genotypically HLA-matched sibling donor hematopoietic stem cell transplantation is highly effective. Centers in North America [Buckley et al. 1999] and Europe [Antoine et al. 2003] can anticipate survival figures of over 80% (Fig. 13-2). However, in the absence of a fully matched donor, HLA-mismatched transplants are much less successful, and in the case of ADA deficiency, survival figures of about 30% might be anticipated. In addition, survivors of mismatched transplants encounter more late complications and have poorer immune reconstitution than do those undergoing fully matched procedures. Thus, this group of patients has the most to gain from alternative therapies based on gene transfer and have been recruited to phase I trials of retroviral gene therapy.

13.2 IMMUNE DISORDERS AS ATTRACTIVE TARGETS FOR GENE THERAPY

There are a number of important reasons why severe combined immune deficiencies have been the first disorders to be corrected by retroviral gene therapy:

1. The molecular basis for over 80% of SCID disorders is now established. The diagnosis can now be made rapidly and causative genetic mutation often identified.
2. Target cell populations and precursor hematopoietic stem cells are easily accessible through peripheral blood or bone marrow harvesting. This allows ex vivo manipulation and genetic modification of cells in the laboratory, followed by return to the host by simple infusion. This approach minimizes off-target effects and virtually eliminates the risk of sensitization against vector particles.
3. SCID disorders usually present in the first few months of life. Infants exhibit remarkable regenerative potential if treated early while the potential for effective thymopoiesis is intact. The cost/benefit ratio of effective therapy in these infants is extremely high, especially when calculated in terms of life years added.
4. Rarely, spontaneous postzygotic reversion mutations may arise and have been documented as leading to partial reconstitution in patients with SCID-X1 [Stephan et al. 1996], ADA SCID [Hirschhorn et al. 1996], Wiskott–Aldrich syndrome [Ariga et al. 2001], and Nemo syndrome [Nishikomori et al. 2004]. These extremely unusual patients highlight the ability of a single precursor cell to repopulate the lymphoid compartment in the context of profound immunodeficiency. This supports the notion

that a small number of gene-corrected stem cells could repopulate and reconstitute affected persons.

5. There are established animal models for these conditions that have been corrected by retroviral gene addition to defective HSCs [Soudais et al. 2000; Kiem et al. 2004].

13.3 CLINICAL GENE THERAPY TRIALS FOR SCID

Retrovirus-mediated gene correction of γc-deficient SCID-X1 was first reported in 2000, in two infants by French investigators [Cavazzana-Calvo et al. 2000]. Autologous HSCs expressing the stem cell marker CD34 were cultured in a combination of interleukin-3 (IL-3), megakaryocyte growth and development factor, stem cell factor, and Flt-3 ligand before exposure to a murine retroviral vector (MFG) encoding the γc transgene and packaged with an amphotropic envelope. Retronectin, a recombinant fibronectin fragment, was used to assist vector–target cell co-localization during three rounds of virus exposure. Transduced cells were reinfused without prior chemotherapeutic preconditioning, and 9 of 10 patients had effective immunological reconstitution [Hacein-Bey-Abina et al. 2002], although as discussed below, there have also been unexpected adverse events in some patients. Subsequently, 10 infants have been treated at our own center using a similar vector, pseudotyped with the gibbon ape leukemia virus (GALV) envelope and transduced using slightly modified culture conditions. All have had sustained immune recovery, with the majority achieving immune recovery sufficient to merit the withdrawal of prophylactic antibiotics and immunoglobulin replacement therapy [Gaspar et al. 2004]. A similar approach was used to treat ADA SCID, and as discussed below, a number of patients have now been enrolled in these trials.

13.4 IMMUNE RECOVERY AFTER GENE THERAPY FOR SCID-X1

The kinetics of immune reconstitution following gene therapy for SCID-X1 closely mirrors that seen following conventional stem cell transplantation (Fig. 13-3). NK cells are detected 2 to 4 weeks after the procedure, and T cells usually within 12 weeks. Detailed serial analysis of immune recovery has revealed the rapid emergence of CD45RA$^+$ CD27$^+$ CCR7$^+$ naive T cells. This is good evidence of new thymic output and is supported by the detection of recent thymic emigrants through the quantification of T-cell receptor excision circles (TRECS). These are by-products generated during T-cell ontogeny following T-cell receptor gene recombination. TRECS are diluted during cell division, and thus quantification is a measure of post-thymic proliferation. Within 6 to 12 months of gene therapy, TREC levels have been found to be within the normal range for age. Analysis of T-cell receptor diversity by spectratype analysis initially detected oligoclonal populations, which over time

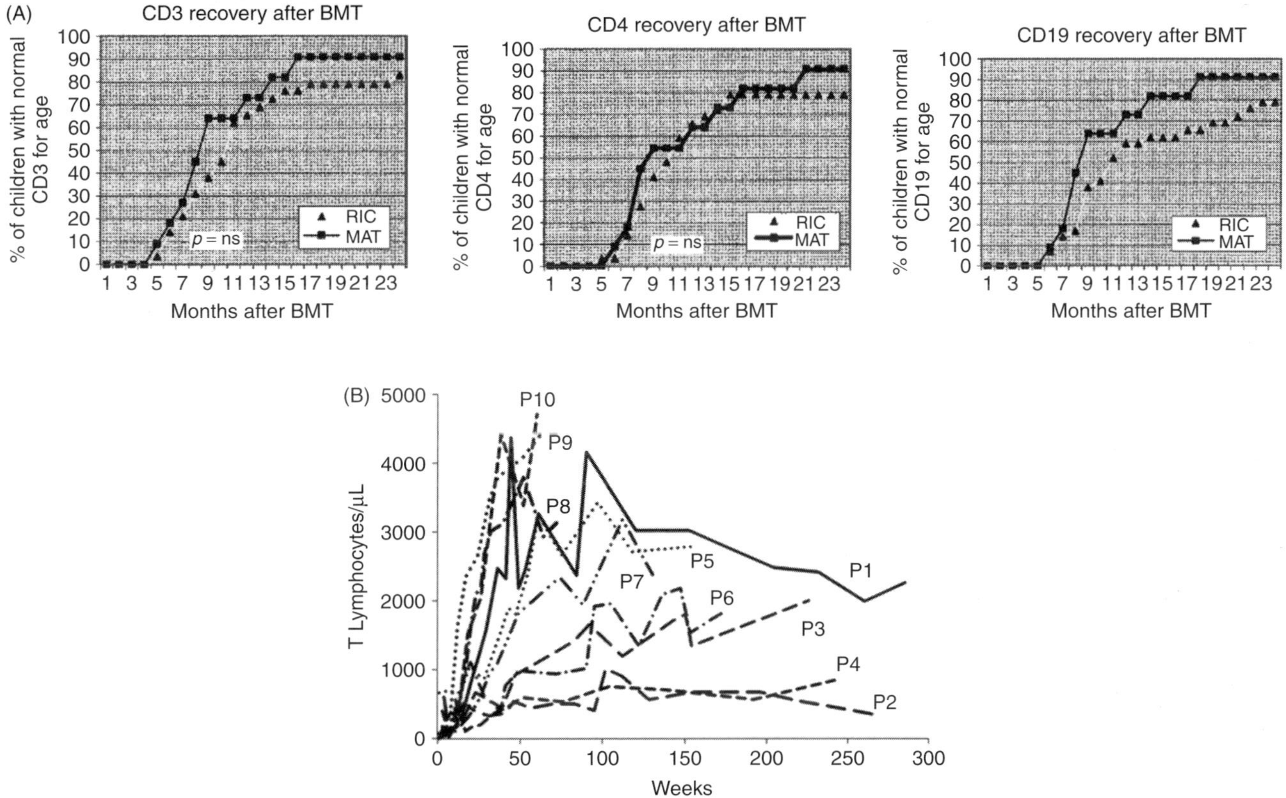

Figure 13-3 (A) Kinetics of immune recovery following allogeneic transplantation for primary immune deficiency using either reduced-intensity conditioning or myeloablative therapy. Between six months and two years post-transplant, recovery of $CD3^+$ T cells, $CD4^+$ helper T cells, and $CD19^+$ B cells develops. (From Rao et al. 2005.) (B) Kinetics of T-lymphocyte recovery following gene therapy in 10 infants treated at our institution mirrors what was seen following conventional transplantation.

become more diverse, leading to a fully Gaussian repertoire distribution in most V-beta families. T-cell responses against mitogens such as conconavalin A (ConA) and staphylococcal eneteroxin B (SEB) confirmed in vitro that the cells were capable of proliferative responses.

B-cell immunity and antibody responses were also restored in a number of patients. Following the detection of autologous IgA and IgM production, immunoglobulin replacement therapy (IgG) was withdrawn in these cases and patients were monitored for evidence of IgG production. Reimmunization with childhood vaccines subsequently confirmed the production of specific antibody responses against tetanus toxoid and *Haemophilus influenzae* type B. The integrity of the reconstituted immune system was challenged through natural exposure to childhood infections in some cases. For example, varicella-zoster virus (VZV) infection resolved naturally in one case, and this provided an opportunity to confirm the generation of T-cell memory responses against VZV on the basis of interferon-γ secretion following exposure of T cells to viral antigen in vitro. Analysis of memory phenotype B cells from this patient revealed editing of the B-cell immunoglobulin receptor repertoire through somatic hypermutation [Gaspar et al. 2004]. This is an essential aspect of humoral immunity that facilitates ongoing diversification of the immunoglobulin receptor in response to antigenic challenges.

13.5 GENE THERAPY FOR ADA DEFICIENCY

Initial attempts to correct ADA-deficient SCID began in the 1990s and targeted peripheral blood mononuclear cells. Patient T cells were stimulated with a combination of recombinant IL-2 and an anti-CD3 antibody. The gene-modified T cells were returned to patients by peripheral infusion and the procedure was repeated about 12 times over a two-year period. Immunity improved in these patients, but because they remained on PEG-ADA replacement therapy, the role of the gene-corrected T cells was not clearly established [Blaese et al. 1995]. In one of the two patients treated in this study, high levels (20%) of genetically modified T cells persisted in vivo for over 10 years [Muul et al. 2003]. Another study used two different retroviral vectors encoding the ADA gene independently to modify marrow stem cells and peripheral blood lymphocytes, and showed long-term survival of T and B cells from the marrow transduction, with eventual normalization of the immune repertoire [Bordignon et al. 1995]. Hoogerbrugge et al. [1996] transduced $CD34^+$ stem cells from three patients, two of whom were receiving enzyme replacement therapy, using retroviral gene transfer. The results of this study were disappointing, with loss of gene expression within six months. ADA cord blood $CD34^+$ cells from affected infants have also been transduced [Kohn et al. 1998], and subsequent analysis of proviral integration sites revealed that a limited number of clones had been modified, and in one patient the majority of the T-cell pool had derived from a single lymphoid progenitor [Schmidt et al. 2003]. In all these studies it has been postulated that continued administration of PEG-ADA reduced the selective advantage of the genetically modified cells and therefore limited their engraftment potential. In rare circumstances, when PEG-ADA was withdrawn there was an improvement in gene-modified T-cell immunity [Aiuti et al. 2002b] and this supported the notion that if enzyme replacement therapy was withdrawn before the reinfusion of ADA-gene corrected cells, the incoming cells would retain a survival advantage. Thus, a strategy to facilitate the engraftment of genetically modified HSC by combining reduced-dose busulfan preconditioning and withholding of PEG-ADA replacement was evaluated. One child, aged 7 months, developed normal T-, B-, and NK-cell counts and normal immunoglobulin production, as well as significantly reducing systemic d-ATP levels. A second child, aged 2 years and 6 months, had slower T-cell reconstitution and remained on immunoglobulin replacement therapy [Aiuti et al. 2002a]. T-cell receptor analysis showed a diverse, polyclonal T-cell repertoire in both patients and there was good evidence of detoxification. At our own center, a similar procedure was undertaken using a retroviral vector modified to encode spleen focus forming virus long terminal repeat sequences and a mutated woodchuck postregulatory element (WPRE) designed to improve transgene expression and increase ADA levels [Gaspar et al. 2006]. An alternative conditioning regimen using melphalan was combined with PEG-ADA withdrawal. Good levels of enzyme expression, with reduced levels of toxic metabolites, supported reconstitution of the T-cell compartment. A diverse T-cell receptor repertoire has been confirmed, along with the presence of naive populations and evidence of thymic output. The use of conditioning chemotherapy to render patients receptive to engraftment with gene-modified stem cells is not without risk. Prolonged pancytopaenia was reported in one patient with ADA SCID after bone marrow cytoreduction with busulfan (3 mg/kg), and necessitated rescue therapy with autologous pre-stored bone marrow [Engel et al. 2006]. Unexpectedly, the patient was found to have trisomy 8 mosaicism on bone marrow examination, and it is likely that this predated the gene therapy procedure or arose following the conditioning regimen. Overall, ADA-SCID has proven an excellent candidate for correction by gene therapy, and systemic detoxification with immune recovery has been documented in over 10 patients.

13.6 INSERTIONAL MUTAGENESIS FOLLOWING RETROVIRAL GENE THERAPY FOR SCID

Risks associated with multiple insertional events following exposure to replicating retroviruses are well documented. In one animal study, hematological malignancies were detected in around one-third of nonhuman primates following autologous transplantation with bone marrow that had been transduced with replication-competent retrovirus [Vanin et al. 1994]. However, non-replication-competent retroviral vectors were thought to carry a greatly reduced, perhaps negligible risk of mutagenic potential. Only very rarely had mutagenesis been reported in animal studies using replication-deficient retroviral vectors. In one study murine bone marrow labeled by retroviral transduction with ΔLNGFR, a truncated form of the low-affinity nerve growth factor receptor [Li et al. 2002], was transplanted to secondary recipients, some of which developed myeloproliferative disease. Investigations revealed that an identical leukemic clone was present in all the affected mice, and a single vector copy was found to have integrated into the first exon of the murine *EVI1* gene. Previous studies had identified this gene as the site of wild-type viral integration in 5/37 mice that had developed retrovirus-induced myeloid leukemias [Morishita et al. 1988]. Thus, both wild-type virus and replication-defective engineered viral vector seemed to have targeted the same host cell oncogene. The risk of similar adverse events was thought to be extremely low in human studies until complications arose in the French SCID-X1 trial in 2002. Two of the youngest children to be treated (aged 3 months, and 12 months) had received a high dose of gene-modified CD34 cells [Hacein-Bey-Abina et al. 2003a,b]. Around 30 months after treatment the older child was found to have increased numbers of γδ T cells and within a further four months there was evidence of leukemic blasts and infiltration into bone marrow and spleen. Subsequently the expanded T-cell population was found to be clonal but with abnormal cytogenetics, indicating a partial trisomy 6 and a t(6;13) translocation. Soon after, the younger child developed a similar lymphoproliferative disorder with three αβ T-cell clones identified. In both children linear amplification (LAM) PCR enabled the site of proviral integration to be mapped close to the site of the LMO2 (LIM domain only-2) gene on chromosome 11 [Hacein-Bey-Abina et al. 2003b] (Fig. 13-4). LMO2 is a cysteine-rich LIM (Lin-11, Isl-1, Mec-3) finger protein essential for normal hematopoiesis [Yamada et al. 1998] but is usually silenced in post-thymic T cells. Importantly, aberrant LMO2 expression is well known to have a role in some spontaneous T-ALL following chromosomal translocations such as t(11;14) [Royer-Pokora et al. 1991].

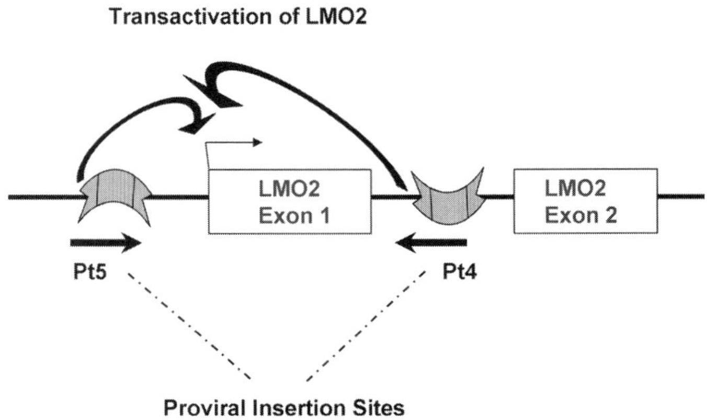

Figure 13-4 Insertion close to the transcription start site of LMO2 in either the sense or reverse orientation was sufficient to transactivate the oncogene, and this in turn precipitated uncontrolled T-cell expansion.

Subsequent to the initial reports of adverse events, a further two children developed mutagenic complications in the same trial, although in these cases the insertion sites varied. There is considerable controversy as to whether retroviral insertional events per se were sufficient to initiate transformational changes in these children. Additional precipitants may have been required, or the growth-promoting nature of the transgene may be relevant. Some groups have argued that because γc plays such a central role in T-cell development and function, unregulated expression may have contributed to leukemogenesis in lymphoid progenitor cells. This could have combined with the "first hit" of oncogene transactivation due to proviral integration. Murine studies have postulated such a link [Dave et al. 2004], and in longer-term tracking of SCID-X1 mice corrected by high-level lentiviral gene transfer of γc, a number of animals developed suspicious lymphoid malignancies [Woods et al. 2006]. Other experiments have not supported such findings despite extended follow-up of treated animals [Thrasher et al. 2006]. Other possible contributing factors should also be noted: The patients all had poor preexisting immunity and this has permitted the evolution of leukemogenic T-cell clones. In such immunodeficiency there may also be increased capacity for homeostatic capacity of T cells, and this environment could support rapid expansion of leukemogenic clones. The high number of genetically modified HSCs returned to some of the patients in the SCID-X1 trial is also relevant. If the chances of integrating into a transcriptionally active gene are estimated to be around 1 in 10^5, it has been estimated that each patient received 1 to 10 T-cell precursors with integration sites close to LMO2 [Hacein-Bey-Abina et al. 2003b]. Such calculations are based on an assumption of random proviral integration patterns, but it is now clear that retroviral integration is biased toward transcriptional start sites of active genes, increasing the likelihood of LTR-mediated transactivation or transcriptional disruption of host genes.

13.7 AGE LIMITATIONS ON GENE THERAPY POTENTIAL IN SCID

A small number of patients with attenuated SCID phenotype and older patients with residual defects or poor immunity following HSCT in infancy have also been treated with somatic gene therapy. A 3-year-old boy without suitable allogeneic HSCT donor underwent gene therapy and had slow reconstitution kinetics and remains on immunoglobulin replacement. A 15-year-old patient treated with autologous gene-modified stem cells failed to reconstitute and subsequently died from infective complications [Thrasher et al. 2005]. Similarly, a 20-year-old man who had undergone a phenoidentical paternal graft in infancy but had poor reconstitution and continued T-cell deficiency, absent NK cells, and low numbers of B cells was treated under a similar protocol. He had developed bronchiectasis, hepatitis, and protein-losing enteropathy, and magnetic resonance imaging had failed to detect the presence of thymic tissue. Despite receiving a high number of gene-corrected autologous $CD34^+$ stem cells, reconstitution was poor, with low numbers of naive T cells and poor TREC levels. Gene therapy in a further three patients who had poor immunity following HSCT in infancy has recently been reported [Chinen et al. 2007]. Only the youngest, aged 10, had any sustained improvement of T-cell immunity. Overall, it appears that older patients are less suitable candidates for gene correction of autologous HSC. This is probably a reflection of reduced thymic potential in older patients, in particular if there has been reduced thymopoiesis over an extended period or chronic graft versus host disease following previous transplantation. These cases highlight the importance of treating patients in early infancy, at a time when thymus is more amenable to seeding with lymphoid progenitors and thymopoiesis can be rescued.

13.8 PROSPECTS FOR GENE THERAPY FOR SCID

Large-scale mapping of over 500 retroviral integration sites from 9 patients with SCID-X1 treated using gene therapy revealed around two-thirds of insertions in, or very near to, genes. Many of these genes were highly expressed in the $CD34^+$ stem cell target population, and there was clear evidence of clustering at common integration sites (CISs) [Deichmann et al. 2007]. In the short term, strategies are being developed to minimize the risk of transactivation events at CIS. Self-inactivating (sin) retroviral vector constructs devoid of their powerful U3 promoter–enhancer elements [Schambach et al. 2006] and reliant on weaker internal promoter sequences have been generated and are undergoing preclinical evaluation. Additional safety maneuvers might include the use of insulator elements such as the chicken β-globin locus cHS4 insulator [Emery et al. 2000]. Inclusion of these sequences would be designed to reduce vector promoter effects on adjacent genes. In the longer term, it may be feasible to exploit an alternative approach based on gene repair (rather than gene addition), correcting a small number of HSCs sufficient to reconstitute immunity in SCID. Recently, zinc finger proteins (ZFPs) linked to a nonspecific DNA cleavage domain of the Fok1-type IIS restriction enzyme have been investigated. The resulting zinc finger nuclease can initiate double-stranded DNA breaks at specific sites, which are then repaired by homologous recombination [Kandavelou et al. 2005]. C2H2 ZFN targeting γc has been used to repair the γc gene and induce repair of human cell lines and primary T cells [Urnov et al. 2005]. The process requires further refinement, and a full evaluation of possible undesired or off-target effects has yet to be established.

13.9 NON-SCID IMMUNE DISORDERS: GENE THERAPY FOR CHRONIC GRANULOMATOUS DISEASE

A number of non-SCID disorders of the immune system are also attractive targets for gene therapy. These can be serious, life-threatening conditions, amenable to curative therapy by allogeneic stem cell transplantation. Chronic granulomatous disease (CGD) is a rare genetic immunodeficiency due to defects of nicotinamide dinucleotide phosphate (NADPH) oxidase function [Heyworth et al. 2003]. Mutations in the CYBB gene, encoding the $gp91^{phox}$ subunit, give rise to X-linked CGD, and less commonly, mutations in CYBA, NCF-1, and NCF-2 (which encode the respective subunits $p22^{phox}$, $p47^{phox}$, and $p67^{phox}$) give rise to recessive forms of CGD. The resulting defects of phagocyte function predispose to serious recurrent bacterial and fungal infections [Goldblatt and Thrasher 2000]. Hematopoietic stem cell transplantation (HSCT) can cure CGD, but is generally considered only if a fully HLA-matched donor is available [Seger et al. 2002]. Fungal infection is a major adverse risk factor in the transplant setting [Martino et al. 2002, 2005], but despite this, successful HSCT has been undertaken in CGD patients with established *Aspergillus* disease [Ozsahin et al. 1998; Watanabe et al. 2001]. For patients without a suitable stem cell donor, alternative approaches are required. Malech et al. [1997] were the first to treat patients with CGD using a gammaretroviral vector to correct autologous $CD34^+$ peripheral blood stem cells (PBSCs). Patients did not receive conditioning, and circulating gene-modified cells were transiently detectable, peaking at 4 to 6 weeks after therapy. After 6 months, gene-modified cells declined to undetectable levels. More recently, reconstitution data from patients treated with retroviral gene therapy for X-CGD following nonmyeloabltive conditioning with busulfan has also been reported [Ott et al. 2006]. Granulocyte colony-stimulating factor–mobilized peripheral blood $CD34^+$ cells were transduced with a retroviral vector expressing $gp91^{phox}$ and reinfused to three patients 5 days later. Gene-modified cells were detected within three weeks, followed by a continuous increase until day 241, by which time 46% leukocytes expressed $gp91^{phox}$. Levels at one year were similar, declining to 27% by 18 months. As well as granulocyte marking, gene-modified B cells were detected and there was low-level T-cell marking. There was sustained superoxide production in neutrophils in the first two patients treated, and clearance of longstanding infections. Proviral integration sites analyzed at multiple time points by linear amplification mediated PCR and demonstrated the presence of polyclonal integrants in both lymphoid and myeloid populations at early time points. Beyond five months the pattern was less random, with evidence of clonal selection. Integration occurred preferentially in gene-coding regions and was highly skewed toward transcriptional start sites. Sequencing of individual integrants detected insertions close to three particular genes: *MDS1*, *EVI1*, and *PRDM16* or *SETP1*. Vector insertion at these CISs appears to have led to proliferation and expansion of neutrophils. Overexpression of *EVI1* in murine bone marrow induces myeloproliferation followed by a myelodysplasia [Buonamici et al. 2004], and *EVI1* expression is associated with human myelodysplasia and myeloid leukemia [Johansson et al. 2002]. Importantly, there was no evidence of frank leukemia in these patients, although the first patient treated went on to develop unexplained cytopenia and died from sepsis. This occurred more than 2 years after the procedure, at a time when around 60% of his circulating neutrophils were gene modified but only around 10% had NADPH oxidase activity.

This finding raised the possibility of transcriptional silencing and consequent reversion to the disease phenotype. Additional patients have been treated at other centers, also using nonmyeloablative conditioning. At our own center one hospitalized patient cleared invasive aspergillosis and is alive and at home over five years later. However, gene-corrected cells were not readily detected in the circulation beyond a few months, raising important issues regarding the intensity of preconditioning required and the possibility of immune-mediated clearance of the gene-modified populations.

Other non-SCID disorders currently under consideration for gene therapy include leukocyte adhesion deficiency, in which defective expression of the β2-integrin CD18 leads to migration failure of neutrophils and T cells. Sustained correction of a canine model of the disease using lentiviral vectors has been described [Bauer et al. 2006]. Similarly, retroviral- and lentiviral-mediated correction of circulating immune cells has been described in murine models of Wiskott–Aldrich syndrome, another potentially life-threatening primary immune disorder [Martin et al. 2005; Boztug et al. 2006; Dupre et al. 2006; Charrier et al. 2007].

13.10 T-CELL GENE THERAPY SUPPORT FOR STEM CELL TRANSPLANTATION

In addition to immunological disorders, a variety of hematological disorders, certain malignancies, and metabolic diseases are amenable to treatment by allogeneic transplantation [Appelbaum 2001]. Gene-based therapies have been used in this arena as part of a strategy to support immune-mediated effects of transplantation and to accelerate immune recovery. In particular, T cells have been manipulated to express a suicide gene to allow their safe in the allogeneic setting. Patients with an HLA-matched sibling donor can usually tolerate infusions of large number of donor T cells, with minimal risk of significant graft versus host disease (GVHD). In contrast, mismatched and haploidentical transplants must be undertaken following T-cell depletion or with heavy immunosuppression. Although the depletion of donor T cells from the graft greatly reduces the risk of significant GVHD, it also causes a loss of graft potency [Ho and Soiffer 2001]. This in turn delays immune reconstitution and is associated with an increased risk of graft failure, relapse of malignancy and infective complications. The dilemma of using T-cell-replete grafts while limiting the possibility of GVHD is usually addressed by combining serotherapy with immunosuppressive agents such as cyclosporin, with additional steroid-based therapy as required. T-cell suicide gene therapy was conceived as a strategy that would allow T cells to be used for their beneficial immunotherapeutic effects while ensuring that they could be eliminated in the event of complications such as GVHD [Tiberghien et al. 1994] This approach relies on the conversion of a nontoxic prodrug into a toxic moiety by a gene-encoded enzyme system. Ideal prodrug-activating systems would be effective at low substrate concentrations and lack cellular homologs capable of eliciting similar responses. The herpes simplex virus thymidine kinase (HSVTK) enzyme has been used in combination with the antiviral prodrugs ganciclovir (GCV) and aciclovir (ACV) The prodrugs are phosphorylated to the monophosphate HSVTK, and further phosphorylation by cellular kinases results in the production of toxic triphosphate derivatives [Greco and Dachs 2001]. The strategy has been widely tested and is most effective when rapidly dividing HSVTK-expressing cells are exposed to high concentrations of GCV. Clinical trials using donor T cells that had been retrovirally transduced to carry the HSVTK gene were first reported almost a decade ago in proof-of-principle studies [Bonini et al. 1997]. A number of centers have now undertaken analogous studies, treating over 100 patients using a variety of retroviral constructs. In all cases it has been necessary to include a selection system (either neomycin resistance or ΔLNGFR expression) to ensure that highly enriched populations of gene-modified T cells are generated [Tiberghien et al. 2001; Burt et al. 2003; Fehse et al. 2004] In addition, robust activation of donor T cells is required to ensure satisfactory transduction, and this has varied from use of the T-cell mitogen phytohemagglutinin (PHA) to activation with anti-CD3 antibody or a combination of anti-CD3 and CD28 antibodies. The original strategy tested the use of gene-modified donor T-cell infusions in the event of leukemic relapse following HLA-matched transplantation [Bonini et al. 1997] Almost 60 patients have been treated using this approach, with documented clinical responses in around one-third [Bonini et al. 2007]. GVHD was controlled in five patients using the prodrug strategy. A further 15 patients received gene-modified T cells at the same time as the infusion of the donor graft—the day 0 strategy [Tiberghien et al. 2001; Fehse et al. 2004] Six cases of GVHD resolved, but in one of these studies, eradiaction of donor T cells was followed by graft failure [Fehse et al. 2004], emphasizing the important role of donor T cells in protecting donor HSC engraftment. Infusions have also been programmed into the post-HSCT schedule following haploidentical transplants. These are high-risk, last-resort procedures that use stringently T-cell-depleted grafts. As such, they are associated with extended periods of immunodeficiency. HSVTK-modified T cells have been administered six weeks after the transplant, at a time when anti-T-cell serotherapy given as part of the transplant conditioning regimen should not affect the infused populations.

Overall, the incidence of GVHD has been lower than anticipated, and in addition, the occurrence of viral complications has raised concerns that the functionality of the gene-modified T-cell populations may be reduced compared to that of nonmanipulated cells. Laboratory investigations have revealed that the process of T-cell activation prior to transduction can skew the T-cell repertoire [Ferrand et al. 2000], shift cells to a memory phenotype, and increase expression regulatory T-cell activity [Mesel-Lemoine et al. 2006; Qasim et al., 2007]. Some of these effects can be minimized by using bead-conjugated anti-CD3/CD28 antibodies and minimizing the period of ex vivo manipulation [Qasim et al. 2003]. Strategies to circumvent the preactivation of T cells prior to transduction are under development, including the use of lentiviral vectors in conjunction with cytokine stimulation [Cavalieri et al. 2003; Qasim et al. 2007]. Such approaches result in a better preserved T-cell inoculum, but are currently limited by limited lentiviral vector production capacities and low yields. There have also been worries about possible host immune responses against the HSVTK transgene [Traversari et al. 2007]. Multiple T-cell epitopes have been described following the characterization of cytotoxic T-cell responses against HSVTK-expressing T cells [Berger et al. 2006]. Although this may be a limited concern in immunosuppressed patients, rapid clearance of gene-modified T cells is likely in a competent host. Efforts are under way to develop humanized forms of the thymidine kinase enzyme, and other prodrug activating systems are being investigated. Examples include fusion of molecules involved in apoptosis pathways such as Fas [Thomis et al. 2001] and caspase 9 [Straathof et al. 2005] with engineered FK506-binding proteins. Designer dimerizer agents have been generated to trigger apotosis in transduced cells. Alternatively, T cells have been engineered to express the CD20 surface molecule and then targeted with Retuximab and anti-CD20 monoclonal antibody [van Meerten et al. 2006].

13.11 SUMMARY

Retroviral gene therapy for a number of inherited immune deficiencies has been demonstrated successfully and offers a valuable alternative to allogeneic stem cell transplantation in the absence of a suitable donor. Robust immune recovery is particularly notable in younger infants with T-cell deficiencies. The likely mechanism of unanticipated side effects has been elucidated, and concerted efforts are under way to reduce the risks of insertional mutagenesis.

REFERENCES

Aiuti A, Slavin S, Aker M, et al. 2002a. Correction of ADA-SCID by stem cell gene therapy combined with nonmyeloablative conditioning. *Science* 296:2410–2413.

Aiuti A, Vai S, Mortellaro A, et al. 2002b. Immune reconstitution in ADA-SCID after PBL gene therapy and discontinuation of enzyme replacement. *Nat Med* 8:423–425.

Antoine C, Muller S, Cant A, et al. 2003. Long-term survival and transplantation of haemopoietic stem cells for immunodeficiencies: report of the European experience 1968–99. *Lancet* 361:553–560.

Appelbaum FR. 2001. Haematopoietic cell transplantation as immunotherapy. *Nature* 411:385–389.

Ariga T, Kondoh T, Yamaguchi K, et al. 2001. Spontaneous in vivo reversion of an inherited mutation in the Wiskott–Aldrich syndrome. *J Immunol* 166:5245–5249.

Bauer TR Jr, Hai M, Tuschong LM, et al. 2006. Correction of the disease phenotype in canine leukocyte adhesion deficiency using ex vivo hematopoietic stem cell gene therapy. *Blood* 108:3313–3320.

Berger C, Flowers ME, Warren EH, and Riddell SR. 2006. Analysis of transgene-specific immune responses that limit the in vivo persistence of adoptively transferred HSV-TK-modified donor T cells after allogeneic hematopoietic cell transplantation. *Blood* 107:2294–2302.

Blaese RM, Culver KW, Miller AD, et al. 1995. T lymphocyte-directed gene therapy for ADA-SCID: initial trial results after 4 years. *Science* 270:475–480.

Bonini C, Ferrari G, Verzeletti S, et al. 1997. HSV-TK gene transfer into donor lymphocytes for control of allogeneic graft-versus-leukemia. *Science* 276:1719–1724.

Bonini C, Bondanza A, Perna SK, et al. 2007. The suicide gene therapy challenge: how to improve a successful gene therapy approach. *Mol Ther* 15:1248–1252.

Bordignon C, Notarangelo LD, Nobili N, et al. 1995. Gene therapy in peripheral blood lymphocytes and bone marrow for ADA- immunodeficient patients. *Science* 270:470–475.

Boztug K, Dewey RA, and Klein C. 2006. Development of hematopoietic stem cell gene therapy for Wiskott–Aldrich syndrome. *Curr Opin Mol Ther* 8:390–395.

Buckley RH. 2004. Molecular defects in human severe combined immunodeficiency and approaches to immune reconstitution. *Annu Rev Immunol* 22625–22655.

Buckley RH, Schiff SE, Schiff RI, et al. 1999. Hematopoietic stem-cell transplantation for the treatment of severe combined immunodeficiency. *N Engl J Med* 340:508–516.

Buonamici S, Li D, Chi Y, et al. 2004. *EVI1* induces myelodysplastic syndrome in mice. *J Clin Invest* 114:713–719.

Burt RK, Drobyski WR, Seregina T, et al. 2003. Herpes simplex thymidine kinase gene-transduced donor lymphocyte infusions. *Exp Hematol* 31:903–910.

Cavalieri S, Cazzaniga S, Geuna M, et al. 2003. Human T lymphocytes transduced by lentiviral vectors in the absence of TCR activation maintain an intact immune competence. *Blood* 102:497–505.

Cavazzana-Calvo M, Hacein-Bey S, de Saint BG, et al. 2000. Gene therapy of human severe combined immunodeficiency SCID-X1 disease. *Science* 288:669–672.

Charrier S, Dupre L, Scaramuzza S, et al. 2007. Lentiviral vectors targeting WASp expression to hematopoietic cells, efficiently transduce and correct cells from WAS patients. *Gene Ther* 14:415–428.

Chinen J, Davis J, De Ravin SS, et al. 2007. Gene therapy improves immune function in preadolescents with X-linked severe combined immunodeficiency. *Blood* 110:67–73.

Dave UP, Jenkins NA, and Copeland NG. 2004. Gene therapy insertional mutagenesis insights. *Science* 303:333.

Deichmann A, Hacein-Bey-Abina S, Schmidt M, et al. 2007. Vector integration is nonrandom and clustered and influences the fate of lymphopoiesis in SCID-X1 gene therapy. *J Clin Invest* 117:2225–2232.

Dupre L, Marangoni F, Scaramuzza S, et al. 2006. Efficacy of gene therapy for Wiskott–Aldrich syndrome using a WAS promoter/cDNA-containing lentiviral vector and nonlethal irradiation. *Hum Gene Ther* 17:303–313.

Emery DW, Yannaki E, and Tubb J, Stamatoyannopoulos G. 2000. A chromatin insulator protects retrovirus vectors from chromosomal position effects. *Proc Natl Acad Sci U S A* 97:9150–9155.

Engel BC, Podsakoff GM, Ireland JL, et al. 2007. Prolonged pancytopenia in a gene therapy patient with ADA-deficient SCID and trisomy 8 mosaicism: a case report. *Blood* 109:503–506.

Fehse B, Ayuk FA, Kroger N, et al. 2004. Evidence for increased risk of secondary graft failure after in vivo depletion of suicide gene-modified T lymphocytes transplanted in conjunction with $CD34^+$-enriched blood stem cells. *Blood* 104:3408–3409.

Ferrand C, Robinet E, Contassot E, et al. 2000. Retrovirus-mediated gene transfer in primary T lymphocytes: influence of the transduction/selection process and of ex vivo expansion on the T cell receptor beta chain hypervariable region repertoire. *Hum Gene Ther* 11:1151–1164.

Fischer A. 2001. Primary immunodeficiency diseases: an experimental model for molecular medicine. *Lancet* 357:1863–1869.

Gaspar HB, Parsley KL, Howe S, et al. 2004. Gene therapy of X-linked severe combined immunodeficiency by use of a pseudotyped gammaretroviral vector. *Lancet* 364:2181–2187.

Gaspar HB, Bjorkegren E, Parsley K, et al. 2006. Successful reconstitution of immunity in ADA-SCID by stem cell gene therapy following cessation of PEG-ADA and use of mild preconditioning. *Mol Ther* 14:505–513.

Goldblatt D and Thrasher AJ. 2000. Chronic granulomatous disease. *Clin Exp Immunol* 122:1–9.

Greco O and Dachs GU. 2001. Gene directed enzyme/prodrug therapy of cancer: historical appraisal and future prospectives. *J Cell Physiol* 187:22–36.

Hacein-Bey-Abina S, Le Deist F, Carlier F, et al. 2002. Sustained correction of X-linked severe combined immunodeficiency by ex vivo gene therapy. *N Engl J Med* 346:1185–1193.

Hacein-Bey-Abina S, von Kalle C, Schmidt M, et al. 2003a. A serious adverse event after successful gene therapy for X-linked severe combined immunodeficiency. *N Engl J Med* 348:255–256.

Hacein-Bey-Abina S, von Kalle C, Schmidt M, et al. 2003b. LMO2-associated clonal T cell proliferation in two patients after gene therapy for SCID-X1. *Science* 302:415–419.

Heyworth PG, Cross AR, and Curnutte JT. 2003. Chronic granulomatous disease. *Curr Opin Immunol* 15:578–584.

Hirschhorn R, Yang DR, Puck JM, Huie ML, Jiang CK, and Kurlandsky LE. 1996. Spontaneous in vivo reversion to normal of an inherited mutation in a patient with adenosine deaminase deficiency. *Nat Genet* 13:290–295.

Ho VT and Soiffer RJ. 2001. The history and future of T-cell depletion as graft-versus-host disease prophylaxis for allogeneic hematopoietic stem cell transplantation. *Blood* 98:3192–3204.

Hoogerbrugge PM, van Beusechem VW, Fischer A, et al. 1996. Bone marrow gene transfer in three patients with adenosine deaminase deficiency. *Gene Ther* 3:179–183.

Husain M, Grunebaum E, Naqvi A, et al. 2007. Burkitt's lymphoma in a patient with adenosine deaminase deficiency–severe combined immunodeficiency treated with polyethylene glycol–adenosine deaminase. *J Pediatr* 151:93–95.

Johansson B, Fioretos T, and Mitelman F. 2002. Cytogenetic and molecular genetic evolution of chronic myeloid leukemia. *Acta Haematol* 107:76–94.

Kandavelou K, Mani M, Durai S, and Chandrasegaran S. 2005. "Magic" scissors for genome surgery. *Nat Biotechnol* 23:686–687.

Kiem HP, Sellers S, Thomasson B, et al. 2004. Long-term clinical and molecular follow-up of large animals receiving retrovirally transduced stem and progenitor cells: no progression to clonal hematopoiesis or leukemia. *Mol Ther* 9:389–395.

Kohn DB, Hershfield MS, Carbonaro D, et al. 1998. T lymphocytes with a normal ADA gene accumulate after transplantation of transduced autologous umbilical cord blood CD34$^+$ cells in ADA-deficient SCID neonates. *Nat Med* 4:775–780.

Li Z, Dullmann J, Schiedlmeier B, et al. 2002. Murine leukemia induced by retroviral gene marking. *Science* 296:497.

Malech HL, Maples PB, Whiting-Theobald N, et al. 1997. Prolonged production of NADPH oxidase-corrected granulocytes after gene therapy of chronic granulomatous disease. *Proc Natl Acad Sci U S A* 94:12133–12138.

Martin F, Toscano MG, Blundell M, et al. 2005. Lentiviral vectors transcriptionally targeted to hematopoietic cells by WASP gene proximal promoter sequences. *Gene Ther* 12:715–723.

Martino R, Subira M, Rovira M, et al. 2002. Invasive fungal infections after allogeneic peripheral blood stem cell transplantation: incidence and risk factors in 395 patients. *Br J Haematol* 116:475–482.

Martino R, Parody R, Fukuda T, et al. 2006. Impact of the intensity of the pre-transplant conditioning regimen in patients with prior invasive aspergillosis undergoing allogeneic hematopoietic stem cell transplantation: a retrospective survey of the Infectious Diseases Working Party of the European Group for Blood and Marrow Transplantation. *Blood* 108:2928–2936.

Mesel-Lemoine M, Cherai M, Le Gouvello S, et al. 2006. Initial depletion of regulatory T cells: the missing solution to preserve the immune functions of T lymphocytes designed for cell therapy. *Blood* 107:381–388.

Morishita K, Parker DS, Mucenski ML, Jenkins NA, Copeland NG, and Ihle JN. 1988. Retroviral activation of a novel gene encoding a zinc finger protein in IL-3-dependent myeloid leukemia cell lines. *Cell* 54:831–840.

Muul LM, Tuschong LM, Soenen SL, et al. 2003. Persistence and expression of the adenosine deaminase gene for 12 years and immune reaction to gene transfer components: long-term results of the first clinical gene therapy trial. *Blood* 101:2563–2569.

Nishikomori R, Akutagawa H, Maruyama K, et al. 2004. X-linked ectodermal dysplasia and immunodeficiency caused by reversion mosaicism of NEMO reveals a critical role for NEMO in human T-cell development and/or survival. *Blood* 103:4565–4572.

Ott MG, Schmidt M, Schwarzwaelder K, et al. 2006. Correction of X-linked chronic granulomatous disease by gene therapy, augmented by insertional activation of MDS1-EVI1, PRDM16 or SETBP1. *Nat Med* 12:401–409.

Ozsahin H, von Planta M, Muller I, et al. 1998. Successful treatment of invasive aspergillosis in chronic granulomatous disease by bone marrow transplantation, granulocyte colony-stimulating factor-mobilized granulocytes, and liposomal amphotericin-B. *Blood* 92:2719–2724.

Qasim W, King D, Buddle J, et al. 2003. The impact of retroviral suicide gene transduction procedures on T cells. *Br J Haematol* 123:712–719.

Qasim W, Mackey T, Sinclair J, et al. 2007. Lentiviral vectors for T-cell suicide gene therapy: preservation of T-cell effector function after cytokine-mediated transduction. *Mol Ther* 15:355–360.

Rao K, Amrolia PJ, Jones A, et al. 2005. Improved survival after unrelated donor bone marrow transplantation in children with primary immunodeficiency using a reduced-intensity conditioning regimen. *Blood* 105:879–885.

Royer-Pokora B, Loos U, and Ludwig WD. 1991. TTG-2, a new gene encoding a cysteine-rich protein with the LIM motif, is overexpressed in acute T-cell leukaemia with the t(11;14)(p13;q11). *Oncogene* 6:1887–1893.

Schambach A, Bohne J, Chandra S, et al. 2006. Equal potency of gammaretroviral and lentiviral SIN vectors for expression of O^6-methylguanine–DNA methyltransferase in hematopoietic cells. *Mol Ther* 13:391–400.

Schmidt M, Carbonaro DA, Speckmann C, et al. 2003. Clonality analysis after retroviral-mediated gene transfer to $CD34^+$ cells from the cord blood of ADA-deficient SCID neonates. *Nat Med* 9:463–468.

Seger RA, Gungor T, Belohradsky BH, et al. 2002. Treatment of chronic granulomatous disease with myeloablative conditioning and an unmodified hemopoietic allograft: a survey of the European experience, 1985–2000. *Blood* 100:4344–4350.

Soudais C, Shiho T, Sharara LI, et al. 2000. Stable and functional lymphoid reconstitution of common cytokine receptor gamma chain deficient mice by retroviral-mediated gene transfer. *Blood* 95:3071–3077.

Stephan V, Wahn V, Le Deist F, et al. 1996. Atypical X-linked severe combined immunodeficiency due to possible spontaneous reversion of the genetic defect in T cells. *N Engl J Med* 335:1563–1567.

Straathof KC, Pule MA, Yotnda P, et al. Spencer DM, Rooney CM. 2005. An inducible caspase 9 safety switch for T-cell therapy. *Blood* 105:4247–4254.

Thomis DC, Marktel S, Bonini C, et al. 2001. A Fas-based suicide switch in human T cells for the treatment of graft-versus-host disease. *Blood* 97:1249–1257.

Thrasher AJ, Hacein-Bey-Abina S, Gaspar HB, et al. 2005. Failure of SCID-X1 gene therapy in older patients. *Blood* 105:4255–4257.

Thrasher AJ, Gaspar HB, Baum C, et al. 2006. Gene therapy: X-SCID transgene leukaemogenicity. *Nature* 443:E5–E6.

Tiberghien P, Reynolds CW, Keller J, et al. 1994. Ganciclovir treatment of herpes simplex thymidine kinase–transduced primary T lymphocytes: an approach for specific in vivo donor T-cell depletion after bone marrow transplantation? *Blood* 84:1333–1341.

Tiberghien P, Ferrand C, Lioure B, et al. 2001. Administration of herpes simplex–thymidine kinase-expressing donor T cells with a T-cell-depleted allogeneic marrow graft. *Blood* 97:63–72.

Traversari C, Marktel S, Magnani Z, et al. 2007. The potential immunogenicity of the TK suicide gene does not prevent full clinical benefit associated with the use of TK-transduced donor lymphocytes in HSCT for hematologic malignancies. *Blood* 109:4708–4715.

Urnov FD, Miller JC, Lee YL, et al. 2005. Highly efficient endogenous human gene correction using designed zinc-finger nucleases. *Nature* 435:646–651.

van Meerten T, Claessen MJ, Hagenbeek A, and Ebeling SB. 2006. The CD20/alphaCD20 "suicide" system: novel vectors with improved safety and expression profiles and efficient elimination of CD20-transgenic T cells. *Gene Ther* 13:789–797.

Vanin EF, Kaloss M, Broscius C, and Nienhuis AW. 1994. Characterization of replication-competent retroviruses from nonhuman primates with virus-induced T-cell lymphomas and observations regarding the mechanism of oncogenesis. *J Virol* 68:4241–4250.

Watanabe C, Yajima S, Taguchi T, et al. 2001. Successful unrelated bone marrow transplantation for a patient with chronic granulomatous disease and associated resistant pneumonitis and *Aspergillus* osteomyelitis. *Bone Marrow Transplant* 28:83–87.

Woods NB, Bottero V, Schmidt M, von Kalle C, and Verma IM. 2006. Gene therapy: therapeutic gene causing lymphoma. *Nature* 440:1123.

Yamada Y, Warren AJ, Dobson C, Forster A, Pannell R, and Rabbitts TH. 1998. The T cell leukemia LIM protein Lmo2 is necessary for adult mouse hematopoiesis. *Proc Natl Acad Sci U S A* 95:3890–3895.

14

GENETICS OF THE IMMUNE RESPONSE TO PROTEINS EXPRESSED AFTER GENE TRANSFER

JAY LOZIER, M.D., PH.D.

Department of Laboratory Medicine, NIH Clinical Center, Bethesda, Maryland

Gene Therapy Immunology, Edited by Roland Herzog

14.1 INTRODUCTION

Gene therapy has been proposed as a method for treatment of various diseases, including hemophilia A and B, immunodeficiencies, urea cycle disorders, sphingolipidoses, glycogen storage diseases, α1-antitrypsin deficiency, HIV/AIDS, cancer, and atherosclerotic cardiovascular disease (Table 14-1). Expression of transgenes following gene transfer is critically important for therapy of both congenital diseases (as permanent replacement therapy) and acquired diseases (often, to kill malignant cells or other undesirable cells). Stable, long-term transgene expression is most critical where permanent replacement of a missing gene function is required. One of many factors that may limit the effectiveness of gene therapy is the immune response to proteins secreted by transduced cells, leading to the elimination or neutralization of the activity of the secreted protein, or elimination of transduced cells necessary to secrete the desired gene product.

TABLE 14-1 Disease States or Conditions for Which Gene Therapy Is Proposed

Disease	Method	References
Hemophilia A/B	Gene transfer of factor VIII/factor IX, to muscle, liver, and other target tissues using various viral vectors	Pierce et al. [2007]
Immuno-deficiencies	Retroviral gene transfer of deficient genes to lymphocytes or granulocyte precursors	Cavazzana-Calvo and Fischer [2007], Malech and Hickstein [2007]
Urea cycle disorders	Adenovirus or AAV vector gene transfer of deficient genes to liver	Michalak and Butterworth [1997]
Sphingolipidoses	Gene transfer to various target cell types	Sevin et al. [2007], Sidransky et al. [2007]
Glycogen storage diseases	Adenovirus or AAV vector gene transfer of deficient genes to liver or kidney	Chou and Mansfield [2007]
α1-Antitrypsin deficiency	Viral and nonviral gene transfer of α1-antitrypsin gene to pulmonary epithelium, liver, or muscle	Cruz et al. [2007]
HIV/AIDS	Gene transfer of small RNA molecules to lymphocytes	Scherer et al. [2007]
Cancer	Gene transfer of various transgenes to various tissues and cell types	Barzon et al. [2006], Glasgow et al. [2006], Stoff-Khalili et al. [2006], Bazan-Peregrino et al. [2007]
Atherosclerosis	Viral and nonviral gene transfer of ApoE lipoprotein gene to liver	Harris et al. [2006]

The immune response to gene product replacement, provided either by gene transfer or infusion of purified protein, may be determined in large part by the mutation that causes the underlying disease. This depends most critically on whether the defective disease protein is present but inactive or is absent altogether (cross-reacting material positive or negative, $CRM^{+/-}$). This factor is obviously determined genetically. The predisposition of the recipient to mount an immune response has long been attributed to genetically determined differences in the major histocompatibility complex (MHC), which controls antigen presentation by class I or class II mechanisms. More recently, other immune-response modifier genes have been shown to be relevant to the production of antibodies to foreign proteins and may contribute to the immune response.

The immune response to transgene products is affected not only by the expressed protein and genetic factors present in the recipient of a gene transfer vector, but also by the adjuvant effects of many, if not all viral vectors used for gene transfer. The route and dose of vector administration, co-expressed genes (e.g., selectable markers, such as neomycin phosphotransferase), and exposure to the transgene product by previous therapy with exogenous therapeutic protein infusions (e.g., factor VIII or factor IX infusions in patients with hemophilia A or B) may influence the immune response.

In this chapter we focus on genetic factors in the recipient that determine the immune response to proteins expressed following gene transfer. Many of the illustrative examples will be drawn from the experience with gene therapy of hemophilia, for which there are perhaps more clinical and preclinical gene transfer data available than for any other disease. Further, we deal exclusively with the long-term immune response that limits the effectiveness of gene therapy and do not address immediate catastrophic immune response to gene transfer vectors that was seen in the Jessie Gelsinger case [Raper et al. 2003].

14.2 ANIMAL MODELS USED TO ASSESS THE IMMUNE RESPONSE TO EXPRESSED TRANSGENES

Development of gene therapy and its translation into clinical use in humans typically takes place in an orderly process where vectors are first constructed and tested for their ability to produce a protein after transducing target cells in vitro. Following characterization of the optimal in vitro conditions for gene transfer, a vector is then tested for its ability to transduce target cells of intact organ systems in living animals to produce the desired protein (e.g., factor VIII, factor IX, α1-antitrypsin). Upon preclinical demonstration of safety and efficacy in animals, a vector is then introduced into humans as an Investigational New Drug under U.S. Food and Drug Administration regulation in the United States or an equivalent paradigm in the European Union under regulation by the European Agency for the Evaluation of Medicinal Products (EMEA). Many animal models have been used for preclinical assessment of the immune response to transgenes, which is one of the most important issues to address before use in humans. Each model has its particular strengths and weaknesses for evaluation of the immune response.

14.2.1 Rodents

Typical entry-level preclinical safety and efficacy studies are done in either mice or rats. This is in large part due to the relatively low cost of doing studies in rodents compared to higher animal species, especially nonhuman primates. Further, the biology and genetics of the immune response to foreign proteins is probably better characterized in mice than even in humans. Finally, the ability to engineer various transgenic or knockout mice that replicate human diseases makes it possible to assess the efficacy of treatment by gene replacement as well as to gather safety data from a mouse study [Kulkarni and Karlsson 1993; Lubahn et al. 1993; Lin et al. 1997; Schastry 1998; Jin et al. 2004]. Not surprisingly, vast amounts of experimental resources are available to study immunity to transgene or vector proteins in mice, and to a lesser extent, rats. The immune system of the mouse is very similar to that of humans, and many basic discoveries regarding the function of the human immune system were first worked out in mice (e.g., MHC, transplantation, humoral and cellular immunity, immune tolerance). One disadvantage of using mice and other rodents (compared to larger animals) is the inability to obtain large volumes of blood or to collect blood frequently. Nevertheless, studies of gene transfer in mice and/or rats is *de rigueur* for preclinical assessment of gene transfer, and considerable insight into the immune response to transgenes has been developed from this model. Larger animal models that have been used in preclinical studies include rabbits, dogs, and nonhuman primates (primarily, rhesus and cynomolgus monkeys).

14.2.2 Rabbits

The rabbit is a model system that has been used extensively for safety testing of gene transfer vectors. There are few spontaneous, well-characterized rabbit models of human genetic diseases, with the notable exception of the Watanabe heritable hyperlipidemic (WHHL) rabbit, which has been used to test retroviral or adenoviral gene therapy of lipid disorders [Kozarsky et al. 1994]. The gene transferred in therapy of this animal disease is the LDL receptor, a transmembrane protein that is missing from diseased animals [Kita et al. 1981]. Most preclinical testing in rabbits is done for assessment of acute toxicity and safety, and little is reported on the immune consequences of gene transfer. Most common transgenes to be expressed in rabbits would be of human origin and therefore would be expected to be immunogenic. Not enough is known about the differential immune response to foreign proteins by different breeds of rabbits, so relatively little is known about the genetics of the immune response in these animals. For the most part, rabbit studies typically address the immediate and chronic toxicity.

14.2.3 Canines

Hemophilia A and B [Hough et al. 2002; Lozier et al. 2002], Leber's congenital amaurosis [Aguirre et al. 1998], and Duchenne's muscular dystrophy [Kornegay et al. 1988] are a few of the diseases for which there are excellent dog models that have been used to test gene therapy. Preclinical testing of gene therapy in dogs has been reported for these and other diseases [Gilbert et al. 2001; Cerletti et al. 2003; Acland et al. 2005; High 2005; Wang et al. 2007]. Purebred dogs fall somewhere between genetically homogeneous mouse strains and humans who are highly heterogeneous due to outbreeding. There are now platforms for high-throughput analysis of hundreds or thousands of known canine genetic polymorphisms recently cataloged in the canine genome project [Lindblad-Toh et al. 2005]. A necessary prerequisite for analysis of genetic factors is that there are enough animals in the study for a statistically meaningful conclusion to be reached. Unfortunately, although the requisite knowledge to analyze the genetics of the immune response to expressed transgenes is rapidly developing in canines, dog studies typically do not have sufficient sample sizes to permit statistical analysis of numerous genetic polymorphisms (i.e., whole genome scanning or analysis). Analysis of individual genetic traits can be done in some studies, despite small sample sizes.

14.2.4 Nonhuman Primates

Preclinical testing of gene therapy in nonhuman primates is desirable since their immune systems and physiology are thought to be most like that of humans. Often, immunologic reagents (e.g., antibodies) that react to human proteins or molecules will often cross-react with their nonhuman primate counterpart, so many reagents and antibodies are available for analysis of human proteins of interest expressed in nonhuman primates. This is due to the fact that there is typically >95% homology between human protein and their nonhuman primate counterparts [Villinger et al. 1995]. Of course, if a human transgene protein is being expressed in a nonhuman primate, it will still be possible to induce an immune response to the protein. One problem with gene expression studies in normal nonhuman primates is that endogenous proteins can make detection of the expressed human protein problematic, especially where a small amount of transgene is expressed in the recipient. In theory, this can be approached by developing specific monoclonal antibodies that can recognize the difference between human and nonhuman primate homologs, or by using polyclonal antibodies derived from the nonhuman primate that will not cross-react with endogenous protein. The latter strategy has been employed with varying degrees of success [Lozier et al. 1999a]. Similar to the situation for dogs, monkey studies are quite expensive to perform and do not typically involve enough animals to draw valid conclusions with respect to genetic influences on the immune response to expressed transgenes. The recent publication of the rhesus macaque genome makes this type of analysis at least a theoretical possibility [Rhesus Macaque Genome Sequencing and Analysis Consortium 2007]. In summary, well-characterized animal models that are relatively inexpensive to perform testing with have led to the most insights on the genetics of the immune response to expressed transgenes.

14.3 NATURE OF THE IMMUNE RESPONSE TO TRANSGENES

The immune response to transgenes expressed following gene transfer proceeds along the same pathways as the immune response to any "foreign" protein. After antigens are presented to T and B lymphocytes by antigen-presenting cells, the T cells are educated to recognize foreign cells having the antigen, and select B lymphocytes are induced to differentiate into antibody-producing plasma cells. Two aspects of the immune response to expressed transgenes are of particular note. First, during gene transfer mediated by viral-based vectors, the vector itself may function as an adjuvant to the immune response. The most potent adjuvant effects appear to be associated with adenovirus vectors, whose capsids are themselves very immunogenic, since they elicit the production of high levels of immunostimulatory cytokines such as IL-6 [Lozier et al. 1999b], although other vectors may have adjuvant properties as well [Yuasa et al. 2007]. Second, following simple injection of a therapeutic protein (e.g., factor VIII or factor IX) antigen-presenting cells presumably take up extracellular protein and process it into peptides for presentation of smaller molecules by class II presentation. It is possible (even likely) that protein expressed by cells that are transduced by viral vectors will be presented by class I mechanisms. Thus, there may be class I and class II antigen presentations that take place following viral-based vector gene transfer. In theory, a therapeutic protein that is expressed from a viral vector–transduced cell may serve to "cross-prime" other antigen-presenting cells that render the protein into peptides for presentation by class II mechanisms. The differing adjuvant properties of viruses may account for the different levels of immunogenicity seen with different vectors used in gene transfer. The immune response to vector-transduced cells may limit the effectiveness of gene therapy, in the case of gene replacement approaches, or may otherwise be a beneficial property in situations where the goal is to kill or inactivate undesirable cells (e.g., antitumor or immunosuppressive approaches).

14.4 EFFECT OF ROUTE OF VECTOR ADMINISTRATION ON THE IMMUNE RESPONSE

Gene transfer using the same vector, but given by different routes of administration, can result in dramatically different immune responses. For example, C57 mice typically mount a minimal immune response to human factor IX when gene transfer vectors are administered by the intravenous route (e.g., AAV or adenovirus vectors) [Michou et al. 1997; Lozier et al. 2005], or when the human factor IX protein itself is administered intravenously [Lozier et al. 2005]. However, when adenovirus vectors that express human factor IX are given via the intramuscular route, a vigorous antibody response can be elicited [Fields et al. 2000]. The basis for this is not known with certainty, but it is possible that antigen-presenting cells in muscle may be substantially better at stimulating immunity than those in liver (where adenovirus vectors preferentially accumulate when given intravenously). The route-dependent differences in immunity in the same inbred mice when using the same vector need to be kept in mind when comparing the immune response to gene therapy vectors in animal models.

14.5 INFLUENCE OF THE UNDERLYING GENE DEFECT ON THE IMMUNE RESPONSE

For hemophilia A and B there is a plethora of information on the effects of factor VIII or factor IX mutation on the immune response to infused therapeutic factor VIII or factor IX. In hemophilia A there is an overall risk of developing neutralizing antibodies to factor VIII that is approximately 20%. The risk, however, is not randomly distributed through all patients with hemophilia A, and inhibitors are found predominantly in those patients with severe disease where there is essentially no factor VIII activity (<1% of normal levels). Within those who have severe hemophilia A, the risk is greatest among those with early nonsense mutations where the protein product is truncated, or in those with complete gene deletions where no factor VIII is transcribed or translated [Oldenburg et al. 2002; Astermark et al. 2005]. In the latter mutation type, inhibitor risk is about 70%, suggesting that there is no early deletion of immune effector clones that bind factor VIII or induction of tolerance to factor VIII by the immune system. Thus, factor VIII in any form is a foreign protein to patients with complete deletions of the factor VIII gene. There is a common inversion of the factor VIII gene in patients having severe hemophilia A in which the first 22 exons are reversed in their orientation with respect to the last four exons [Lakich et al. 1993; Naylor et al. 1993a]. This results in severe hemophilia A, where there is no detectable circulating factor VIII antigen or activity. It is interesting that the risk for inhibitors in patients with the gene inversion is approximately 20%, in contrast to the much higher rate for patients with complete deletion of the factor VIII gene, suggesting that the immune system in patients with the inversion is in some way "educated" as to what normal factor VIII looks like. It is known that factor VIII mRNA is transcribed from the inverted gene in patients with the inversion, and also that lymphocytes express the factor VIII transcript [Naylor et al. 1993b]. Thus, it is plausible that there is sufficient translation of factor VIII peptides to mediate immune tolerance by whatever mechanism is relevant.

In hemophilia B, there are no common prototypical mutations, and there is, instead, a very wide range of "private" gene defects, most of which are mis-sense mutations [Haemophilia B Mutation Database, Version 13, 2004]. The overall inhibitor rate during replacement therapy is on the order of 3% [Lozier and Kessler 2005] (substantially less than for hemophilia A)], although in the rare patients with complete gene deletions, the rate is substantially higher. An unexplained finding is that factor IX inhibitors, although less common than factor VIII inhibitors, are more commonly associated with anaphylaxis and complement-mediated immune adverse effects such as nephritis than are factor VIII inhibitors [Constantinescu et al. 1997; Ewenstein et al. 1997; Warrier et al. 1997; Jadhav and Warrier 2000]. This may be the consequence of complement-fixing IgG1 and IgG2 isotype antibodies found more commonly in factor IX inhibitors than in factor VIII inhibitors that are predominantly of the IgG4 isotype [Fulcher et al. 1987; Casper 1991].

Animal models for hemophilia A and B suggest that both the underlying mutation type as well as other genetic differences may contribute to the immune response to factor VIII or factor IX. For instance, there are two colonies of hemophilia A dogs in Chapel Hill, North Carolina and Ontario, Canada, where in both dogs the disease appears to be due to a factor VIII gene inversion such as that seen commonly in humans [Lozier et al. 2003; Hough et al. 2003]. However, the rate of inhibitor development in the Chapel Hill colony during replacement therapy for trauma or spontaneous bleeding is quite rare, but in the Canadian colony approaches the "typical" 20% frequency seen in humans with the gene inversion and severe hemophilia A [Timothy C. Nichols and David Lillicrap, personal communications]. Clearly, other genetic factors may bear upon the immune response. There are lhasa apso hemophilia B dogs where the factor IX protein is missing due to a small deletion leading to an early stop codon and no functional or immunologically detectable protein [Mauser et al. 1996]. This colony is prone to inhibitor development, in contrast to a different colony of hemophilia B dogs with a mis-sense mutation that is not particularly inhibitor prone [Evans et al. 1989]. Both hemophilia B colonies have been used for testing of various gene transfer strategies, including AAV, retrovirus, and adenovirus gene transfer, in anticipation of clinical gene therapy trials.

Thus far, the immune response to factor VIII or factor IX following gene transfer in humans with hemophilia has not been seen, although so far patients have been selected for extensive previous exposure to factor VIII or factor IX (and in the case of factor IX, also selected for mis-sense mutations less prone to inhibitor development) [Kay et al. 2000; Roth et al. 2001; Manno et al. 2003, 2006; Powell et al. 2003]. Thus, we do not have a full understanding of the relative immunogenicity of gene transfer of hemophilia A or B compared with conventional protein replacement therapy. For gene therapy to realize its maximum potential benefit to patients, previously untreated patients and/or those with "high-risk" mutations will ultimately need to be treated by gene therapy methods.

14.6 EVIDENCE FOR GENETIC FACTORS IN ANIMALS THAT INFLUENCE THE IMMUNE RESPONSE TO EXPRESSED TRANSGENES

Animals subjected to gene transfer or even protein infusions show differential immune responses to various proteins (manifest primarily by antibody titers). This has perhaps been most characteristic of inbred mouse strains for α-1-antitrypsin, coagulation factor VIII, and coagulation factor IX. The antibody response to α-1-antitrypsin after gene transfer depends critically on the inbred strain of mouse [Barr et al. 1995]. It is well known that C57BL/6J mice typically do not respond to human factor IX with antibodies after protein injection or viral-mediated gene transfer with adenovirus or AAV-based vectors, whereas other inbred strains of mice do respond with varying levels of anti-human factor IX antibodies [Michou et al. 1997; Lozier et al. 2005]. Similarly, inbred mice have differential responses to human factor VIII whether administered as protein or expressed from adenovirus vectors [Rawle et al. 2004; Lozier and Zhang 2005]. Due to the existence of genetically well characterized recombinant inbred mouse strains derived from parental strains of mice with high or low responsiveness to human factor VIII or human factor IX, it is possible to measure the antibody response to human factor VIII or factor IX proteins expressed from viral gene transfer vectors to assess the genetic factors that influence the immune response.

14.6.1 Recombinant Inbred Mice

A resource of inestimable value for genetic analysis of diseases or phenotypic traits has been recombinant inbred mice, developed primarily at the Jackson Laboratories [Paigen 2003]. These lines are created, as shown in Fig. 14-1, by mating mice of two different inbred mouse strains to create F_1 progeny that are uniformly heterozygous for the two parental mouse strains' DNA throughout their genome. Then, when F_1 progeny are mated, all the F_2 progeny will have a random distribution of the original parental strains' DNA throughout the genome, due to homologous recombination between differing strands of DNA throughout the F_1 parental DNA. They therefore will have a random distribution of any polymorphic sites found in the original inbred parental mouse strains' DNA. Each F_2 can be bred with littermates and progeny re-bred with littermates in successive generations to converge on a set of inbred mouse strains, each of which is unique in the distribution of the genetic polymorphisms found in the original parental strains. It takes about 20 generations of breeding to establish a congenic line that is genetically homogeneous. Several sets of recombinant inbred mice have been developed laboriously using parental strains that are commonly studied by researchers (e.g., C57BL/6J, A/J, DBA, C3H). These sets of mice have also been cataloged at numerous sites where genetic polymorphisms are found in the parental strains. For example, for the AXB and BXA recombinant inbred mouse strains that have been derived by the initial mating of an A/J female and C57BL/6J male, or C57BL/6J female and A/J male, respectively, there are more than 750 polymorphic sites in the parental genomes that have been cataloged for more than a dozen AXB strains and more than a dozen BXA strains [Sampson et al. 1998]. Where the original inbred parental strains differ in a trait that can be measured or observed, knowledge of these polymorphisms in DNA in all involved strains permits an analysis of the association of the trait with genetic polymorphisms that differ in the mice. This is a powerful tool for mapping of genes in mice that influence the immune response and has been exploited for the study of many different conditions or diseases found in mice.

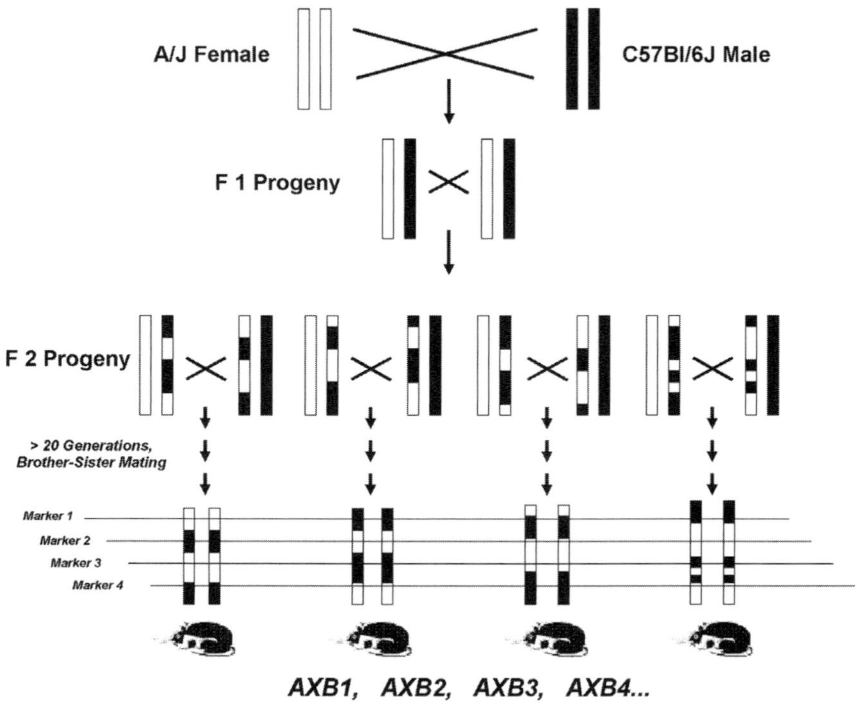

Figure 14-1 Generation of recombinant inbred mouse strains for genetic analysis of phenotypes. When two strains of inbred mice (e.g., A/J and C57BL/6J) are mated, the F_1 progeny are identical obligate heterozygotes for DNA from each parental strain throughout its genome. During meiosis following breeding of the F_1 progeny, there is sister chromatid exchange by homologous recombination. At this step random differences begin to appear in the DNA content of the F_2 progeny. By repeated brother–sister mating for at least 20 generations, congenic recombinant inbred mouse strains are generated that are unique. With enough time and effort, enough unique recombinant inbred mice can be generated such that there are polymorphic sites that are randomly distributed within the genome that association studies can be performed to see which polymorphic marker(s) correlate with a phenotypic trait under study. For the sake of simplification, only one hypothetical chromosome and four markers are depicted in this example. However, the same recombination process occurs on all mouse chromosomes, and there are many more polymorphic markers known than shown; in fact, more than 750 markers have been cataloged for the AXB/BXA recombinant inbred strains derived from A/J and C57BL/6J parental strains.

14.6.2 Quantitative Trait Locus Mapping with Recombinant Inbred Mice

Statistical analysis of a quantifiable trait in well-characterized recombinant inbred mice to infer the position of a causative gene is termed quantitative trait locus (QTL) mapping. This method requires that the two parental founder strains of a series of recombinant inbred lines of mice must differ significantly with respect to the trait under study. If there is no difference between the two parental strains, analysis of the recombinant inbred mice derived from them will be uninformative and QTL mapping will not be possible. Once a series of recombinant inbred mice are identified whose parental strains differ with respect to a trait of interest, QTL mapping can be undertaken. Since each recombinant inbred strain derives half of its genetic information from each parental strain, and each recombinant inbred strain is a random assortment of genetic information from the parental strains, expression of the strain in each mouse will vary according to the parental gene(s) they contain. By analyzing enough unique recombinant inbred mice, it is possible to infer which polymorphic site is associated with that trait. The greater the association of a polymorphic site with the trait under study, the closer the controlling gene is to the polymorphic site. The statistical association is commonly referred to by a parameter called the linkage relatedness score (LRS) or logarithmic odds (LOD) score. The LRS is proportional to the LOD score, and either term may be used in describing genetic linkage. A site with a high LOD score may be in the gene of interest or may simply be close to the actual gene that controls the trait. Once a strong association between a polymorphic site and expression of a trait is established, the local region can be analyzed in detail to see if plausible candidate genes are located within. A causal hypothesis can then be constructed and tested for any candidate gene that has intentionally been modified by creation of transgenic or knockout mice.

Experimental linkage analysis in mice is simpler than clinical studies in humans, since human studies require analysis of numerous polymorphisms in persons from families with large enough informative pedigrees to establish linkage with a particular traits. In contrast, an investigator can observe or manipulate mice in which polymorphisms throughout the genome have already been cataloged to estimate linkage with a trait.

Genetics of Mouse Immune Response to Human Factor IX One quantitative trait that can readily be observed in mice is the antibody response to a foreign protein, including those expressed following experimental gene transfer. This approach has been pursued for the immune response to human factor IX expressed from adenovirus vectors in recombinant inbred mice derived from the A/J and C57BL/6J strains. As mentioned previously, the antibody response to human factor IX in C57BL/6J is low, and the response to human factor IX in the A/J mouse is higher, in fact, than for any other strain of mouse (Fig. 14-2). Therefore, recombinant inbred mice derived from these two parental strains should vary in antibody response according to which parental genes they have inherited. Analysis of the response using readily available software [Wang et al. 2003] has shown a very good correlation between the antibody response to human factor IX in these mice and polymorphisms near the MHC locus on chromosome 17, as well as other polymorphisms near immune response modifiers such as IL-22 and interferon-γ (Fig. 14-3). These are genes that may plausibly control the immune response to "foreign" proteins, and probably account for the differential immune response seen in the C57BL/6J and A/J strains. Results of experiments in B10.A congenic mice (Fig. 14-4) has been

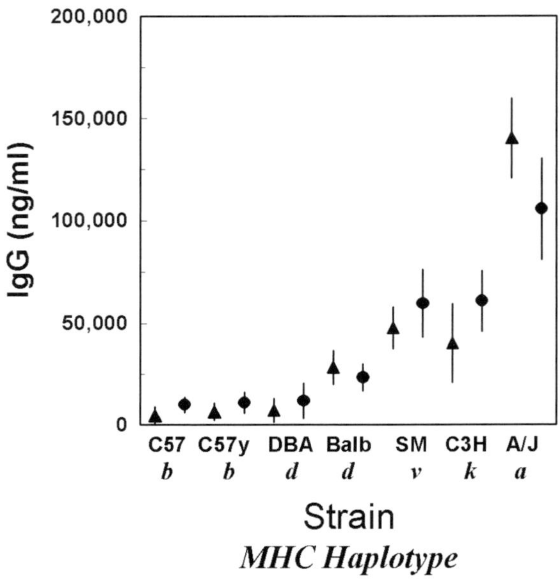

Figure 14-2 Differential antibody response to human factor IX after adenovirus gene transfer in various inbred mouse strains. Seven strains of inbred mice were injected with 6.8×10^{11} vector particles per kilogram of AVC3FIX5 adenovirus vector and levels of anti-human FIX IgG were measured one month later. Mean IgG anti-human factor IX levels are shown with 95% confidence intervals indicated by vertical lines (triangles, males; circles, females; 10 mice per group). *p* Values for comparison of antibody levels between C57 and A/J mice by one-way ANOVA were highly significant for both males and females ($p < 0.0001$ for each analysis). Statistically significant differences were also seen for comparisons of C57 mice with C3H, SM, and BALB mice (males or females), but nonsignificant *p* values (>0.45) were observed for one-way ANOVA comparisons of C57 with C57y or DBA mice. MHC H-2 haplotype designations (in italic) are shown below each strain. (Data from Lozier et al. [2005].)

consistent with the hypothesis that the antibody response is dictated by class II presentation. B10.A mice have the same MHC genes as A/J mice, within a C57BL/10J background, and demonstrate an antibody response to human factor IX that is half that of the A/J strain (Fig. 14-4). This suggests that the A/J MHC complex is sufficient for a strong antibody response to human factor IX and other non-MHC genes impart additional response to human factor IX in A/J mice.

When B10.A5R mice are challenged with factor IX vector, the antibody response is minimal, like that of the C57BL/6J strain. The B10.A5R strain is an MHC chimera where the genes for K class I-a and Aβ and Aα class II genes are identical to those found in C57BL/10J, while Eα class II genes and the rest of the MHC genes are identical to A/J. This response suggests that class II genes are critical to the A/J immune response to human factor IX, though

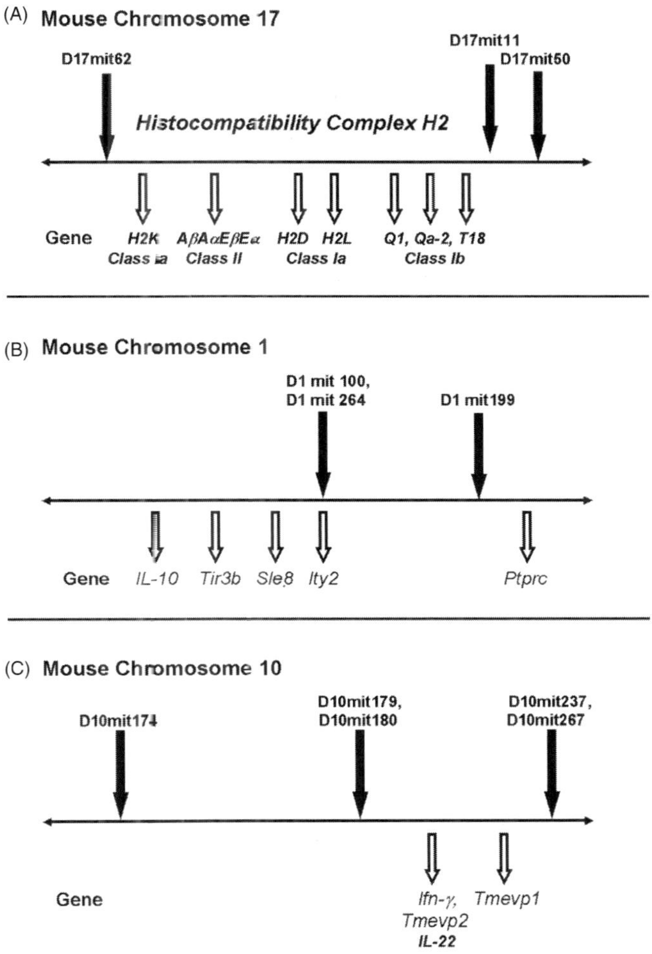

Figure 14-3 Markers associated with anti-human factor IX antibody response in mice. (A) D17mit62 is the polymorphic marker with the highest association with anti-human factor IX antibody levels in AXB and BXA recombinant inbred mouse strains, and is near the MHC H-2 gene cluster on chromosome 17. Mouse chromosome 17 is depicted with a horizontal line. Polymorphic markers associated with antibody development are shown as a solid arrow above the line depicting chromosome 17, and genes of the histocompatibility locus are shown as open arrows below the line. (B) The polymorphic markers D1mit100, D1mit264, and D1mit199 (indicated by solid arrows) are near various immunoregulatory genes on chromosome 1 (depicted with a horizontal line). The genes found near these markers include *IL-10*: interleukin-10, *Tir3b*: trypanosomiasis infection response gene 3b, *Sle8*: systemic lupus erythematosis susceptibility gene 8, *Ity2*: immunity to *S. typhimurium* 2 gene, and *Ptprc*: protein tyrosine phosphatase, receptor type, C (a.k.a. CD45, B220). (C) The polymorphic markers D10mit174, D10mit 179, D10mit180, D10mit237, and D10mit267 (indicated by solid arrows) are near the mouse interferon-γ gene on chromosome 10 (depicted with a horizontal line). Genes on chromosome 10 that are near these markers include *Ifn-γ*: interferon-γ, *Tmevp1&2*: Theiler's murine encephalomyelitis virus persistence 1 and 2, *IL-22*: interleukin-22. (Data from Lozier et al. [2005].)

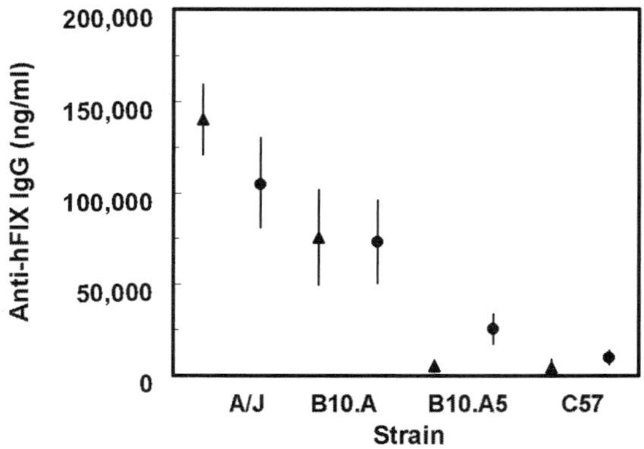

Strain	MHC-H2 Genes									
	K class I-a	Aβ class II	Aα class II	Eβ class II	Eα class II	S class III	D class I-a	L class I-a	Qa-2 class I-b	T18 class I-b
A/J	k	k	k	k	k	d	d	d	a	a
B10.A	k	k	k	k	k	d	d	d	a	a
B10.A5	*b*	*b*	*b*	*b*/k	k	d	d	d	a	a
C57BL/6J	*b*	*b*	*b*	^	*b*	*b*	*b*	^	*a*	*b*

Figure 14-4 Anti-human factor IX IgG levels following intravenous injection of AVC3FIX5 in B10.A congenic mice: role of MHC H-2 genes. B10.A$-H2^a\ H2 - T18^a$/SgSnJ and B10.A-$H2^{i5}H2 - T18^a$(5R)/SgSnJ mice were injected with weight-adjusted doses of AVC3FIX5 adenovirus vector, and anti-human factor IX IgG levels were measured one month later. Mean IgG levels are shown with 95% confidence intervals indicated by vertical lines (triangles, males; circles, females; ten mice for each group). Mouse strains: A/J (A/J), B10.A$-H2^a\ H2 - T18^a$/SgSnJ (B10.A), B10.A-$H2^{i5}H2 - T18^a$(5R)/SgSnJ (B10.A5R), and C57BL/6J (C57). The genes at the Eβ class II and L class I-a loci (indicated by) are absent from the C57BL/6J strain. Alleles common to C57BL/6J mice are shown in italic. (Data from Lozier et al. [2005].)

the contribution of K class I-a genes cannot be ruled out. Unfortunately, there are no congenic mice where only the MHC class II genes from A/J mice are found within C57BL/6J class I genes that flank the class II genes in the complex. Therefore, the evidence for class II genes being solely responsible for the MHC contribution to the immune response is not conclusive. However, the fact that human factor IX protein injections induce antibodies in A/J mice but not C57BL/6J mice is consistent with the idea that class II presentation is critical (since class I presentation is less likely in this setting).

Genetics of Mouse Immune Response to Human Factor VIII Mapping of genes that influence the immune response to human factor VIII in mice has been done, by methods similar to the work on human factor IX. CXB recombinant inbred mice were used due to the fact that the parental strains BalbC/ByJ and C57BL/6ByJ have significantly different antibody responses to human factor VIII whether expressed from an adenovirus vector [Rawle et al. 2004] or by injection of purified protein [Lozier and Zhang 2005] (Fig. 14-5). In contrast to the work on factor IX, the linkage studies in CXB mice showed association between the antibody response to factor VIII with different genes in males and females. For male mice there was significant association (LOD scores of about 3.0) with three polymorphic markers on chromosome 8 that are near various genes that control T-lymphocyte subsets, chemokine ligands, and the immune response seen in various autoimmune diseases (Fig. 14-6). In females, the MHC locus on chromosome 17 is implicated, as for the antibody response to factor IX, and there is significant linkage with a polymorphic site on mouse chromosome 5 (D5Mit31) that is near the gene for zinc α2-glycoprotein I (AZGP-1). The plausibility that AZGP-1 protein is relevant to the immune response to factor VIII is increased by the fact that it has structural homology to class I protein at its amino terminus and immunoglobulin constant region domains at its carboxyl terminus. Although

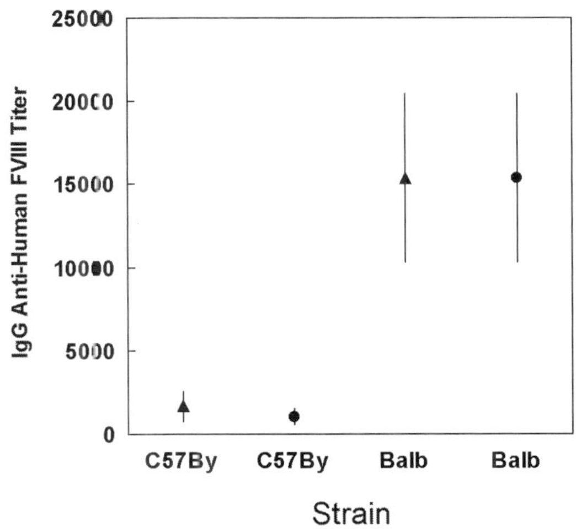

Figure 14-5 Differential antibody response to human factor VIII after adenovirus gene transfer in C57BL/6ByJ and BALB/cByJ mice. Seven strains of inbred mice were injected with 6.8 $\times$ 10^{11} vector particles per kilogram of AVPGKf8mg adenovirus vector, and levels of anti-human FIX IgG were measured one month later. Mean IgG anti-human factor IX levels are shown with 95% confidence intervals, indicated by vertical lines (triangles, males; circles, females; five mice per group). *p* Values for comparison of antibody levels between C57 and A/J mice by one-way ANOVA were highly significant for both males and females ($p < 0.001$ for each analysis). Statistically significant differences were also seen for comparisons of the antibody response of C57BL/6ByJ mice with that of Balb/cByJ mice (males or females) following injection of purified protein ($p < 0.02$, data not shown). (Based on data from Lozier and Zhang [2005] and unpublished data from Lozier.)

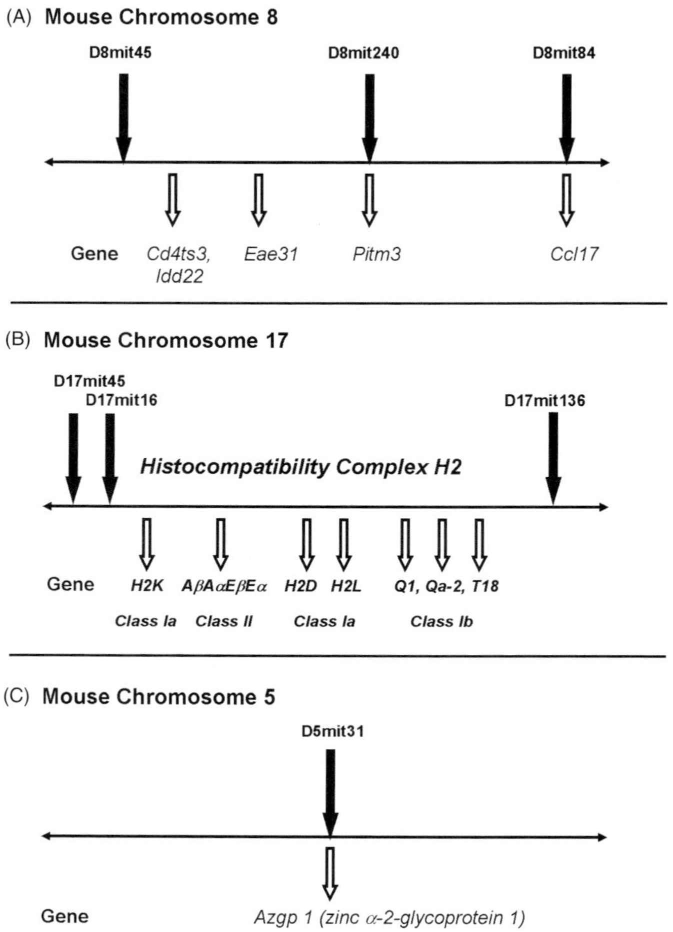

Figure 14-6 Markers associated with anti-human factor VIII antibody response in mice. (A) D8mit45, D8mit240, and D8mit84 are the polymorphic markers with the highest association with anti-human factor VIII antibody levels in male CXB recombinant inbred mice. These are near various genes that are associated with control of T-lymphocyte subsets, various autoimmune syndromes of mice, and a chemokine ligand. Mouse chromosome 8 is depicted with a horizontal line. Polymorphic markers associated with antibody development are shown as a solid arrow above the line depicting chromosome 8, and genes of the histocompatibility locus are indicated by open arrows below the line. Cd4ts3, CD4 T-cell subset 3; Iddm22, insulin-dependent diabetes susceptibility 22; Eae31, experimental allergic encephalitis susceptibility 31; Pitm3, prion incubation time 3; Ccl17, chemokine ligand 17. (B) The polymorphic marker D17mit16 is the polymorphic marker (indicated by solid arrows) that has the greatest association with the antibody response to human factor VIII in female CXB mice. It is near the MHC gene cluster on chromosome 17 (depicted with a horizontal line) that contains class I, II, and III genes. (C) The polymorphic marker D5mit31 (indicated by solid arrows) is a marker with a LOD score of 2.4 for association with the antibody response to human factor VIII in female mice. It is near the mouse zinc α-2 glycoprotein I gene on mouse chromosome 5 (indicated by the solid horizontal line.)

AZGP-1 does not bind β2 microglobulin and apparently does not present antigens as would a class I molecule, it binds lipids important for lipid metabolism, and binds zinc, a transition metal [Sanchez et al. 1999]. Notably, factor VIII binds copper, a transition metal (a transition metal like zinc) and binds lipids. Binding of AZGP-1 to factor VIII can be shown by ELISA methodology (Lozier, unpublished data). It therefore is plausible that AZGP-1 may both bind common molecules or one another, and in some way influence the interaction of factor VIII with the immune system.

14.7 EVIDENCE FOR GENETIC COMPONENTS TO THE HUMAN IMMUNE RESPONSE TO EXOGENOUS PROTEINS, AND IMPLICATIONS FOR GENE TRANSFER

Traditional replacement therapy of protein deficiencies in humans has long been known to be complicated by neutralizing antibodies to the infused protein for a long time. As might be expected, the best example is hemophilia A, where inhibitor antibodies are seen in about 20% of patients with severe disease (<1% of normal activity). The nature of the underlying mutation in the factor VIII gene clearly contributes to the risk of inhibitor [Oldenburg et al. 2002; Astermark et al. 2005]. The highest incidence occurs in patients whose mutation renders them not only deficient in functional activity but also without any immunologically detectable protein (CRM negative), where the inhibitor rate is about 70%. This phenomenon of an extremely high inhibitor rate in CRM-negative patients is also seen in Pompe's disease and Gaucher's disease [Amalfitano et al. 2001].

Studies have shown increased inhibitor risk in certain racial groups [Aledort and DiMichelle 1998], and studies of related patients with hemophilia suggest a genetic component to inhibitor development [Gill 1999]. Studies of the genetics of the immune response to replacement therapy have shown for patients with severe hemophilia A that specific polymorphisms in the IL-10, TNF-α, and CTLA4 genes are associated with increased risk for factor VIII inhibitor development [Astermark et al. 2006a,b, 2007]. Typically, the polymorphic variants associated with increased inhibitor risk result in two- to threefold increased risk of inhibitor development. Surprisingly, HLA haplotypes do not predict hemophilia A inhibitors very well, nor do polymorphic markers in IL-1β or IL-4 cytokine genes [Hay et al. 1997; Oldenburg et al. 1997; Astermark et al., 2006b].

14.8 CONCLUSIONS

To reach its full potential, gene therapy will ultimately have to solve the same immunologic issues as protein replacement therapy pertaining to predicting and treating inhibitor antibodies that develop in response to expressed proteins. Thus far, clinical gene therapy trials for hemophilia A and B have been performed in patients who have proven themselves to be quite unlikely to develop inhibitors based on extensive prior therapy with protein replacement without inhibitors. Once a successful treatment approach is developed in patients treated previously, it will be interesting to see whether the immune response is different for gene therapy as opposed to protein replacement approaches. In theory, continuous presentation of a protein (as might be expected with gene transfer) might be less immunogenic than intermittent protein exposure seen in traditional replacement therapy (however, see reports of immunogenicity of factor IX in the context of continuous infusions). On the other hand, viral vector proteins may serve as adjuvants for the immune response, and their presence may prove to be deleterious [Lozier et al. 1999b; Yuasa et al. 2007].

As always, empirical data will confirm or deny hypothetical predictions of immunogenicity. If robust gene expression can bring about significant sustained levels of a protein, it might be possible to pursue gene transfer as a method to induce tolerance to existing inhibitor antibodies. However, the more immediate goal remains demonstration of replacement of missing proteins at therapeutic levels. Hopefully, as the significance of genetic diversity becomes more clear and the methods to ascertain polymorphisms throughout the human genome become faster and more economical, we may be able to make truly useful predictions as to which patients treated by gene transfer will develop an unwanted immune response and which patients will not. Until then, we remain in a period of slow empirical progress to the goal of understanding immune processes that will determine the success of gene therapy.

REFERENCES

Acland GM, Aguirre GD, Bennett J, et al. 2005. Long-term restoration of rod and cone vision by single dose rAAV-mediated gene transfer to the retina in a canine model of childhood blindness. *Mol Ther* 12:1072–1082.

Aguirre GD, Baldwin V, Pearce-Kelling S, Narfstrom K, Ray K, and Acland GM. 1998. Congenital stationary night blindness in the dog: common mutation in the RPE65 gene indicates founder effect. *Mol Vis* 4:23–29.

Aledort LM and DiMichele DM. 1998. Inhibitors occur more frequently in African-American and Latino haemophiliacs. *Haemophilia* 4:68.

Amalfitano A, Bengur AR, Morse RP, et al. 2001. Recombinant human acid alpha-glucosidase enzyme therapy for infantile glycogen storage disease type II: results of a phase I/II clinical trial. *Genet Med* 3:132–138.

Astermark J, Oldenburg J, Escobar M, White GC II, and Berntorp E, (MIBS Study Group). 2005. The Malmo International Brother Study (MIBS): Genetic defects and inhibitor development in siblings with severe hemophilia A. *Haematologica* 90:924–930.

Astermark J, Oldenburg J, Carlson J, et al. 2006a. Polymorphisms in the TNFA gene and the risk of inhibitor development in patients with hemophilia A. *Blood* 108:3739–3745.

Astermark J, Oldenburg J, Pavlova A, Berntorp E, and Lefvert AK (MIBS Study Group). 2006b. Polymorphisms in the IL10 but not in the IL1beta and IL4 genes are associated with inhibitor development in patients with hemophilia A. *Blood* 107:3167–3172.

Astermark J, Wang X, Oldenburg J, Berntorp E, and Lefvert AK (MIBS Study Group). 2007. Polymorphisms in the CTLA-4 gene and inhibitor development in patients with severe hemophilia A. *J Thromb Haemost* 5:263–265.

Barr D, Tubb J, Ferguson D, et al. 1995. Strain related variations in adenovirally mediated transgene expression from mouse hepatocytes in vivo: comparisons between immunocompetent and immunodeficient inbred strains. *Gene Ther* 2:151–155.

Barzon L, Zanusso M, Colombo F, and Palu G. 2006. Clinical trials of gene therapy, virotherapy, and immunotherapy for malignant gliomas. *Cancer Gene Ther* 13:539–554.

Bazan-Peregrino M, Seymour LW, and Harris AL. 2007. Gene therapy targeting to tumor endothelium. *Cancer Gene Ther* 14:117–127.

Casper CK. 1991. Complications of hemophilia A treatment: factor VIII inhibitors. *Ann NY Acad Sci* 614:97–105.

Cavazzana-Calvo M and Fischer A. 2007. Gene therapy for severe combined immunodeficiency: Are we there yet? *J Clin Invest* 117:1456–1465.

Cerletti M, Negri T, Cozzi F, et al. 2003. Dystrophic phenotype of canine X-linked muscular dystrophy is mitigated by adenovirus-mediated utrophin gene transfer. *Gene Ther* 10:750–757.

Chou JY and Mansfield BC. 2007. Gene therapy for type I glycogen storage diseases. *Curr Gene Ther* 7:79–88.

Constantinescu AR, Weiss LS, Saidi P, Eisele J, and Ettinger LJ. 1997. Nephrotic syndrome associated with hypocomplementemia in a 4-year-old boy with hemophilia B. *J Pediatr Hematol Oncol* 19:345–347.

Cruz PE, Mueller C, and Flotte TR. 2007. The promise of gene therapy for the treatment of alpha-1 antitrypsin deficiency. *Pharmacogenomics* 8:1191–1198.

Evans JP, Brinkhous KM, Brayer GD, Reisner HW, and High KA. 1989. Canine hemophilia B resulting from a point mutation with unusual consequences. *Proc Natl Acad Sci U S A* 86:10095–10099.

Ewenstein BM, Takemoto, Warrier I, et al. 1997. Nephrotic syndrome as a complication of immune tolerance induction in hemophilia B. *Blood* 89:1115–1116.

Fields PA, Kowalczyk DW, Arruda VR, et al. 2000. Role of vector in activation of T cell subsets in immune responses against the secreted transgene product factor IX. *Mol Ther* 1:225–235.

Fulcher CA, de Graaf MS, and Zimmerman TS. 1987. FVIII inhibitor IgG subclass and FVIII polypeptide specificity determined by immunoblotting. *Blood* 69:1475–1480.

Gilbert R, Nalbantoglu J, Howell JM, et al. 2001. Dystrophin expression in muscle following gene transfer with a fully deleted ("gutted") adenovirus is markedly improved by *trans*-acting adenoviral gene products. *Hum Gen Ther* 12:1741–1755.

Gill JC. 1999. The role of genetics in inhibitor formation. *Thromb Haemost* 82:500–504.

Glasgow JN, Everts M, and Curiel DT. 2006. Transductional targeting of adenovirus vectors for gene therapy. *Cancer Gene Ther* 13:830–844.

Haemophilia B Mutation Database, Version 13. 2004. http://www.kcl.ac.uk/ip/petergreen/haemBdatabase.html.

Harris JD, Evans V, and Owen JS. 2006. ApoE gene therapy to treat hyperlipidemia and atherosclerosis. *Curr Opin Mol Ther* 8:275–287.

Hay CR, Ollier W, and Pepper L (UKHCDO Inhibitor Working Party) 1997. HLA class II profile: a weak determinant of factor VIII inhibitor development in severe haemophilia A. *Thromb Haemost* 77:234–237.

High KA. 2005. Gene transfer for hemophilia: can therapeutic efficacy in large animals be safely translated to patients? *J Thromb Haemost* 3:1682–1691.

Hough C, Kamisue S, Cameron C, et al. 2002. Aberrant splicing and premature termination of transcription of the FVIII gene as a cause of severe canine hemophilia A: similarities with the intron 22 inversion mutation in human hemophilia. *Thromb Haemost* 87:659–665.

Jadhav M and Warrier I. 2000. Anaphylaxis in patients with hemophilia. *Semin Thromb Hemost* 26:205–208.

Jin DY, Zhang TP, Gui T, Stafford DW, and Monahan PE. 2004. Creation of a mouse expressing defective human factor IX. *Blood* 104:1733–1739.

Kaiser J. 2007. Gene therapy: questions remain on cause of death in arthritis trial. *Science* 317:1665.

Kay MA, Manno CS, Ragni MV, et al. 2000. Evidence for gene transfer and expression of factor IX in haemophilia B patients with an AAV vector. *Nat Genet* 24:257–261.

Kita T, Brown MS, Watanabe Y, and Goldstein JL. 1981. Deficiency of low density lipoprotein receptors in liver and adrenal gland of the WHHL rabbit, an animal model of familial hypercholesterolemia. *Proc Natl Acad Sci U S A* 78:2268–2272.

Kornegay JN, Tuler SM, Miller DM, and Levesque DC. 1988. Muscular dystrophy in a litter of golden retriever dogs. *Muscle Nerve* 11:1056–1064.

Kozarsky KF, McKinley DR, Austin LL, Raper SE, Stratford-Perricaudet LD, and Wilson JM. 1994. In vivo correction of low density lipoprotein receptor deficiency in the Watanabe heritable hyperlipidemic rabbit with recombinant adenoviruses. *J Biol Chem* 269:13695–13702.

Kulkarni AB and Karlsson S. 1993. Transforming growth factor-beta 1 knockout mice. A mutation in one cytokine gene causes a dramatic inflammatory disease. *Am J Pathol* 143:3–9.

Lin HF, Maeda N, Smithies O, Straight DL, and Stafford DW. 1997. A coagulation factor IX–deficient mouse model for human hemophilia B. *Blood* 90:3962–3966.

Lindblad-Toh K, Wade CM, et al. 2005. Genome sequence, comparative analysis and haplotype structure of the domestic dog. *Nature* 438:803–819.

Lozier JN and Kessler CM. 2005. Clinical aspects and therapy of hemophilia. In *Hematology: Principles and Practice*, R Hoffman, Ed. Churchill-Livingstone, New York, pp. 2047–2069.

Lozier JN and Zhang P. 2005. Mapping of genes that control the antibody response to human factor VIII in mice. *Blood* 106(Suppl 1):536a.

Lozier JN, Metzger ME, Donahue RE, and Morgan RA. 1999a. The rhesus macaque as an animal model for hemophilia B gene therapy. *Blood* 93:1875–1881.

Lozier JN, Metzger ME, Donahue RE, and Morgan RA. 1999b. Adenovirus-mediated expression of human coagulation factor IX in the rhesus macaque is associated with dose-limiting toxicity. *Blood* 94:3968–3975.

Lozier JN, Dutra A, Pak E, et al. 2002. The Chapel Hill hemophilia A dog colony exhibits a factor VIII gene inversion. *Proc Natl Acad Sci U S A* 99:12991–12996.

Lozier JN, Tayebi N, and Zhang P. 2005. Mapping of genes that control the antibody response to human factor IX in mice. *Blood* 105:1029–1035.

Lubahn DB, Moyer JS, Golding TS, Couse JF, Korach KS, and Smithies O. 1993. Alteration of reproductive function but not prenatal sexual development after insertional disruption of the mouse estrogen receptor gene. *Proc Natl Acad Sci U S A* 90:11162–11166.

Malech HL and Hickstein DD. 2007. Genetics, biology and clinical management of myeloid cell primary immune deficiencies: chronic granulomatous disease and leukocyte adhesion deficiency. *Curr Opin Hematol* 14:29–36.

Manno CS, Chew AJ, Hutchison S, et al. 2003. AAV-mediated factor IX gene transfer to skeletal muscle in patients with severe hemophilia B. *Blood* 101:2963–2972.

Manno CS, Pierce GF, Arruda VR, et al. 2006. Successful transduction of liver in hemophilia by AAV-factor IX and limitations imposed by the host immune response. *Nat Med* 12:342–347.

Mauser AE, Whitlark J, Whitney KM, and Lothrop CD Jr. 1996. A deletion mutation causes hemophilia B in lhasa apso dogs. *Blood* 88:3451–3455.

Michalak A and Butterworth RF. 1997. Ornithine transcarbamylase deficiency: pathogenesis of the cerebral disorder and new prospects for therapy. *Metab Brain Dis* 12:171–182.

Michou AI, Santoro L, Christ M, Juillard V, Pavirani A, and Mahtali M. 1997. Adenovirus-mediated gene transfer: influence of transgene, mouse strain and type of immune response on persistence of transgene expression. Gene Ther 4:473–482.

Naylor J, Brinke A, Hassock S, Green PM, and Giannelli F. 1993a. Characteristic mRNA abnormality found in half the patients with severe haemophilia A is due to large DNA inversions. *Hum Mol Genet* 2:1773–1778.

Naylor JA, Green PM, Rizza CR, and Giannelli F. 1993b. Analysis of factor VIII mRNA reveals defects in everyone of 28 haemophilia A patients. *Hum Mol Genet* 2:11–17.

Oldenburg J, Picard JK, Schwaab R, Brackmann HH, Tuddenham EG, and Simpson E. 1997. HLA genotype of patients with severe haemophilia A due to intron 22 inversion with and without inhibitors of factor VIII. *Thromb Haemost* 77:238–242.

Oldenburg J, El-Maarri O, and Schwaab R. 2002. Inhibitor development in correlation to factor VIII genotypes. *Haemophilia* 8(Suppl 2):23–29.

Paigen K. 2003. One hundred years of mouse genetics: an intellectual history: I. The classical period. *Genetics* 163:1–7.

Pierce GF, Lillicrap D, Pipe SW, and Vandendriessche T. 2007. Gene therapy, bioengineered clotting factors and novel technologies for hemophilia treatment. *J Thromb Haemost* 5:901–906.

Powell JS, Ragni MV, White GC 2nd, et al. 2003. Phase 1 trial of FVIII gene transfer for severe hemophilia A using a retroviral construct administered by peripheral intravenous infusion. *Blood* 102:2038–2045.

Raper SE, Chirmule N, Lee FS, et al. 2003. Fatal systemic inflammatory response syndrome in a ornithine transcarbamylase deficient patient following adenoviral gene transfer. *Mol Genet Metab* 80:148–158.

Rawle FE, Shi CX, Brown B, et al. 2004. Heterogeneity of the immune response to adenovirus-mediated factor VIII gene therapy in different inbred hemophilic mouse strains. *J Gene Med* 6:1358–1368.

Rhesus Macaque Genome Sequencing and Analysis Consortium (Gibbs RA, Rogers J, Katze MG, et al.). 2007. Evolutionary and biomedical insights from the rhesus macaque genome. *Science* 316:222–234.

Roth DA, Tawa NE, O'Brien JM, Treco DA, and Selden RF (Factor VIII Transkaryotic Therapy Study Group). 2001. Nonviral transfer of the gene encoding coagulation factor VIII in patients with severe hemophilia A. *N Engl J Med* 344:1735–1742.

Sampson SB, Higgins DC, Elliot RW, et al. 1998. An edited linkage map for the AXB and BXA recombinant inbred mouse strains. *Mamm Genome* 9:688–694.

Sanchez LM, Chirino AJ, and Bjorkman PJ. 1999. Crystal structure of human ZAG, a fat-depleting factor related to MHC molecules. *Science* 283:1914–1918.

Schastry BS. 1998. Gene disruption in mice: models of development and disease. *Mol Cell Biochem* 181:163–179.

Scherer L, Rossi JJ, and Weinberg MS. 2007. Progress and prospects: RNA-based therapies for treatment of HIV infection. *Gene Ther* 14:1057–1064.

Sevin C, Auborg P, and Cartier N. 2007. Enzyme, cell and gene-based therapies for metachromatic leukodystrophy. *J Inherit Metab Dis* 30:175–183.

Sidransky E, LaMarca ME, and Ginns EI. 2007. Therapy for Gaucher's disease: Don't stop thinking about tomorrow. *Mol Genet Metab* 90:122–125.

Stoff-Khalili MA, Dall P, and Curiel DT. 2006. Gene therapy for carcinoma of the breast. *Cancer Gene Ther* 13:633–647.

Villinger F, Brar SS, Mayne A, Chikkala N, and Ansari AA. 1995. Comparative sequence analysis of cytokine genes from human and nonhuman primates. *J Immunol* 155:3946–3954.

Wang J, Williams RW, and Manly KF. 2003. WebQTL: Web-based complex trait analysis. *Neuroinformatics* 1:299–308.

Wang Z, Kuhr CS, Allen JM, et al. 2007. Sustained AAV-mediated dystrophin expression in a canine model of Duchenne muscular dystrophy with a brief course of immunosuppression. *Mol Ther* 15:1160–1166.

Warrier I, Baird-Cox K, and Lusher JM. 1997. Use of central venous catheters in children with haemophilia: one haemophilia treatment centre experience. *Haemophilia* 3:194–198.

Yuasa K, Yoshimura M, Urasawa N, et al. 2007. Injection of a recombinant AAV serotype 2 into canine skeletal muscles evokes strong immune responses against transgene products. *Gene Ther* 14:1249–1260.

15

IMMUNE MODULATION AND TRANSIENT SUPPRESSION STRATEGIES

VALDER R. ARRUDA, M.D., PH.D

Department of Pediatrics, University of Pennsylvania School of Medicine, The Children's Hospital of Philadelphia, Philadelphia, Pennsylvania

15.1 INTRODUCTION

The unwanted immune responses to the vector and to the transgene may hamper the success of many human gene therapy strategies. Immune responses in gene

Gene Therapy Immunology, Edited by Roland Herzog

therapy are the result of complex interactions of host, target tissue, vector, vector delivery method, and transgene. Harnessing the innate and adaptive immune systems to provide long-lasting therapeutic effects following gene transfer is the major goal of immunotherapy [Strom 2007]. Effective treatment of an established immune response is much more difficult to achieve than prevention of a response before it has had a chance to develop. Therefore, the development of safe and efficacious prophylactic immune modulatory regimens is critical to achieving the full potential of gene-based therapy.

The balance between host and infection agents tends to evolve toward a state of mutual survival. For the host, survival depends on mechanisms of innate resistance and the repertoire of T and B lymphocytes responsible for providing adaptive immunity [Zinkernagel 1996]. Innate immunity is the first line of defense of the body to acute injury and occurs within the first 12 hours of invasion; it is a primitive response that operates by pattern recognition receptors and does not induce immunological memory [Zinkernagel 1996; Zinkernagel and Hengartner 2001]. The adaptive immunity is activated next and represents a complex system that responds to specific antigens. It evolves, operates by determining self from nonself, and has memory. Innate immune response is an essential prerequisite for the adaptive immune response because co-stimulatory molecules that are induced on the cells of the innate immune system during their initial interaction with the microorganisms activate the antigen-specific lymphocytes of the adaptive immune response [Zinkernagel and Hengartner 2001]. The innate immune response is desirable in the context of therapeutic vaccines or for mediating a tumor-destructive local response (which is not the subject of this chapter). However, innate immunity could be detrimental if tissue injury created at a target organ or site of cell implant produces a "danger signal" that stimulates these potent natural defense mechanisms and targets the host cells, which are presenting viral proteins and/or expressing the transgene, for destruction by the immune system.

The central safety issue in gene-based strategies remains tolerance induction to the transgene. Most of the gene therapy trials for genetic diseases are aimed at sustained expression of therapeutic genes by introducing the vector in the target tissue with minimal or no tissue damage. Vectors are designed to contain no viral coding genes and no pathogenic genes. Transgene expression restricted to the target tissue by using tissue-specific promoters has also been exploited extensively to avoid immune responses to the transgene. In addition, the host immune status and its previous exposure to the transgene and to the wild-type viruses that originate in the recombinant vectors will influence the immune response outcome of a gene-based strategy.

In this chapter we focus on drug-based strategies to avoid immune responses to the vector and transgene following in vivo delivery of recombinant vectors. This differs from strategies based on stem cell therapies, in which the host cells are transduced ex vivo by vectors prior to reimplantation, as described in Chapters 5 and 12. The prototype of this approach is the use of hematopoietic stem cell therapy transduced by retroviral vectors in which myelocytotoxic drugs (cyclophosphamide and busulfan) are given to the host to create space in the bone marrow for the homing and expansion of gene-corrected cells.

Transduced cells and/or the therapeutic transgene expression following delivery of vectors are prone to trigger alloimmune responses involving both naive and memory lymphocytes, including lymphocytes previously stimulated by viral antigens cross-reacting with HLA antigens [Halloran 2004]. This creates, to a certain extent, a clinical parallel to the immune responses following organ transplantation, in which neoantigens in the graft are presented to the host immune system. To avoid allograft rejection, immunosuppression is required during the induction phase, followed by a long-term maintenance regimen. There are major differences in organ transplantation, such as the amounts of antigen presented, the nature of antigen (eukaryote DNA), the generation of exclusive effector versus memory T cells, and vascular rejection, which requires intense immunosuppression for induction that probably is not needed for a gene-based modified target tissue. In contrast, the full potential of organ transplantation has not yet been realized, due to the hazard associated with long-term immunosuppression, whereas in gene-based strategies, control of the immune responses is likely to be transient in nature.

15.2 IMMUNE MODULATION STRATEGIES

The immune system has the remarkable ability to defend against diverse microbial pathogens and yet not respond to self. T cells are key mediators of the immune response, and their activation is tightly regulated to prevent autoreactivity. The process of T-cell activation and self-tolerance are therefore potential targets for manipulation by drugs.

15.2.1 Model of Alloimmune Response

Whether the immune system reacts to antigen depends on (1) the relative frequencies of responding T and B cells and on the thresholds of binding affinity that their receptor displays, (2) the levels of antigen present, and (3) the period during which the antigen remains in secondary organized lymphatic tissue, where primary immune responses are initiated [Zinkernagel 1996; Zinkernagel and Hengartner 2001].

T-cell activation requires two signals that are derived from antigen-presenting cells (APCs) (Fig. 15-1). Signal 1 is the antigen displayed on the surface of APCs in the form of peptides bound to histocompatibility molecules and triggers T cells with cognate T-cell receptors transduced through the CD3 complex. The recognition of antigen by T-cell receptors provides specificity to the response. APCs provide co-stimulation, signal 2, delivered when CD80 (B7-1) and CD86 (B7-2) on the surface of dendritic cells engage CD28. This is the best-characterized T-cell co-stimulatory pathway. CD28 is constitutively expressed on 95% of $CD4^+$ T cells and 50% of $CD8^+$ T cells in humans [Bluestone and Abbas 2003].

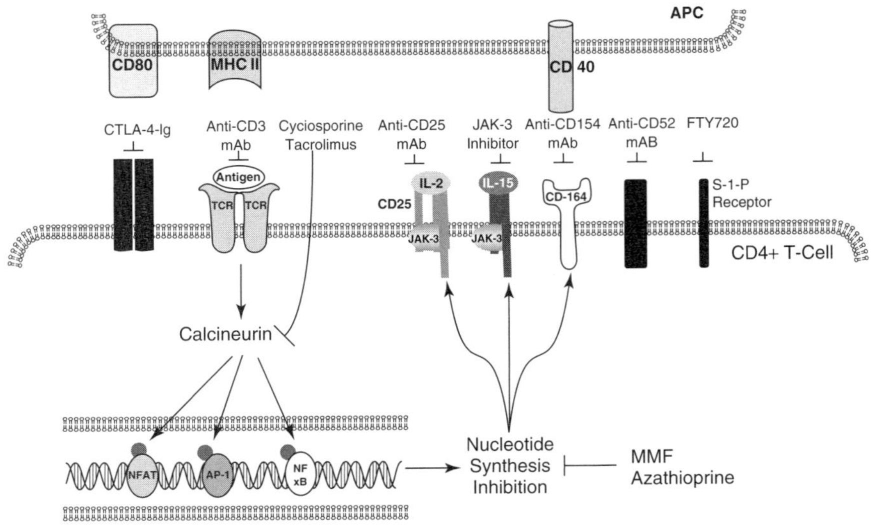

Figure 15-1 Immunosuppressive drugs and their respective target on a CD4$^+$ T cell. APC, antigen-presenting cell; small-molecule drugs: mycophenolate mofetil (MMF) and azathioprine; calcineurin inhibitors: cyclosporine and tacrolimus; FTY720: sphingosie-1-phosphate-receptor antagonist (S-1-P receptor); monoclonal antibodies: anti-CD3, anti-CD25 (daclizumab, basiliximab), and anti-CD52; fusion protein: cytotoxic T-lymphocyte-associated antigen (CTL4-Ig, LEA29Y).

Signals 1 and 2 activate three signal transduction pathways: (1) the calcium–calcineurin pathway, (2) the RAS-mitogen-activated protein transcription factor (MAP) kinase pathway, and (3) the nuclear factor-κB pathway. The pathways activate transcription factors that trigger the expression of others molecules, including interleukin-2 (IL-2), CD154, and CD25. Signal 3 triggers cell proliferation, which is provided by activation of the target-of-rapamycin pathway by IL-12 and IL-15. Lymphocyte proliferation also requires nucleotide synthesis. Proliferation and differentiation lead to a large number of effector and memory T cells. B cells are activated when antigen engages their antigen receptor to form alloantibodies. Thus, within days, the immune response generates the agents for tissue damage recognition, activated T cells, and alloantibodies.

15.2.2 Model of Immune Tolerance

Immunological tolerance can be defined as a state in which the immune system, in the absence of ongoing immunosuppression, does not mount a pathological response against a specific antigen, whereas responses to others antigens are intact. In several models of immune tolerance, the presence of antigen is required to maintain the tolerant state, such as by frequent infusion of the protein antigen or by sustained transgene expression in gene-based strategies (reviewed in Chapters 8, 12, and 16).

Modern research into mechanisms of immune tolerance offers the promise of reprogramming the immune system to harness the natural tolerance mechanisms of the body. There is growing evidence that pharmacological therapies provide a novel area for the treatment of immune-mediated diseases and may induce immune tolerance by diverting the T-cell activation pathways (thereby augmenting the apoptosis rates of activated T cells), or by up-regulating regulatory T cells [Roncarolo and Battaglia 2007; Tao et al. 2007].

Regulatory T cells (Tregs) are well-characterized T-cell subsets that play a central role in inducing and maintaining immunologic tolerance. One subset of Tregs is present in 5 to 10% of unstimulated $CD4^+$ T cells and expresses the IL-2 receptor α-chain (CD25). $CD4^+CD25^+$ Tregs are generated in the thymus and are part of the normal peripheral T-cell repertoire where they potently suppress proliferation and cytokine production of both $CD4^+$ and $CD8^+$ T cells [Kang et al. 2007; Mays and Chen 2007]. The majority of $CD4^+$ $CD25^+$ Treg cells express cytotoxic T-lymphocyte antigen 4 (CTLA-4), a surface marker of T cells that outcompetes CD28 for binding to CD80/86 (B7) on APCs. The binding of CTLA-4 to B7 sends inhibitory signals to T cells. In addition, suppressor $CD4^+CD25^+$ Treg cells also express glucocorticoid-induced tumor necrosis factor receptor (GITR). The identification of a specific suppressive Treg population within a pool of T cells remained elusive for many years until the characterization of a more specific Treg marker, the transcription factor forkhead box P3 (FoxP3), which appears to be a master switch for development of $CD4^+CD25^+$ Tregs [Mays and Chen 2007]. Expression of FoxP3 is necessary and sufficient for suppressor function of $CD4^+CD25^+$ Treg cells, and it is present in low to undetectable levels in both naive and activated $CD4^+CD25^-$ T cells as well as in other T, B, and NK cells. FoxP3 has been shown to repress IL-2 and IL-4 gene transcription, and to up-regulate the expression of CD25 and CTLA-4. $CD4^+CD25^+$ T cells play critical roles in the prevention of organ-specific autoimmunity and allograft rejection in the maintenance of self-tolerance and in the regulation of humoral responses. Thus, preservation of these natural Tregs as well as augmentation of inducible subsets may provide an alternative for successful immune modulation without the side effects of immunosuppressive drugs [Kang et al. 2007].

15.3 IMMUNOSUPPRESSIVE DRUGS

Current treatment for immunological disorders are nearly all empirical in origin, using immunosuppressive drugs identified by screening large numbers of natural and synthetic compounds. Immunosuppression can be achieved by depleting lymphocytes, blocking lymphocyte response pathways, or diverting lymphocyte traffic. Immunosuppressive drugs include the following (see Fig. 15-1):

1. Glucocorticoids
2. Small-molecule drugs
   a. Immunophilin-binding drugs
      (1) Calcineurin inhibitors
         - Cyclophilin-binding drugs [cyclosporine, ISA(X)247]
         - FKBP12-binding drugs (tacrolimus, modified-release tacrolimus)
      (2) Target-of-rapamycin inhibitors (sirolimus, everolimus)
   b. Inhibitors of nucleotide synthesis
      - Mycophenolate mofetil
      - Cyclophosphamide
      - Azathioprine
      - FTY720
3. Protein drugs
   a. Depleting antibodies (against T cells, B cells, or both)
      - Polyclonal antibody (horse or rabbit antithymocyte globulin)
      - Mouse monoclonal anti-CD3 antibody (muromonab-CD3)
      - Humanized monoclonal anti-CD52 antibody (alemtuzumab)
      - B-cell-depleting monoclonal anti-CD20 antibody (rituximab)
   b. Nondepleting antibodies and fusion proteins
      - Humanized or chimeric monoclonal anti-CD25 antibody (daclizumab, basiliximab)
      - Fusion protein with natural binding properties [CTLA-4-Ig (LEA29Y)]
   c. Intravenous immunoglobulin (IVIg)

15.3.1 Glucocorticoids

Corticosteroid drugs are nonspecific anti-inflammatory agents. The primary action of these drugs is receptor-mediated, which results in inhibition of cytokine gene transcription. In addition, the leukocyte and macrophage functions are also depressed. By inhibiting cytokine production, steroids prevent T-cell recruitment and activation and are thus potent immunosuppressants. Receptor-mediated effects are mainly transcriptional through DNA-binding and protein–protein interactions of the steroid–receptor complex targeting nuclear factor-κB and activator protein 1 (AP-1) [Karin 1998]. At high doses, glucocorticoids have receptor-independent effects. However, there are also many adverse effects, including fluid retention, weight gain, diabetes, bone mineral loss, dyslipidemia, and personality changes. Corticosteroids used in transplant recipients and in inflammatory autoimmune disease are often administered in combination with other drugs to keep the dose and toxic effects to a minimum. Most recent immunosuppressive regimens do not include long-term corticosteroid therapy. However, pulse therapy with intravenous methylprednisolne remains a feasible option to acutely down-regulate pathological immune responses.

15.3.2 Small-Molecule Drugs

Azathioprine Azathioprine is derived from 6-mercaptopurine, which interferes with DNA synthesis, exerts a negative feedback on purine metabolism, and reduces nucleotide synthesis. These actions result in inhibition of T-cell activation and convert a co-stimulation signal into an apoptotic signal. Azathioprine was the first immunosuppressive agent to achieve widespread use in organ transplantation. It is usually well tolerated in therapeutic doses but has significant side effects, such as bone marrow suppression and, less commonly, hepatotoxicity, pancreatitis, and possibly increased risk of cancer.

Cyclosphosphamide Cyclophosphamide is a member of the nitrogen mustard family and, similar to azathioprine, interferes with DNA synthesis and has major effects on dividing cells. The side effects include myelosuppression, vomiting and nausea, gastrointestinal discomfort, hemorrhagic cystitis, and hair loss. In addition, there is an increased risk of tumor formation, especially in patients treated for long periods.

Mycophenolate Mofetil Mycophenolate mofetil (MMF) is an antiproliferative immunosuppressant agent in the same class as azathioprine and sirolimus. MMF is a selective inhibitor of the de novo pathway of purine biosynthesis, thereby providing more specific and potent inhibition of T- and B-cell proliferation [Allison and Eugui 2005]. MMF is an ester prodrug of mycophenolic acid (MPA), a potent inhibitor of the enzyme inosine monophosphate dehydrogenase (IMPDH), which is essential in the metabolic pathway of de novo purine synthesis. When administered orally, MMF is converted to MPA and finally secreted in the bile. The main side effects are gastrointestinal (diarrhea) and hematological (anemia, leukopenia). MMF may increase cytomegalovirus disease. However, MMF exhibits in vitro anti-pneumocystic activity and inhibition of human immunodeficiency virus (HIV) replication in vitro as well as in vivo [Chapuis et al. 2000].

Calcineurin Inhibitors Calcineurin is a key enzyme in the production of IL-2 by T cells. IL-2 is critical for the recruitment and activation of $CD4^+$ T cells via the induction of other cytokines. IL-2 modulates the activity of cytotoxic $CD8^+$ cells, natural killer cells, and B cells. The two calcineurin inhibitors, cyclosporine and tacrolimus (FK506), have become the cornerstone of immunosuppressive therapy in solid organ transplantation. Each agent forms complexes with a cytosolic protein called immunophilin [Mueller 2004a]. Cyclosporine binds to a group of immunophilins called cyclophilins, which are present in all tissues. Tacrolimus binds with FK506-binding protein 12 (FKBP12) to form a complex that inhibits calcineurin with greater molar potency than does cyclosporine. These complexes bind to calcineurin and inhibit cytokine transcription by $CD4^+$ T cells. Blockage of cytokine production and cytokine-receptor expression inhibits T-cell proliferation and differentiation. Compared with nonimmune cells, lymphocytes show greater sensitivity to cyclosporine and tacrolimus, which may be due to the limiting amounts of calcineurin in nonimmune cells [Mueller 2004a]. The adverse effects of cyclosporine correlate directly with the drug level and include nephrotoxicity, hypertension, hyperlipidemia, hirsutism, gingival hyperplasia, and tremor. Tacrolimus resembles cyclosporine in terms of nephrotoxicity, but it is less likely to cause the other side effects. Although tacrolimus is the dominant calcineurin inhibitor, cyclosporine is better for patients with a high risk of diabetes (older age or obesity) [Halloran 2004].

Target-of-Rapamycin Inhibitors Sirolimus engages FKBP12 to create complexes that bind and inhibit the target of rapamycin but not calcineurin. Inhibition of the target of rapamycin blocks signal 3 by preventing cytokine receptors from activating the cell cycle. Thus, it acts at a point distinct from calcineurin inhibitors, MMF or azathioprine, and therefore could be used synergistically with either group. The main side effects of sirolimus include hyperlipidemia, thrombocytopenia, diarrhea, and poor wound healing [Abraham and Wiederrecht 1996]. Sirolimus has been combined with tacrolimus to avoid the toxicity (nephrotoxicity and hypertension) observed in combined sirolimus and cyclosporine treatment. Everolimus is a sirolimus derivative with improved bioavailability and shorter half-life than sirolimus. Because these drugs may have antineoplastic [Guba et al. 2002] and arterial protective effects [Morice et al. 2002], it has been proposed that sirolimus may be the best drug to control or prevent long-term immunosuppression post-transplantation, such as increased risk of cancer and occlusive cardiovascular disease.

15.3.3 Depleting Antibodies

Antithymocyte Globulin Polyclonal antithymocyte globulin (ATG) is produced by immunizing horses or rabbits with human lymphoid cells. ATG is used as an induction agent for a short period of time resulting in profound lymphopenia that lasts for months [Brennan et al. 1999]. There are several side effects, such as immunodeficiency, increased risk of infection, thrombocytopenia, cytokine-release syndrome, and occasionally, serum sickness [Halloran 2004].

Muromonab-CD3 Anti-CD3 monoclonal antibodies have been used for decades [Norman et al. 2000]. This drug induces a massive cytokine-release syndrome before both depleting and functionally altering T cells. Humans can develop neutralizing antibodies against muromonab-CD3 that limit its clinical use.

Alemtuzumab Alemtuzumab is a humanized monoclonal antibody against CD52 that massively depletes T-cell, B-cell, natural killer, and monocyte markers. It is approved for the treatment of refractory B-cell chronic lymphoid leukemia. However, experience with alemtuzumab in organ transplantation or other clinical situations is limited [Halloran 2004]. The combination of alemtuzumab and sirolimus in kidney transplants did not prevent allograft rejections. Side effects of this drug include neutropenia, anemia, and autoimmunity.

Rituximab Rituximab is an anti-CD20 monoclonal antibody that eliminates most B cells. It was originally developed for the treatment of non-Hodgkin's B-cell lymphoma. Rituximab is used in combination with other immunosuppressive drugs, plasmapheresis, and intravenous immunoglobulin to control deleterious alloantibody responses in transplants [Halloran 2004; Kessel et al. 2008]. However, this drug has been used to eradicate antibodies to coagulation FVIII (inhibitors) in hemophilia as well as non-hemophilia patients, for the treatment of rheumatoid arthritis, immune thrombocytopenic purpura, and other benign diseases with an acceptable safety profile [Kessel et al. 2008].

15.3.4 Nondepleting Proteins

Daclizumab and Basilixumab The anti-CD25 monoclonal antibodies daclizumab and basilixumab are commonly used in transplantation for immunosuppression induction regimens. Because expression of CD25 (IL-2 receptor α-chain) requires T-cell activation, anti-CD25 antibodies cause minimal depletion of T cells [Yabu and Vincenti 2007]. Since there is redundancy within the IL-2 receptor complex that permits IL-2R signaling in the presence of high levels of IL-2, anti-CD25 antibodies are often associated with calcineurin inhibitors to induce immunosuppression effectively [Halloran 2004; Mueller 2004b]. Daclizumab is a humanized antibody with a half-life of about 11 days, whereas basilixumab is a chimeric antibody with a half-life of 6.5 days. However, their effect remains for several weeks. These antibodies are well tolerated and reduce the incidence of infection and other complications in organ transplantation [Vincenti et al. 1998].

CTLA-4 CTLA4-Ig is a fusion protein combining the extracellular domain of CTLA4, which engages CD80 and CD86 with the Fc portion of IgG blocking the co-stimulation of the T cells, thus initiating a potent down-modulatory effect [Bluestone et al. 2006]. CTLA4-Ig has been used successfully in an immunosuppressive regimen in humans with rheumatoid arthritis and in animal models of transplantation and, at least transiently, blocks the inhibitor formation in hemophilia A models. Although an immunoglobulin fusion protein construct of CTLA4 suppressed rejection in rodents, it lacked efficacy in primate transplant models. However, LEA29Y [Yabu and Vincenti 2007], a second-generation variant of CTL4-Ig, exhibits increased avidity for both CD80 and CD86, resulting in a 10-fold increase in potency in vitro and significant prolongation of renal allograft survival in a preclinical primate model. Ongoing kidney transplant clinical trials on the combination of repeated injection of LEA29Y with MMF and anti-CD25 antibody test the novel concept of repeating injections of nondepleting proteins while avoiding the use of calcineurin inhibitors [Halloran 2004].

Intravenous Immune Globulin Human intravenous immunoglobulin (IVIG) preparations are manufactured with pooled human plasma from several thousand screened volunteer donors and contain highly purified polyvalent immunoglobulin G (i.e., $IgG > 90\%$). Developed initially for the treatment of patients with immune deficiencies, the majority of IVIG use is accounted for within hematology and neurology clinics [Darabi et al. 2006]. Growing use in rheumatology, dermatology, and nephrology subspecialties has also contributed to the increase in IVIG utilization. The mechanisms of action of IVIG are complex, involving modulation of expression and function of Fc receptors; interference with activation of complement and the cytokine and idiotype network; regulation of cell growth; and effects on the activation, differentiation, and effector functions of dendritic, T, and B cells. IVIG is associated with several potential adverse effects such as acute renal toxicity, hypersensitivity reactions, hemolytic anemia, urticarial rashes, hemolysis, and cytopenias. One important consideration in gene therapy is that IVIG contains high levels of neutralizing antibodies to some of the most commonly used recombinant viral vectors such as AAV and adenovirus. Therefore, the use of IVIG will result in a passive immunization against these viruses, which consequently bears the risk of hampering the efficacy of gene transfer by these vectors.

15.3.5 Other Drugs

There are several other targets of therapeutic interest to achieve more specific immunosuppression (Fig. 15-1). FTY720 is in development as a novel immunosuppressant aimed at the sequestration of T and B cells into peripheral lymph nodes and mesenteric lymph nodes by a mechanism involving shyngosine-1-phosphate receptor on lymphocytes [Schwab and Cyster 2007]. FTY720 has no effect on T-cell activation, cytokine production, or B-cell proliferation. Janus kinase 3 (JAK3) is a tyrosine kinase associated with the cytokine receptor γ-chain, which participates in the signaling of many cytokine receptors (IL-2, 4, 7, 9, 12, and 21). JAK3 inhibitors are in development, and an oral drug is currently undergoing preclinical testing [Changelian et al. 2007]. Interestingly, another tyrosine kinase inhibitor (imatinib mesylate) developed originally for the treatment of chronic myeloid leukemia (CML) and other malignancies also plays a role in T-cell receptor signaling [Mumprecht et al. 2006]. This drug is now the first line for the treatment of CML and it is well tolerated with mild to moderate hematological side effects. Recently, studies in a lymphocytic choriomeningitis virus (LCMV) model demonstrated that imatinib efficiently targets the memory CTLs post reexposure to LCMV infection without compromising responses to other viruses, a highly desirable safety aspect of an immunosuppressive drug. In addition, the use of imatinib also delayed the onset of diabetes in a CTL-induced diabetes model [Mumprecht et al. 2006].

15.4 IMMUNOSUPPRESSIVE REGIMENS

Several immunosuppression regimens consist of a combination of distinct agents to minimize the side effects of any single drug while maintaining adequate immunosuppression by targeting multiple steps in T-cell activation. Standard combinations include calcineurin inhibitor and an antiproliferative agent with a short-term course of corticosteroids [Halloran 2004; Mueller 2004b; Perry and Neuberger 2005; Post et al. 2005]. In organ transplantation, induction therapy often requires the use of monoclonal or polyclonal antibodies to effect sustained immunosuppresssion at an early phase. However, the intensity of such induction therapy varies according to the risk of graft rejection. In organ transplantation models, tipping the balance from donor-specific immunity toward tolerance and away from rejection is the main goal of an ideal immune tolerance protocol. The unusually large number of T cells that are responsive to transplant tissues (5 in 20 T cells), as compared with the response to a foreign protein (one in 1 million), is remarkable and points out that pharmacological tolerogenic regimens (see below) may be feasible for the immune modulation required for successful gene-based strategies [Strom 2007]. This may argue against the need for intensive induction therapy with monoclonal or polyclonal antibodies in a gene therapy setting.

In all three major organ transplantation settings, including heart [Mueller 2004b], kidney [Halloran 2004], and liver [Perry and Neuberger 2005; Post et al. 2005], there is not a single regimen that is most used, and even within an organ-specific group the ongoing and planned trials consist of heterogeneous drug combinations. Therefore, it is prudent to consider all major characteristics of the underlying disease to be treated by gene therapy in the light of the organ transplantation experience to evaluate both the efficacy and side effects of all available drugs. Notably, most of these immunosuppressive drugs have been used in the context of other alloimmune, primary autoimmune, and benign diseases. Because the growing tendency to enroll patients with relatively long life expectancy in gene therapy clinical studies, the safety outcome of a given immunosuppressive therapy is better evaluated than by assessing the long-term complications of specific conditions associated with organ transplantation.

The most common risk of immunosuppression therapy after organ transplantation is the increased susceptibility to opportunistic infection [Fishman 2007] within the initial two years, followed by cancer and cardiovascular disease in the long-term follow-up [Dantal and Soulillou 2005]. Although allograft rejection is still a considerable complication in the early years following transplantation, infection is also a common complication. The main long-term complications following organ transplant include cardiovascular disease and cancer. Because sirolimus has been clinically associated with a protective effect on the development of occlusive arterial disease and antitumor effects, its use is an attractive option for late-maintenance immunosuppressive regimens [Guba et al. 2002; Morice et al. 2002].

Regarding gene therapy using adeno-associated viral (AAV) vectors and tacrolimus, it has been proposed that cellular factors exist that bind to the ends of the AAV genome and inhibit second-strand synthesis. One such protein is the immunophilin, FK506-binding protein, that also targets and may block conversion of the single-stranded AAV genome to a transcriptional active double-stranded form [Zhao et al. 2006]. FKBP52 is also the binding immunophilin for tacrolimus. Thus, it is possible that tacrolimus and AAV vectors may compete for binding to FKBP52; if this hypothetical situation occurs, the expression by AAV vectors may be enhanced.

Some immunosuppressive drugs present antiviral activity and therefore could be an attractive strategy in patients with chronic viral infection. Experience with MMF and tacrolimus in HCV-positive recipients of liver transplants demonstrated that recurrence of HCV infection is lower than in regimens with corticosteroids [Fasola et al. 2002]. In addition, MMF exhibits antiviral activity in HIV-infected patients [Chapuis et al. 2000]. To date, there is no evidence that these drugs could also interfere with the infectivity of recombinant viral vectors.

The efficacy of MMF, tacrolimus, and cyclosporin in various regimens has been tested extensively in solid organ transplantation, including liver, kidney, lung, and heart among adult [Halloran 2004; Mueller 2004b; Perry and Neuberger 2005; Post et al. 2005] and pediatric patients [Kari and Trompeter 2004]. Unlike cyclosporine, tacrolimus does not interfere with the absorption of MMF; this leads to greater MPA exposure when MMF and tacrolimus are co-administered. Thus, the combination of tacrolimus and MMF requires a lower dose of the drugs, which improves the safety of this regimen. The safety of these drugs is also supported by long-term follow-up of patients receiving tacrolimus or MMF for the treatment of benign diseases such as psoriasis, rheumatoid arthritis, lupus nephritis, and autoimmune gastrointestinal disorders [Chan et al. 2000; Yocum et al. 2004].

The combination of MMF and sirolimus has also being tested in organ transplantation, including transplantation in patients with HCV infection. However, the combination of sirolimus and cyclosporine is associated with nephrotoxicity and hypertension [Grinyo and Cruzado 2006]. Notably, sirolimus has been associated with selective expansion of $CD4^{+}CD25^{+}FoxP3^{+}$ Tregs in distinct models of immunity [Battaglia et al. 2006]. Sirulimus induces FoxP3 expression in activated $CD4^{+}$ $CD25^{+}$, induces in vivo conversion of naive T cells into Tregs, and promotes activation-induced cell death of T effector cells [Roncarolo and Battaglia 2007]. Thus, protocols using sirolimus could shift the balance of alloimmunity toward tolerance.

15.4.1 Considerations when Coupling Immunosuppressive Therapy with Gene Therapy

It is anticipated that distinct immunosuppressive regimens will be developed for each particular gene therapy strategy. There are unique safety aspects on the use of immunosuppressive drugs during gene transfer to a specific target tissue that need to be addressed in preclinical and epidemiological clinical studies. A number of factors need to be taken into consideration:

1. Interference with vector internalization, stability, and transduction efficiency

2. Modification of the biodistribution of vector to nontarget tissues
3. Compromising host-defense mechanisms that may facilitate infection by opportunistic pathogens and probably altering vector transduction efficacy and/or immunological profile
4. Higher susceptibility of tissue damage by the combination of vector and/or drug, especially in strategies targeting tissues with underlying diseases (primary or iatrogenic liver disease, renal diseases, inflammatory status of skeletal muscle in patient with muscular dystrophy, inflammatory joint diseases, and bone marrow failure)
5. Drug side effects could exacerbate underlying metabolic complications, such as lipid disorders, glucose metabolism, and others
6. Long-term complications such as increased risk of malignancies, impairing gonadal function, and infertility

15.4.2 Transient Immunosuppressive Therapy in Gene Therapy

The duration of the immunosuppression required to prevent or to ameliorate undesirable immune responses following gene therapy is not yet defined. There is evidence in several large-animal models of disease, suggesting that transient (short-duration) immunomodulation would allow sustained transgene expression and correction of the disease phenotype.

For those gene therapy studies requiring invasive procedures (surgery, intravascular catheterization) for vector delivery to the target organ, a higher risk of nosocomial infection within the first weeks is expected than with minimally or noninvasive approaches. The delivery of vector to immune-privileged organs such as the eye and the brain [Lowenstein et al. 2007] often requires an invasive procedure to reach the target tissue; it is therefore possible that changes in the environmental conditions may also affect the immune status of this site, and anti-inflammatory or immunosuppressive therapies may be required transiently.

Proper screening and installment of prophylactic therapeutics could also minimize the risk of activation of latent infection such as cytomegalovirus, *Pneumocystis carinii*, herpes simplex virus, hepatitis B virus, *Mycobacterium tuberculosis*, and others. These complications often occur in, but are not restricted to, the first month of immunosuppressive therapy. The main determinants of the risk of infection are the dose, duration, and sequence of immunosuppressive therapies. This complication can be minimized by monitoring drug levels and by using a short duration of immunosuppression.

Intravascular delivery of AAV2 vectors to skeletal muscle has been achieved successfully in hemophilia B dogs (clotting factor IX, FIX, deficiency), and sustained transgene expression (>5 years) has been achieved at levels >10-fold higher than delivery by the direct intramuscular route (IM) [Arruda et al. 2005]. In these experiments, immune responses to the neotransgene (FIX) were prevented by transient immunosuppression with cyclophosphamide starting one week before vector injection for a total of six doses total (once a week up to day 42 post-injection). This regimen was also effective in preventing the formation of antibody to canine FIX following IM injection of AAV-FIX in another model of hemophilia B with a high risk of developing FIX antibody [Herzog et al. 2001]. Notably, cyclophosphamide was ineffective in inducing tolerance to FIX once the antibody to FIX was present after IM injection of AAV-FIX in the dog model [Arruda et al. 2004], which reinforces the idea that preventive rather than therapeutic immunosuppressive strategies are likely to control immune responses following gene transfer.

In a feline model of lipoprotein lipase (LPL) deficiency, the expression of human LPL by AAV1 vectors in skeletal muscle resulted in transient transgene expression due to anti-hLPL immune responses [Ross et al. 2006]. The level and duration of the transgene expression were improved significantly, while the animals from a low-dose cohort were on oral administration of cyclophosphamide. However, in cats treated with higher vector doses, the formation of antibody against the human LPL was not completely ablated. The use of non-species-specific transgene is a limitation of this study but demonstrates that preventive immunosuppression therapy has a potential effect in avoiding immune responses to the transgene.

Studies in the golden retriever muscular dystrophy (GRMD) model are encouraging, with the potential of cell- and/or gene-based therapy coupled with immunosuppression for the treatment for muscular dystrophy. One study demonstrated T-cell-mediated immune responses following IM injection of AAV2 or AAV6 in naive normal dogs. Thus, in experiments using the GRMD model, the authors sought to prevent immune responses by short-term immune suppression (up to three months post-vector injection) [Wang et al. 2007]. The regimen, containing cyclosporin, MMF, and ATG, was effective in sustaining expression of canine microdystrophin after discontinuation of the drugs without local $CD8^+$ T-cell infiltrates. Data from a recent study on the use of mesangioblast stem cells in the GRMD model also reinforce the importance of method of delivery and immunosuppression for DMD [Sampaolesi et al. 2006]. Following delivery of the mesangioblasts by intraarterial (femoral) injection, dystrophin expression was associated with remarkable improvement in both muscle morphology and function. It is possible that immunosuppression required for the use of heterologous mesangioblasts was playing a coadjuvant role in the improvement of the disease phenotype.

The use of CTLA4-Ig fusion protein in the context of gene therapy has been reported in adenoviral vectors in murine models [Kay et al. 1997] and more recently in a feline model of lysossomal disease. The latter study proves that transient administration of CTLA-4Ig prevents a CTL-mediated immune response to the liver of cats injected with retroviral vectors during the neonatal period, and long-term sustained transgene expression was documented [Ponder et al. 2006]. CTLA4-Ig, in combination with anti-CD40L was the most effective strategy to prevent immune responses to the transgene following hepatic delivery of non-viral-vector-encoding human factor VIII (FVIII) in a murine model of hemophilia A [Miao et al. 2006].

A combination of methylprednisolone and cyclosporine for four weeks was tested in a provocative rabbit model for lentiviral vector transfer of a gene encoding enhanced green fluorescent protein (EGFP) [Doi et al. 2004]. While all control rabbits developed antibodies against EFGP and showed signs of rejection, no such evidence was observed with animals that received immunosuppression. One month of systemic immunosuppression permanently prevented rejection of RPE with EGFP expression. This study illustrates that even at immunoprivilege sites, immune responses could be triggered if the environment is perturbed.

Recent findings in a clinical trial, in which an AAV vector expressing FIX was introduced into the liver of hemophilia B subjects, highlighted a new issue previously not identified in animal studies. Two subjects enrolled in this trial developed transient elevation of liver enzymes, a likely consequence of immune rejection of transduced hepatocytes mediated by AAV2 capsid-specific $CD8^+$ T cells (but not formation of antibodies to FIX) [Manno et al. 2006]. Studies in healthy donors showed that humans carry a population of capsid-specific memory $CD8^+$ T cells, probably originating following wild-type AAV2 infections [Mingozzi et al. 2007b]. Several possible solutions for this problem include the administration of a short-term anti-T-cell immunosuppression regimen concomitant to gene transfer and/or using alternative serotypes of AAV vectors. Because these findings in human subjects were not documented in preclinical studies using AAV2 or other serotypes, there has not yet been an animal model to test the efficacy of immunosuppression therapy in preventing capsid-mediated immune responses, but the safety of distinct therapeutic regimens with vector administration was determined in nonhuman primates. Overcoming the immune response against AAV capsid will probably require only transient immunosuppression since the input capsid proteins are slowly degraded and thus present only transiently in the transduced cells.

Different groups carried out studies in nonhuman primates (NHP) for the safety of AAV vectors consisting of MMF with tacrolimus (AAV8) or MMF and rapamycin (AAV2) over a period of 10 weeks [Jiang et al. 2006; Mingozzi et al. 2007a]. The findings of these studies showed that these immunosuppressive regimens do not interfere with parameters of gene transfer, vector biodistribution, and transgene expression following delivery of vector to the hepatic artery of NHP. The use of NHP has an additional advantage over other preclinical models, because one can use immunosuppressive drugs such as monoclonal antibodies designed to target human proteins, which are highly conserved among primates.

The current evidence of the high efficacy of nondepleting anti-CD25 monoclonal antibodies daclizumab and basiliximab for induction of immunosuppression in organ transplantation suggested that such a strategy could also prevent the early onset of immune response following gene transfer. However, studies in NHP injected with AAV-FIX showed that adding daclizumab to an MMF–rapamycin regimen caused an increased risk of neutralizing antibody formation to FIX [Mingozzi et al. 2007a]. Earlier data demonstrate that sustained transgene expression by AAV-mediated, liver-directed gene transfer induces antigen-specific tolerance, and in mice, this effect is mediated in part by $CD4^+CD25^+$ Tregs [Cao et al. 2007].

The monitoring of peripheral mononuclear cells of AAV-injected NHP revealed that following daclizumab injection (one day prior to and 15 days post-vector injection) the population of $CD4^{+}CD25^{+}FoxP3^{+}$ Tregs diminished to almost undetectable levels, to return to baseline levels after week 11. Therefore, it is possible that the pool of Tregs involved in inducing and/or sustaining immune tolerance to FIX was severely affected by the anti-CD25 regimen. In addition, daclizumab also enhances the humoral response to the vector capsid [Mingozzi et al. 2007a]. These effects on $CD4^{+}CD25^{+}FoxP3^{+}$ Tregs and in the humoral responses were also observed in humans receiving daclizumab plus MMF and rapamycin to avoid allograft rejection. In experimental models, tolerance to the allograft was also severely compromised by the use of T-cell-depleting antibodies, which alters the balance in favor of effector and memory T cells compared to a Treg population [Neujahr et al. 2006]. Despite the relative efficacy of inhibition of immune responses by blockage of T-cell co-stimulation in naive rodent models, it is difficult to suppress such responses in animals with memory cells. Thus, the preservation of Tregs following an immunosuppressive regimen is of fundamental importance in the induction of immune tolerance.

15.4.3 Gene Transfer in the Presence of Neutralizing Antibodies to Vectors

The presence of neutralizing antibodies to parent wild-type viruses imposes important limitations on the in vivo transduction efficacy of the cognate recombinant vector. Use of an AAV vector in NHP with neutralizing antibodies to AAV capsid proteins at titers equal or higher than 1 : 5 failed to achieve transgene expression, in contrast to animals with low or undetectable antibody titers [Jiang et al. 2006]. In humans, AAV2 hepatic gene expression was ablated in the presence of neutralizing antibodies against the AAV serotype 2 capsid at titers of 1 : 17 [Manno et al. 2006]. In contrast, in human subjects with hemophilia B, the presence of neutralizing antibodies to AAV2 did not prevent local FIX gene transfer and transgene expression following IM injection of AAV2 vector-encoding human FIX, as evidenced by muscle biopsies collected at early and late time points [Manno et al. 2003]. The use of immunosuppression targeting B cells prior to vector delivery to subjects with a high titer of antibodies to the vector has not yet been tested. One possibility is the removal of circulating specific IgG by extracorporeal absorption into affinity columns combined with transient immunosuppression or anti-CD20 monoclonal antibody, as usually carried out for the treatment of autoimmune diseases. However, the limited capacity of IgG removal and the high cost of this approach are the major obstacles to widespread use of this approach.

REFERENCES

Abraham RT and Wiederrecht GJ. 1996. Immunopharmacology of rapamycin. *Annu Rev Immunol* 14:483–510.

Allison AC and Eugui EM. 2005. Mechanisms of action of mycophenolate mofetil in preventing acute and chronic allograft rejection. *Transplantation* 80:S181–S190.

Arruda V, Schuettrumpf J, et al. 2004. Safety and efficacy of factor IX gene transfer to skeletal muscle in murine and canine hemophilia B models by adeno-associated viral vector serotype 1. *Blood* 103:85–92.

Arruda VR, Stedman HH, Nichols TC, Haskins ME, Nicholson M, Herzog RW, Couto LB, High KA. 2005. Regional intravascular delivery of AAV-2-F.IX to skeletal muscle achieves long-term correction of hemophilia B in a large animal model. *Blood* 105:3458–3464.

Battaglia M, Stabilini A, et al. 2006. Rapamycin promotes expansion of functional $CD4^{+}CD25^{+}FOXP3^{+}$ regulatory T cells of both healthy subjects and type 1 diabetic patients. *J Immunol* 177:8338–8347.

Bluestone JA and Abbas AK. 2003. Natural versus adaptive regulatory T cells. *Nat Rev Immunol* 3:253–257.

Bluestone JA, St Clair EW, et al. 2006. CTLA4Ig: bridging the basic immunology with clinical application. *Immunity* 24:233–238.

Brennan DC, Flavin K, et al. 1999. A randomized, double-blinded comparison of thymoglobulin versus Atgam for induction immunosuppressive therapy in adult renal transplant recipients. *Transplantation* 67:1011–1018.

Cao O, Dobrzynski E, et al. 2007. Induction and role of regulatory $CD4^{+}CD25^{+}$ T cells in tolerance to the transgene product following hepatic in vivo gene transfer. *Blood* 110:1132–1140.

Chan TM, Li FK, et al. (Hong Kong–Guangzhou Nephrology Study Group). 2000. Efficacy of mycophenolate mofetil in patients with diffuse proliferative lupus nephritis. *N Engl J Med* 343:1156–1162.

Changelian PS, Moshinsky D, et al. 2007. The specificity of JAK3 kinase inhibitors. *Blood* 111:2155–2157.

Chapuis AG, Paolo Rizzardi G, et al. 2000. Effects of mycophenolic acid on human immunodeficiency virus infection in vitro and in vivo. *Nat Med* 6:762–768.

Dantal J and Soulillou JP. 2005. Immunosuppressive drugs and the risk of cancer after organ transplantation. *N Engl J Med* 352:1371–1373.

Darabi K, Abdel-Wahab O, et al. 2006. Current usage of intravenous immune globulin and the rationale behind it: the Massachusetts General Hospital data and a review of the literature. *Transfusion* 46:741–753.

Doi K, Kong J, et al. 2004. Transient immunosuppression stops rejection of virus-transduced enhanced green fluorescent protein in rabbit retina. *J Virol* 78: 11327–11333.

Fasola CG, Netto GJ, et al. 2002. Recurrence of hepatitis C in liver transplant recipients treated with mycophenolate mofetil. *Transplant Proc* 34:1563–1564.

Fishman JA. 2007. Infection in solid-organ transplant recipients. *N Engl J Med* 357:2601–2614.

Grinyo JM and Cruzado JM. 2006. Mycophenolate mofetil and sirolimus combination in renal transplantation. *Am J Transplant* 6:1991–1999.

Guba M, von Breitenbuch P, et al. 2002. Rapamycin inhibits primary and metastatic tumor growth by antiangiogenesis: involvement of vascular endothelial growth factor. *Nat Med* 8:128–135.

Halloran PF. 2004. Immunosuppressive drugs for kidney transplantation. *N Engl J Med* 351:2715–2729.

Herzog RW, Mount JD, et al. 2001. Muscle-directed gene transfer and transient immune suppression result in sustained partial correction of canine hemophilia B caused by a null mutation. *Mol Ther* 4:192–200.

Jiang H, Couto LB, et al. 2006. Effects of transient immunosuppression on adeno-associated virus-mediated, liver-directed gene transfer in rhesus macaques and implications for human gene therapy. *Blood* 108:3321–3328.

Kang SM, Tang Q, et al. 2007. $CD4^+CD25^+$ regulatory T cells in transplantation: progress, challenges and prospects. *Am J Transplant* 7:1457–1463.

Kari JA and Trompeter RS. 2004. What is the calcineurin inhibitor of choice for pediatric renal transplantation? *Pediatr Transplant* 8:437–444.

Karin M. 1998. New twists in gene regulation by glucocorticoid receptor: is DNA binding dispensable? *Cell* 93:487–490.

Kay MA, Meuse L, et al. 1997. Transient immunomodulation with anti-CD40 ligand antibody and CTLA4Ig enhances persistence and secondary adenovirus-mediated gene transfer into mouse liver. *Proc Natl Acad Sci U S A* 94:4686–4691.

Kessel A, Rosner I, et al. 2008. Rituximab: beyond simple B cell depletion. *Clin Rev Allergy Immunol.*

Lowenstein PR, Mandel RJ, et al. 2007. Immune responses to adenovirus and adeno-associated vectors used for gene therapy of brain diseases: the role of immunological synapses in understanding the cell biology of neuroimmune interactions. *Curr Gene Ther* 7:347–360.

Manno CS, Chew AJ, et al. 2003. AAV-mediated factor IX gene transfer to skeletal muscle in patients with severe hemophilia B. *Blood* 101:2963–2972.

Manno CS, Pierce GF, et al. 2006. Successful transduction of liver in hemophilia by AAV-factor IX and limitations imposed by the host immune response. *Nat Med* 12:342–347.

Mays LE and Chen YH. 2007. Maintaining immunological tolerance with Foxp3. *Cell Res* 17:904–918.

Miao CH, Ye P, et al. 2006. Immunomodulation of transgene responses following naked DNA transfer of human factor VIII into hemophilia A mice. *Blood* 108:19–27.

Mingozzi F, Hasbrouck NC, et al. 2007a. Modulation of tolerance to the transgene product in a nonhuman primate model of AAV-mediated gene transfer to liver. *Blood* 110:2334–2341.

Mingozzi F, Maus MV, et al. 2007b. CD8(+) T-cell responses to adeno-associated virus capsid in humans. *Nat Med* 13:419–422.

Morice MC, Serruys PW, et al. 2002. A randomized comparison of a sirolimus-eluting stent with a standard stent for coronary revascularization. *N Engl J Med* 346:1773–1780.

Mueller XM. 2004a. Drug immunosuppression therapy for adult heart transplantation: 1. Immune response to allograft and mechanism of action of immunosuppressants. *Ann Thorac Surg* 77:354–362.

Mueller XM. 2004b. Drug immunosuppression therapy for adult heart transplantation: 2. Clinical applications and results. *Ann Thorac Surg* 77:363–371.

Mumprecht S, Matter M, et al. 2006. Imatinib mesylate selectively impairs expansion of memory cytotoxic T cells without affecting the control of primary viral infections. *Blood* 108:3406–3413.

Neujahr DC, Chen C, et al. 2006. Accelerated memory cell homeostasis during T cell depletion and approaches to overcome it. *J Immunol* 176:4632–4639.

Norman DJ, Vincenti F, et al. 2000. Phase I trial of HuM291, a humanized anti-CD3 antibody, in patients receiving renal allografts from living donors. *Transplantation* 70:1707–1712.

Perry I and Neuberger J. 2005. Immunosuppression: towards a logical approach in liver transplantation. *Clin Exp Immunol* 139:2–10.

Ponder KP, Wang B, et al. 2006. Mucopolysaccharidosis I cats mount a cytotoxic T lymphocyte response after neonatal gene therapy that can be blocked with CTLA4-Ig. *Mol Ther* 14:5–13.

Post DJ, Douglas DD, et al. 2005. Immunosuppression in liver transplantation. *Liver Transplant* 11:1307–1314.

Roncarolo MG and Battaglia M. 2007. Regulatory T-cell immunotherapy for tolerance to self antigens and alloantigens in humans. *Nat Rev Immunol* 7:585–598.

Ross CJ, Twisk J, et al. 2006. Correction of feline lipoprotein lipase deficiency with adeno-associated virus serotype 1–mediated gene transfer of the lipoprotein lipase S447X beneficial mutation. *Hum Gene Ther* 17:487–499.

Sampaolesi M, Blot S, et al 2006. Mesoangioblast stem cells ameliorate muscle function in dystrophic dogs. *Nature* 444:574–579.

Schwab SR and Cyster JG. 2007. Finding a way out: lymphocyte egress from lymphoid organs. *Nat Immunol* 8:1295–1301.

Strom TB. 2007. 2006 Homer W. Smith Lecture: taming T cells. *J Am Soc Nephrol* 18:2824–2832.

Tao R, de Zoeten EF, et al. 2007. Deacetylase inhibition promotes the generation and function of regulatory T cells. *Nat Med* 13:1299–1307.

Vincenti F, Kirkman R, et al. (Daclizumab Triple Therapy Study Group). 1998. Interleukin-2-receptor blockade with daclizumab to prevent acute rejection in renal transplantation. *N Engl J Med* 338:161–165.

Wang Z, Kuhr C, et al. 2007. Sustained AAV-mediated dystrophin expression in a canine model of Ducchene muscular dystrophy with a brief course of immunosuppression. *Mol Ther* 15:1160–1166.

Yabu JM and Vincenti F. 2007. Novel immunosuppression: small molecules and biologics. *Semin Nephrol* 27:479–486.

Yocum DE, Furst DE, et al. 2004. Safety of tacrolimus in patients with rheumatoid arthritis: long-term experience. *Rheumatology (Oxford)* 43:992–999.

Zhao W, Zhong L, et al. 2005. Role of cellular FKBP52 protein in intracellular trafficking of recombinant adeno-associated virus 2 vectors. *Virology* 353:283–293.

Zinkernagel RM. 1996. Response: Immunology taught by Darwin. *Science* 272:635a.

Zinkernagel RM and Hengartner H. 2001. Regulation of the immune response by antigen. *Science* 293:251–253.

16

GENE THERAPY FOR AUTOIMMUNE DISEASES

MASSIMO M. TRUCCO, M.D.

Diabetes Institute, Rangos Research Center, Children's Hospital of Pittsburgh, and Department of Pediatrics, University of Pittsburgh School of Medicine, Pittsburgh, Pennsylvania

PAUL D. ROBBINS, PH.D.

Department of Molecular Genetics and Biochemistry, University of Pittsburgh School of Medicine, Pittsburgh, Pennsylvania

NICK GIANNOUKAKIS, PH.D.

Diabetes Institute, Rangos Research Center, Children's Hospital of Pittsburgh, and Department of Pathology, University of Pittsburgh School of Medicine, Pittsburgh, Pennsylvania

Gene Therapy Immunology, Edited by Roland Herzog

16.1 INTRODUCTION

Autoimmunity describes a group of diseases in which the immune system chronically attacks specific cells, tissues, and organs of the host. Genetics play an important role in susceptibility and progression, while environmental triggers have often been proposed as initiating factors [Concannon et al. 1998; Bach et al. 2001; Eisenbarth 2003]. In humans, the most common autoimmune disorders are type I diabetes mellitus, rheumatoid arthritis, multiple sclerosis, Hashimoto's thyroiditis, lupus erythematosus, and Crohn's disease. The age at onset of these diseases varies, as does the target cell type. In type 1 diabetes, also referred to as insulin-dependent diabetes mellitus (T1DM), the specific cellular target is the insulin-producing beta cell of the pancreatic islets of Langerhans. Similarly, in rheumatoid arthritis (RA) it is the synovial membrane that is targeted for immune destruction. Additionally, the thyroid and nerve myelin are the targets in Hashimoto's thyroiditis and multiple sclerosis, respectively. The cell specificity of autoimmune disease suggests that these disorders are self-protein-driven. Unlike T1DM, thyroiditis, and RA, Crohn's disease (an inflammatory disorder of the bowel) and lupus erythematosus (in which multiple visceral tissues are targeted for immune destruction) exhibit immune reactivities against diverse cell types and self-proteins, with no evidence of a specific antigen or a set of related antigens driving the disease. Thus, the etiology of lupus and Crohn's disease will be more difficult to unravel and antigen-directed therapy even more challenging.

What is clear, however, is that a defect in educating the immune system to recognize cell- and tissue-restricted proteins as "self" during ontogeny lies at the root of the etiology of most autoimmune disorders. The central tenet of autoimmunity is that the defect lies in "tolerance" to cell- and tissue-restricted antigens. Broadly defined, *tolerance* refers to recognition by the immune system of self-tissue-restricted antigens in the absence of any efficient encounter between the antigens and the immune system during ontogeny. Tolerance can be central or peripheral. Central tolerance results from the negative selection (deletion), in the thymus gland, of immune cells with antigen receptors that would otherwise recognize self-tissue-restricted antigens. Peripheral tolerance can be better explained as a form of postnatal "ignorance" by the immune system, where circulating immune cells with antigen receptors that would otherwise recognize tissue-restricted antigens of the self remain ignorant of the antigen. Alternatively, they may be rendered and maintained inactive by unknown physiological processes and signals, in a phenomenon termed *anergy*, or are otherwise eliminated by apoptosis, or silenced by networks of regulatory immune cells.

There are currently no satisfactory modalities to control the evolution of autoimmunity or its progression. Insulin replacement therapy maintains reasonable control of blood glycemia in T1DM, but it is unable to prevent the long-term renal, neurologic, visual, and cardiovascular complications. Anti-inflammatory agents can slow down the processes involved in synovial membrane destruction in RA but cannot cure the disease. Other than pharmacologic immunosuppression, little else is available to treat Crohn's disease and lupus. In most autoimmune diseases, tissue destruction has already occurred at the moment of the clinical onset, and there is very little that can be done, other than transplantation of replacement cells, which in itself is immunologically challenging. It would be far easier to manipulate the immune system, in genetically at-risk individuals, in a manner by which tolerance to tissue-restricted antigens of the self could be achieved well in advance of disease onset. To achieve this, however, will require a thorough understanding of the genetics of susceptibility for each disorder as well as a very reliable predictive approach and complete knowledge of the autoantigens involved. Although it is beyond the scope of this review to discuss susceptibility genetics or autoantigens [Eisenbarth et al. 2002; Eisenbarth 2003], we will focus on strategies by which gene and cell therapy can control inflammation in a site-specific manner. Also, we will describe the current state of gene- and cell-based methods that aim to induce tolerance to self-tissue-restricted antigens. Finally, we discuss T1DM and RA as model autoimmune diseases for which a considerable number of options are ready to be translated clinically.

16.2 BIOTHERAPEUTIC APPROACHES FOR AUTOIMMUNITY

Gene and cell therapy are two specific applications of an ever-broadening area of pharmacology that can be termed *biotherapeutics*. The armamentarium of the biotherapist currently includes monoclonal antibodies, small molecules, proteins, cell and tissue transplants, gene vectors, and genes themselves. Proteins and antibodies are commonly used therapeutics (e.g., antibody-mediated cytokine and cell–cell interaction blockade; cell/tissue expansion-suppression via bioactive polypeptides), but they are expensive to produce and often exhibit short half-lives requiring frequent administration through inefficient routes. Proteins require a high concentration to achieve site-specific bioactivity, and this often involves high systemic levels that result in side effects in other organs. Furthermore, a number of protein-based approaches often result in disease recurrence once the administration is stopped.

Gene delivery can overcome many of the limitations associated with proteins and small molecules. It can provide stable, safe, long-term, and controllable production of one or many genes at specific sites. Conceptually, gene therapy is a means of delivering drugs, where the drug is in fact cDNA encoding molecules of biological importance. Just like many pharmacologic agents, there are a number of strategies that one can utilize to deliver the gene(s) to the intended site of action. The choice of delivery vehicle depends on the intended outcome: (1) systemic release of a gene product, (2) site-specific gene delivery and localized production; and (3) administration of gene-engineered cells. Gene therapy has so far only been applied to experimental models of autoimmune disease [Furlan et al. 2004]. Only one human phase I trial has been completed, and this is for RA [Evans et al. 1996], but four protocols are currently filed with the NIH

Recombinant DNA Advisory Committee (one for diabetes, three for RA, and one for multiple sclerosis; NIH: www.gemcris.od.nih.gov).

To deliver genes into cells and tissues, it is necessary to identify the "engineerability" of a cell: whether it is a dividing cell, a differentiating cell, a cell with limited lifespan, or a cell with high metabolic activity. These factors will determine the choice of vector system that will facilitate the conferring of an exogenously demanded activity to a cell. Currently, vector systems fall into two broad categories, each with its advantages and limitations. We describe these in the context of gene therapy for autoimmunity. Table 16-1 illustrates the general properties of the two vector categories: viral and nonviral.

16.3 VIRAL VECTORS

The generation of viral gene delivery vectors requires two major components: vectors encoding a complete sequence or components of a viral genome sequence engineered in such a manner that no replication-competent particles can be generated. Additionally, the gene or genes that achieve the desired therapeutic or prophylactic objective are supplied as part of the viral sequence or separately in another DNA sequence. The second component is a cell line that can efficiently produce recombinant virions that do not have the capacity to replicate once they infect a host. A number of strategies are currently employed to generate replication-defective adenoviral vectors, and many of these are now commercially available or readily accessible by contract companies. Adenoviruses are versatile for the reasons outlined in Table 16-1. Their most important feature is the ability to generate these vectors in high titers and to infect a broad range of cell types [Robbins and Ghivizzani 1998; Robbins et al. 1998]. It is therefore not surprising that the greatest number of gene therapy approaches in vitro and in vivo have been carried out with adenoviruses. The major limitation of these vectors is their immunogenicity, very likely dependent on the presence of expressed sequences in the vector backbone [Robbins and Ghivizzani 1998; Robbins et al. 1998]. If the aim is to generate a state of localized immunosuppression, such a feature is intuitively counterproductive. A number of strategies have succeeded in generating "gutless" adenoviral vectors, but to date, it has been challenging to grow these vectors to high titer without the presence of contaminating helper virus [Robbins and Ghivizzani 1998; Robbins et al. 1998]. Adeno-associated vectors offer advantages over adenoviruses, and recent data suggest their potential benefits [Jindal et al. 2001; Yang et al. 2002]. What is clear is that the utility and versatility of novel viral vectors is ultimately compared to that of adenoviruses; adenoviruses generally are the benchmark.

Retroviral vectors were among the earliest chosen for use in gene therapy models. They easily infect replicating cells, and they integrate into the host genome. Actively replicating immune cells, especially T cells, were among the first cell types to be transduced by retroviruses. Their generation is straightforward and a number of cell lines and processes are currently commercially available. Based

TABLE 16-1 General Properties of Gene Delivery Vehicles with Proven In Vivo Utility

Gutless adenovirus	
	Large transgene capacity (37 kb)
	Low immunogenicity
	Does not integrate into host genome
	Intermediate duration of gene expression (about one year)
	Targets dividing and differentiated nondividing cells
	Difficult to generate; requirement for replication-competent helper adenovirus for production
Adeno-associated virus	
	Transgene capacity limited to 4 kb
	Low immunogenicity
	Rare genomic integration events (mostly does not integrate)
	Intermediate duration of gene expression (about one year)
	Targets dividing and differentiated nondividing cells
	One-third of the human population has preformed neutralizing antibodies
Herpes simplex virus	
	Large transgene capacity (35 kb)
	Highly immunogenic
	Rare genomic integration events (mostly does not integrate)
	Intermediate duration of gene expression (6 to 9 months)
	Targets dividing and differentiated nondividing cells
	Toxic to some cell types; induces inflammation in some tissues
	Highly neurotropic
Plasmid DNA	
	Unlimited transgene capacity
	Low immunogenicity
	Does not integrate into host genome
	Short-term duration of gene expression
	Targets dividing and differentiated nondividing cells
	Easy and inexpensive to produce
Retrovirus	
	Transgene capacity limited to 7 to 8 kb
	Low immunogenicity
	Stable integration into host genome
	Long-term duration of gene expression
	Targets dividing cells
	May cause oncogenesis via insertional *cis*-acting mechanisms
Adenovirus	
	Transgene capacity limited to 8 kb
	High immunogenicity
	Does not integrate into host genome
	Short-term duration of gene expression
	Targets dividing and differentiated nondividing cells
	Lymphocytes not readily transduced; humans have preformed neutralizing antibodies

primarily on the Moloney murine leukemia virus genome, retroviral vectors have evolved into embodiments of avian, bovine, feline, equine, and human retroviruses [Vigna and Naldini 2000; Walther and Stein 2000; Pandya et al. 2001].

The properties of HIV-1 were exploited to develop the first of the vectors of the Lentiviridiae family. Lentiviral vectors offer low to no immunogenecity, but the cell type they can transduce is limited and the titers achievable on a packaging cell basis are significantly fewer than for the adenoviruses. On the other hand, they can infect some cells that are poorly transducible by adenoviral vectors, especially T cells and dendritic cells, and they offer the advantage of stable genomic integration. This is a desired feature in approaches aimed at engineering cells that do not divide, that differentiate, and that are long-lived.

One limitation of all the aforementioned vectors is the transgene size that can be accommodated inside the vector backbone. Where strategies envisage multicistronic transgenes and/or promoters of complex (and long-length) structure, solutions are provided by the herpes simplex viruses [Walther and Stein 2000]. Whereas earlier generations of these vectors were toxic to transduced cells, current embodiments do not promote significant levels of cell toxicity in vitro or in vivo [Goins et al. 2002; Burton et al. 2003]. One disadvantage is the cumbersome process required to generate significant titers, but ongoing efforts at large-scale vector production promise to overcome this limitation.

16.4 NONVIRAL VECTORS

Whereas viral vectors are versatile for almost all gene therapy applications, the immunogenicity, toxicity, potential for replication competency, potential for wild-type helper virus carryover during production, and the sheer logistics required to maintain good manufacturing procedures/good laboratory procedures (GMP/GLP) facilities for clinical-grade vectors are considered to offer more challenges than solutions. Nonviral vectors offer an inexpensive alternative. Traditionally, transfer of naked DNA plasmids was synonymous with nonviral vectors; however, a number of recent developments have welcomed new types of gene transfer vehicles that contain no viral elements.

Naked recombinant DNA plasmid generation is rapidly scalable at considerably lower cost than that of viral vectors. Newer-generation plasmid vectors have been designed either to stimulate immune responses or to have a low immunogenic profile [Liu and Huang 2002]. Additionally, multicistronic vectors are easily achievable compared to challenges to generate the same in viral vectors. Nonetheless, naked DNA cannot attain stable transgene persistence in transduced cells, and high concentrations are often required in multiple dosings.

Newer approaches have succeeded in exploiting amino acid sequences that act as a cell-entry facilitator of intact proteins. These peptide transduction domains (PTDs) are derived from viral nuclear import proteins, and unlike viral and plasmid DNA vectors that require gene transcription and translation for transgene expression, the PTDs are fused to the protein of interest. PTD-fused proteins can be generated readily in high yield with relatively minimal logistical requirements [Rehman et al. 2003]. The nature of the PTD domain can be modified to improve cell-type targeting. Their limitation, however, lies in their relatively short half-life, as they are subject to proteasome-dependent proteolysis. Tables 16-2 to 16-4 outline gene therapy approaches in a number of autoimmune animal models and is current as of the time of writing.

TABLE 16-2 Gene Therapy Vectors and Transgenes Used in Autoimmune Disease Models: T1DM

Vectors for Ex Vivo and In Vivo Islet Transduction	Genes That Promote Islet Allograft Survival In Vitro and In Vivo and/or Beta-Cell Survival in Culture	Other Gene/Cell Therapy Approaches to Prevent/Abrogate Autoimmunity and/or Promote Islet Allograft Survival
Plasmid DNA	Anti-apoptotic genes	Antigen-presenting cell transfer
Adenovirus	bcl-2	Class I MHC
Adeno-associated virus	bcl-x_L	Autologous dendritic cell transfer
MoLV retrovirus	Heme oxygenase-1	Co-stimulation blockade
Lentivirus	Dominant negative protein kinase C delta	Soluble ICAM-1-Ig
Herpes simplex virus	Dominant negative MyD88	CTLA-4Ig
Cationic liposomes	IGF-I	OX40Ig
Peptide fusion domains	IκBα super-repressor	Cytokines
	Hsp70	IL-10
	A20	IL-4
	PEA-15	Soluble IFN-γ receptor TGF-β
	Catalase	Autoantigen transfer
	Manganese superoxide dismutase	GAD
	Cytokines	Others
	IL-4 (although one report demonstrated no protection)	Adenovirus E3 proteins
	Interleukin-1 receptor	Orally administered putative autoantigens (insulin, GAD)
	Antagonist protein	CD152
	IL-12p40	α1-Antitrypsin
	Viral IL-10	
	IL-10	
	TGF-β	
	Immunoregulatory genes	
	Indoleamine 2,3-dioxygenase	
	CTLA-4Ig	
	Fas ligand	
	Adenoviral E3 genes	
	Soluble TNF receptor-Ig	
	VEGF	

TABLE 16-3 Gene Therapy Vectors and Transgenes Used in Autoimmune Disease Models: RA

Gene Vectors Used Systemically or In Situ	Therapeutic Genes
Plasmid DNA	Cytokines/cytokine inhibitors
Adenovirus	IFN-b
Adeno-associated virus	IRAP
MoLV retrovirus	IL-4
Lentivirus	IL-10
Herpes simplex virus	vIL-10
	IL-12p40
	IL-13
	TGF-b
	Soluble IL-1 type II receptor
	Soluble TNF type I receptor-Ig fusion
	Soluble TNF type I receptor
	Others
	Angiostatin
	$P16^{INK4A}$
	P21CIP1
	Thymidine kinase
	MMP-1, TIMP-1, TIMP-3 ribozymes
	Soluble VEGF receptor

16.5 T1DM AND RA AS MODEL AUTOIMMUNE DISEASES: CELLULAR AND MOLECULAR PLAYERS

One of the most prevalent autoimmune diseases with considerable morbidity due to its long-term complications is type 1 diabetes mellitus (T1DM). A disorder of glucose homeostasis, T1DM results due to an insufficient amount of insulin, consequent to a chronic inflammation of the islets of Langerhans in the pancreas. The disease is T-cell-mediated targeting of the insulin-producing beta cells for eventual destruction. Clinical onset of hyperglycemia can occur before the entire beta-cell mass is eradicated [Weets et al. 2006]. In fact, the more advanced inflammation consists of macrophages and T cells that secrete cytokines which are known to suppress glucose sensing and insulin production even though the beta-cell mass remains viable [Arnush et al. 1998b]. Islet cell-specific T cells have been demonstrated in newly diagnosed T1DM patients [Roep and De Vries 1992] and are present in the islet infiltrate at disease onset. This infiltrate contains both $CD4^+$ as well as $CD8^+$ T cells. Such islet cell–specific cells have also been observed in the circulation of healthy persons, albeit in lower numbers and with less reactivity than in diabetics, indicating that other factors are required to trigger disease onset. In addition, diabetogenic T-cell clones are not limited to a particular antigen, but to a plethora of molecules that may not be beta-cell-specific, such

TABLE 16-4 Gene Therapy Vectors and Transgenes Used in Autoimmune Disease Models: EAE/MS

Gene Vectors Used Systemically or In Situ	Therapeutic Genes
Liposomes	Cytokines/cytokine inhibitors
Plasmid DNA	IFNβ
MoLV retrovirus	IFNγ
Herpes simplex virus	IL-1β
Vaccinia virus	IL-2
	IL-4
	IL-6
	IL-10
	TGF-β
	Soluble TNF type I receptor-Ig fusion
	Soluble TNF type I receptor
	Immunoregulatory genes
	IP-10
	Fas ligand
	Others
	PLP
	MOG
	MOG-Ig fusion
	PDGF
	FGF2
	NGF

as glutamate decarboxylase, which is expressed in other islet cells as well as in neurons, $CD4^+$ as well as $CD8^+$ T lymphocytes are the major constituents of the autoimmune infiltrate. An examination of the T-cell receptor (TCR) type present on $CD8^+$ autoreactive T-cell clones indicated that the TCR variable segments, V-β, were heterogeneous, reflecting the heterogeneity of these cells in the infiltrate.

How T cells are attracted to the beta cells and how they initiate beta-cell destruction is still unclear, although there is strong evidence that cytokines and death effectors are active mechanisms. IL-1β and IFN-γ have been shown to activate the expression of pro-inflammatory molecules in beta cells as well as Fas [Stassi et al. 1997; Arnush et al. 1998a]. Activated T cells would then engage Fas through Fas ligand (FasL) and initiate apoptosis. Additionally, TNF-α and perforin/granzyme B actions on beta cells in vivo and in in vitro have also been shown to be important death effector pathways [Dahlen et al. 1998]. Finally, cytokines can also initiate a vicious cycle of oxidative stresses in beta cells by activating endogenous nitric oxide and superoxides that perturb beta cell function and render the cell susceptible to further damage and destruction [Arnush et al. 1998a].

16.5.1 Cells and Signals Triggering RA

In RA, an immune response to self-antigens clearly is important at the early stages of disease. Although the main site of disease pathology is the joint, where leukocytic infiltration results in induction of synovial cell hyperplasia and eventually bone and cartilage erosion, the specific autoantigen is not defined clearly [Kotzin et al. 2000]. A small percentage of patients have reactive T cells against collagen, whereas gp39 has been implicated as an important autoantigen in certain other patients [Kotzin et al. 2000]. Thus, it appears that multiple autoantigens are involved in disease initiation. How the induction of autoimmunity is initiated is unclear, but several lines of evidence suggest that viral or bacterial infection may contribute to the induction of RA, dependent in part on expression of specific HLA DR4 alleles [Fugger and Svejgaard 2000]. In contrast to T1DM, RA is not necessarily a T-cell-driven disease in that treatment of patients with either CD3 or CD4 antibodies has not shown a significant, long-term therapeutic effect. Instead, it appears as if elevated cytokines such as IL-1 and TNF-α produced by both leukocytes and synovial fibroblasts are important for disease progression [Gabay 2000]. Treatment of patients with anti-IL-1 or anti-TNF has shown significant therapeutic effects, reducing inflammation, pain, and possibly even cartilage and bone erosion [Gabay 2000]. Thus, the pathogenesis of arthritis is complex, involving not only T cells but also additional cell types such as B lymphocytes and antigen-presenting cells (APCs) and even activated, hyperplastic synovial fibroblasts. Indirect evidence in this regard is the benefit seen in RA patients treated with Rituximab, an anti-CD20 antibody that targets B cells primarily.

16.5.2 Gene Therapy Strategies Insulin Production Replacement

Given the pivotal role of beta-cell mass in determining whether a person will progress to type 1 diabetes [Faideau et al. 2005], serious efforts have been under way for 20 years to identify alternative means of improving glycemic control in diabetic patients. The major advance that is now clinically acceptable and, to a degree, successful, offering a potential cure for type 1 diabetes, is the transplantation of islets of Langherans [Bottino and Trucco 2005]. Islet transplants are, however, limited by the availability of donors, and their initial function following transplantation is challenged by apoptotic cell death, which generally occurs during the isolation process and immediately following transplantation. Furthermore, transplant patients have to receive long-term—probably lifetime—immunosuppression therapy with all its associated side effects.

A considerable number of studies demonstrate the feasibility of using viral gene delivery vehicles to import transgenes into intact islets ex vivo with the aim of facilitating their transplantation, function, and resilience against alloimmune rejection and autoimmune impairment and destruction [Giannoukakis and Trucco 2003]. The transgenes fall into three broad categories: those that encode soluble proteins interacting with infiltrating immune cells, those that encode intracellular pro-survival/anti-apoptotic proteins, and those that encode differentiation factors for beta-cell progenitors. At the other end of the spectrum are methods that rely on systemic production of factors that promote immune cell regulation (either by enhancing the number and activity of regulatory T cells or by attenuating the effects of antigraft immune cells, for example). Table 16-2 lists transgenes successfully employed to date in facilitating islet allograft survival and/or promoting networks of immune cell hyporesponsiveness to allografts or autoimmunity suppression (also reviewed by Giannoukakis and Trucco [2003]).

There are two key concerns that previous safety trials in humans raise: vector toxicity to transduced tissue and antivector responses [Volpers and Kochanek 2004]. These two concerns are crucial for attempts to administer transgenes systemically in humans. We believe, however, that ex vivo transduction of cells and tissues followed by transplantation may not carry the risks and dangers associated with systemic administration. First, the ex vivo approach involves considerable washing of the vector, along with cells that may be apoptotic and dysfunctional. This has the twofold effect of removing much of the nonspecifically adherent vector that has not been internalized and removes the "danger" signals that the host immune system sees in apoptotic cells of allogeneic origin. Therefore, we propose that ex vivo transduction of allogeneic islets of Langerhans with adenoviral vectors is ready for prime time.

AAV, on the other hand, offers additional attractive features in that some serotypes are less immunogenic than others and certainly less so than adenoviral vehicles [Zaiss and Muruve 2005]. The possibility of AAV integration into the host genome is also an attractive feature that could ensure long-term transgene persistence in vivo following transplantation of ex vivo–engineered islets of Langerhans, for example.

Although limited, recent studies are beginning to confirm the utility of direct intrapancreatic vector administration for diabetes therapy, originally reported a decade ago [Raper and DeMatteo 1996] and improved more recently [Wang et al. 2006]. Along these lines, a recent study by Bosch and colleagues [Ayuso et al. 2006] is important in two respects. First, it confirmed those few early reports [Raper and DeMatteo 1996; McClane et al. 1997; Shifrin et al. 2001] demonstrating that direct in vivo delivery of a viral vector into the pancreas achieves reasonable transduction of pancreatic cells (which may include potential stem cells developing into endocrine cells), and second, and most important, it should raise serious considerations that it is time for the field to move away from mice and into larger animals. Embedded in the study by Bosch and colleagues is preliminary reassurance that adenoviral vector transduction of the endogenous pancreas may not be associated with the inflammatory and toxic effects shown in a plethora of liver-directed gene therapies and the Gelsinger case a few years ago [Somia and Verma 2000; Couzin and Kaiser 2005]. It is no secret that the biochemistry and the physiology of the immune system are not identical in mice and humans. Extrapolating therapeutic success from mouse models to humans can be misleading without an intermediate step of testing the therapy in large animals. In fact, it may be time to consider bypassing rodents completely when the in vitro data are overwhelmingly convincing.

Transplantation of gene-modified islets and direct intrapancreatic gene transfer fall inside this category of "rodent-bypassing" lines of investigation. Chemical immunosuppression required to prevent allogeneic islet rejection has been implicated directly in beta cell functional impairment [Shapiro et al. 2002; Uchizono et al. 2004] and impedes the immune capacity of the recipient significantly at a systemic level. Gene-engineered islets may offer local immunregulatory effects without impairing the immune system systemically, although this has not yet been formally proven completely and convincingly. Furthermore, islets may be engineered in such a way as to direct local immune hyporesponsiveness in addition to providing trophic stimuli for endocrine stem cell differentiation, especially if the transplant is placed into a site with endocrine stem cell potential. Direct intrapancreatic administration of gene vectors may not result in as precise a distribution of transgene product as that produced by a transplant, but it offers the potential for minimal trauma to the transduced tissue (unlike ex vivo–transduced islets, which are often infected by many particles per cell). In this context, large animals offer procedural ease; the liver of a rhesus monkey is considerably larger than that of a mouse, and monkey pancreata are more readily manipulatable.

New accumulating evidence suggests that once autoimmunity is abrogated, the endocrine pancreas properties may be sufficient to allow the physiological regenerative process to restore endogenous insulin production [Bonner-Weir and Sharma 2002; Bonner-Weir et al. 2004; Seaberg et al. 2004; Suzuki et al. 2004; Trucco 2005] even after the disease has become manifest clinically [Zorina et al. 2003]. The physiological regenerative potential of the endocrine pancreas still seems to be quite high immediately after (or very close to) the onset of the disease, when, in general, there still are some insulin-producing cells able to secrete sufficient insulin to make C-peptide testing possible (i.e., over the minimum level detectable by the appropriate assays) [von Herrath and Homann 2004]. In the mouse and possibly in the monkey (e.g., cynomolgus), to substitute enough beta cells during the regenerative process to allow the detection of an influence on the control of the glycemia of the animal seems to take more than three months. Even at this point in time, both of these animals do not yet have perfect control of the glycemia, since intravenous glucose tolerance tests (IVGTTs) are still far from normal. However, this result would already constitute a great advantage for the diabetic patient, even if we do not know definitely whether the reparative process may still work longer after clinical onset, and at the same speed as observed immediately after onset. Preliminary studies in animals seem to indicate that the regenerative process works proportionally more slowly as the time from onset of the disease increases [Rood et al. 2005].

To help the system to activate the regenerative process or to speed up a possibly very slow physiologic recovery, even after protracted diabetes insulin therapy, it would be useful to test different factors that have proven to be efficient in better achieving this goal [Baeyens et al. 2005; Suarez-Pinzon et al. 2005]. For other factors, such as PAX4 [Heremans et al. 2002], HGF [Garcia-Ocana et al. 2000], IGF-1 [George et al. 2002; Guo et al. 2005], or GLP-1 [Farilla et al. 2002], the insulin promoter should be used to construct the cassettes eventually introduced into the vector. In a recent study [Wang et al. 2006], the capacity of adeno-associated virus (AAV)–mediated pancreatic gene transfer was reexamined using the recently available, novel serotypes of AAV coupled with an improved double-stranded AAV vector DNA cassette, which facilitates rapid and stronger transgene expression [Rehman et al. 2005]. It has been shown that robust and long-term gene transfer can be achieved by these vectors in the vast majority, if not all, of the islets. Gene transfer efficiency and vector distribution in the islets are determined by the choice of AAV serotype vectors as well as by the delivery methods. The pancreatic exocrine acinar cells are highly susceptible to AAV8 infection. To minimize the unwanted gene transfer to nonendocrine pancreatic and nonpancreatic tissues seen after intraperitoneal or intravenous delivery, we explored a topical route by retrograde delivery into the pancreatic duct, similar to the technique ERCP (endoscopic retrograde cholangiopancreatography) commonly used in patients with pancreatitis. Since the pancreatic beta cell is, by definition, the most important target in gene transfer and therapy for diabetes, we explored the use of the insulin promoter to minimize nonspecific transgene expression in unintended cells, such as the pancreatic acinar cells and those beyond the pancreas. As expected, two weeks after delivery of AAV8-insulin-promoter-GFP vector in adult mice, strong GFP expression was readily detected exclusively in the islets but not in the exocrine acinar cells [Wang et al. 2006].

In the rapidly shifting priorities of research support for diabetes, translational research toward therapy has not kept pace with the explosive discoveries in the field of molecular investigation. This is most true for gene therapy for diabetes. Third- and fourth-generation viral vectors are now available with low-to-zero potential for immunogenicity. A large array of transgenes awaits to be transferred into islets for subsequent transplantation and/or injected directly into the pancreas to promote the survival of residual beta cell mass and to direct the differentiation of stem cells into endocrine cells in situ. The mouse will always serve its function as the proving ground, however, the large animal will validate this proving ground. In this regard, the study by Bosch and colleagues [Ayuso et al. 2006] should at the very least challenge the diabetes gene therapy community to consider seriously bypassing the mouse when it is obvious that a large-animal model offers a physiological and immunological environment closer to humans and a rational host for human-directed therapies.

16.5.3 T1DM: Tolerance Strategies

There is now no debate about the importance of dendritic cells (DCs) in tolerance. DCs are the body's sentinels par excellence. They are responsible largely for host surveillance against microenvironmental anomalies, including sensing damaged tissue architecture, sensing foreign pathogen invasion and infection, and serving the role of key orchestrator of mechanisms of self-tolerance [Steinman et al. 2000; Vlad et al. 2005]. DCs are in steady-state flux throughout all body tissues, constantly sampling molecules from the environment they encounter.

Under steady-state conditions, having acquired environmental material, they transit through the draining lymphoid organs, where it is believed that they maintain potentially autoreactive immune cells in quiescence either directly or via indirect regulatory immune cell networks [Steinman and Nussenzweig 2002; Steinman et al. 2003; Smits et al. 2005a,b]. When DCs encounter microenvironmental anomalies (e.g., viral infections), the local disruption of tissue architecture, along with an increase in the output of pro-inflammatory signals by infected cells, will prime the DCs to undergo a series of internal changes that are referred to as *maturation*. While thought of conceptually as a series of discrete checkpoint-like events, maturation is rapid and often nonlinear [Liu 2001; Kubach et al. 2005]. Maturation is coupled to migration toward the proximal draining lymph node with concomitant production of cytokines such as TNF-α and chemokines. This production helps to establish a gradient that will be sought and followed by other immune cells, especially activated T cells once triggered out of quiescence inside the lymph node into which also migrate the maturing DCs [Steinman et al. 2000, 2003; Vlad et al. 2005]. Within the lymph node, the DCs will interact with naive T cells through class I and class II MHC/peptide/T-cell receptor (TCR) contacts, where this interaction is stabilized by coincident contact between accessory co-receptors on DCs and T cells, collectively termed co-stimulatory molecules. It is now established that any mechanism that interrupts co-stimulation leads to impaired activation of the responding T cells, possibly leading to functional anergy or apoptosis. This is indeed the outcome of many immunosuppressive strategies aimed at co-stimulation blockade [Sayegh and Turka 1995; Bluestone 1996; Lenschow et al. 1996; Kishimoto et al. 2000; Rothstein and Sayegh 2003; Clarkson and Sayegh 2005].

The distinction between a functional state of immaturity and the tolerogenic state is not yet clear. Some investigators favor a system where tolerogenic DCs possess specific properties, either as a consequence of natural development during ontogeny, or acquired during their lifetime in circulation (Table 16-5). Other investigators offer models where DCs are metastable and can acquire a broad spectrum of functional capacities, ranging from potently immunostimulatory to highly immunosuppressive, depending on their microenvironmental location (and local effects from tissue-derived soluble factors), or their interactions with other physically proximal cells; immune and/or nonimmune [Manz et al. 2001a,b]. Although it is not at all clear which of these models is operative in DC-based tolerance to tissue-restricted antigens, what is clear is that DCs are prominent in promoting the breakdown in tolerance: the hallmark of autoimmune diseases [Kubach et al. 2005; Manfredi et al. 2005; Suciu-Foca et al. 2005].

16.5.4 Dendritic Cell Therapy for T1DM

In the very early stages of diabetes, the inflammation consists of an influx of DCs into the islets, apparently in response to an as yet not-defined anomaly, which may be a consequence of impaired remodeling of the islet architecture through apoptosis, cross-presentation of endogenous epitopes following viral infections

TABLE 16-5 Phenotypes of Human DC Subsets

CD11c^{+} DCs (Myeloid DCs; DC1)	CD11c- DC (Plasmacytoid DC; DC2)
CD13^{+} CD14^{+} CD33^{+} CD11b^{+} TLR2^{+} TLR3^{+} GM-CSF-receptor^{+} HLA-DR^{high}	CD4^{+} CD13^{low} CD14^{low} CD33^{low} CD11b^{low} TLR7^{+} TLR9^{+} IL-3-receptor^{+} HLA-DR^{+}
Produce TNF-α, IL-6, IL-12, IFN-α, IFN-β in response to activation Poorly developed dendrites (veils) Can acquire veiled morphology after a period in culture in absence of exogenous cytokines Induce vigorous proliferation of allogeneic T cells in vitro Potent antibacterial responses/highly phagocytic Mainly immunostimulatory when activated Tolerogenic potential when engineered in vitro/ex vivo	Produce IFN-α, IFN-β in response to activation Exhibit plasmacytoid morphology Well-developed rough ER and Golgi Require exogenous cytokines for survival in vitro Can develop into myeloid DC types in the presence of monocyte-conditioned medium or IL-3 Induce poor proliferation of allogeneic T cells in vitro Potent antiviral responses Potentially tolerogenic

or superantigen-driven immune responses [Oldstone 1989; Conrad and Trucco 1994; Trudeau et al. 2000]. In the genetically diabetes-prone nonobese diabetic (NOD) mouse strain, whose immunopathology is widely held to parallel that believed to occur in humans, insulitis starts very early (3 to 4 weeks of age) with peri-islet inflammation, followed by a slow and progressive impairment and destruction of beta cells by 4 to 6 months of age. DCs and macrophages are the first immune cells detectable at 3 to 4 weeks of age in the islets of NOD mice [Lo et al. 1993; Jansen et al. 1996]. These cells have been shown to acquire antigen and very likely present it to T cells in the pancreatic lymph nodes [Clare-Salzler and Mullen 1992; Shimizu et al. 1995; Hoglund et al. 1999]. Among a number of transgenic mice, two in particular stand out to demonstrate how a microenvironmental anomaly (that is islet-restricted) requires antigen-presenting cells, and DCs in particular, to provoke and exacerbate islet autoimmunity. The first is an NOD mouse expressing TNF-α inside the beta cells under the control of the rat insulin promoter. These mice exhibit accelerated diabetes with strongly destructive insulitis [Green et al. 1998]. Local TNF-α expression enhanced the accumulation of DCs, which then presented antigens from apoptotic cells to

$CD4^+$ T cells [Green et al. 1998]. Indeed, the accumulating DCs produced TNFa, which exacerbated apoptosis and amplified a vicious cycle [Dahlen et al. 1998]. To determine more precisely the relevance of DCs in the initiation and maintenance of T1DM, an elegant set of studies were undertaken by Zinkernagel and colleagues [Ehl et al. 1998; Ludewig et al. 1998a,b] and by von Herrath and colleagues [Christen and von Herrath 2002; von Herrath 2002; Christen and von Herrath 2004a,b]. These studies all point to the central role of DCs in acquiring tissue-restricted antigens and under an environment of inflammatory and anomalous "danger" [Matzinger 1994, 1998; 2001, 2001; Gallucci and Matzinger 2001], would be predicted to undergo maturation, migrate into the pancreatic lymph nodes, and activate self-reactive and specifically, beta cell–targeted T cells.

A question has arisen about the potential that DCs are defective in T1DM immunopathogenesis. Some studies suggest that DCs derived from the only two genetic strains of naturally occurring diabetes are functionally abnormal, ranging from observations that DCs are hyperactivated [Weaver et al. 2001; Marleau and Singh 2002; Sen et al. 2003; Wheat et al. 2004] to those showing evidence that DCs are hypofunctional [Strid et al. 2001; Boudaly et al. 2002; Nikolic et al. 2004]. Diabetes patients, in contrast, do not exhibit any dramatic impairment in responses to infection, recall to vaccination antigens, or ability to mount hypersensitivity reactions [Wheat 1980; McMahon and Bistrian 1995; Eibl et al. 2002], thereby creating more obscurity about potential defects in DC development and function, even though some recent reports suggest that potential deficiencies may exist in humans [Peng et al. 2003; Summers et al. 2003, 2006]. What is abundantly clear, however, is that DCs are potent regulators of the immune system and can be mobilized to orchestrate antitumor activities as well as to induce hyporesponsiveness in order to facilitate allotransplantation and to prevent autoimmunity [Di Nicola et al. 1998; Hackstein et al. 2001; Coates and Thomson 2002; Paul et al. 2002; Davis et al. 2003; Morelli and Thomson 2003; Hardin 2005; Nouri-Shirazi and Thomson 2006].

With the exception of the observations of Morel and colleagues [Feili-Hariri et al. 1999], many other lines of investigation support the concept where DCs exit in a functionally immature state (characterized by low to absent co-stimulation) as agents of immune hyporesponsiveness [Steinman et al. 1999, 2003; Hackstein et al. 2001; Coates and Thomson 2002; Steinman and Nussenzweig 2002; Morelli and Thomson 2003; Nouri-Shirazi and Thomson 2006]. Exogenous administration of functionally immature DCs (Table 16-6) achieves long-term and stable allograft survival in a variety of mouse and rat models and prevents a number of autoimmune diseases [Giannoukakis et al. 1999a,b; Chen et al. 2002; Tarner and Fathman 2002; Trucco et al. 2002; Bottino et al. 2003; Tarner et al. 2003; Giannoukakis and Trucco 2005]. Mechanistically, functionally immature DCs act by inducing anergy either via direct cell contact and/or cytokines [Harnaha et al. 2006; Hugues et al. 2006; Nouri-Shirazi and Thomson 2006], and as more recently shown, by up-regulating the number and function of immune cell subsets, especially the regulatory populations, which include $Foxp3^+$ $CD25^+$ T cells and a class of $CD8^+$ immunosuppressive T cells [Beissert et al. 2006; Enk 2006;

TABLE 16-6 Models of Immunotherapeutic DC Administration to Prolong Graft Survival and to Treat Autoimmunity

Autoimmune Disease	Allotransplantation/Xenotransplantation
Type 1 diabetes	Administration of bone marrow–derived DCs from transplant organ donor
Pancreatic lymph node DCs (untreated)	DC propagated in low-concentration GM-CSF
Mature bone marrow–derived DCs (GM-CSF/IL-4 propagated); or transduced with IL-4 vector	DC propagated in GM-CSF, IL-10, TGF-β, and matured with LPS
NF-κB oligonucleotide decoy propagated	In vitro blockade of NF-κB by adding aspirin, vitamin D_3 metabolites/analogs, glucosamine, *N*-acetylcysteine, corticosteroids, cyclosporin A, rapamycin, deoxyspergualin, mycophenolate mofetil
Antisense oligonucleotide (CD40, CD80, CD86)-propagated	Gene-engineering in vitro: DCs expressing IL-10, TGF-β, CTLA-4Ig, indolamine-2,3 dioxygenase, Fas ligand
Vitamin D receptor ligands	Administration of transplant recipient–derived DCs prior to transplantation:
Other DC embodiments	DCs pulsed with class I MHC allopeptide rapamycin and donor tissue lysate
Thyroiditis	
In vitro generation with TNF-α and supernatant of a GM-CSF-transduced cell line	
GM-CSF-generated followed by in vivo administration of GM-CSF	
Experimental encephalomyelitis (multiple sclerosis model)	
In vitro generation with TNF-α and supernatant of a GM-CSF-transduced cell line	
VIP and GM-CSF in vitro propagation	
TGF-β and MBP antigen	
Arthritis	
VIP and GM-CSF in vitro propagation	
IL-4 or IL-10-expressing bone marrow–derived DC and derivative exosome preparations	
CD95 (Fas ligand) expressing bone marrow–derived DCs	

Huber and Schramm 2006; Lohr et al. 2006; Roncarolo et al. 2006; Shevach et al. 2006; Tang and Bluestone 2006; Verhagen et al. 2006; Zhang et al. 2006]. Table 16-6 lists models in which immature DC administration has been successful and will be the focal point from which potential therapies can emerge, as discussed in the next section.

Anergy has been a well-studied mechanism during the past two decades and is not considered further here [Balomenos and Martinez 2000; Lechler et al.

2001a,b; Brennan et al. 2003; Saouaf et al. 2003; Anderson and Chan 2004; Goodnow et al. 2005; Singh and Schwartz 2006]. We would like to focus on potential networks of immune regulatory cells evoked by DCs stabilized in a functionally immature state: in particular, on Foxp3$^+$CD25$^+$ T cells, whose number is observed to be increased in many recent studies involving the exogenous supply of tolerogenic DCs [Vigouroux et al. 2004; Watanabe et al. 2005; Battaglia et al. 2006; Mennechet and Uze 2006; Rutella et al. 2006]. Immature or semimature DCs can induce the differentiation of naturally occurring (thymic) T regulatory cells (CD4$^+$CD25$^+$) as well as IL-10-producing CD4$^+$ T cells in vitro and in vivo [Vigouroux et al. 2004; Battaglia et al. 2006]. Overexpression of Jagged-1 in DCs results in the augmentation of antigen-specific TGF beta-producing CD4$^+$CD25$^+$ T cells [Yvon et al. 2003]. Functionally immature DCs convert naive T cells into IL-10-secreting cells in vitro, and antigen-pulsed DCs injected subcutaneously into humans augment the number of IL-10-producing CD8$^+$ T cells and trigger a reduction in IFN-γ^+ T cells [Jonuleit et al. 2000; Dhodapkar et al. 2001]. Despite the abundance of data in support of immature DCs as functional inducers of regulatory immune cells, other investigators have discovered that the state of maturity may not be relevant for the induction of immunosuppressive endogenous T cells. For example, similar to the studies by Morel and colleagues [Feili-Hariri et al. 1999], mature DCs were shown to expand CD4$^+$CD25$^+$ T cells, which were functionally suppressive and capable of preventing diabetes in the NOD mouse [Yamazaki et al. 2003; Tarbell et al. 2004; Brinster and Shevach 2005]. Whether this reflects a restimulation of existing CD4$^+$CD25$^+$ T cells or their expansion is unknown.

CD4$^+$CD25$^+$ regulatory T cells expressing the Foxp3 transcription factor (Tregs) are thought to derive from the thymus (natural Tregs) and to differentiate from peripheral CD4$^+$ precursors (peripheral Tregs). Steinman and colleagues have established elegantly that DCs are alone capable of augmenting antigen-specific Tregs in diabetic mouse models [Yamazaki et al. 2003; Tarbell et al. 2004], and that this requires cell contact. Despite their comprehensiveness, these studies did not indicate the precise state of DC maturation, and this will be an interesting feature to identify. We have shown that DCs maintained in a functionally immature state following in vitro treatment with NF-κB decoys and antisense oligodeoxyribonucleotides (AS-ODN) to the CD40, CD80, and CD86 co-stimulatory molecules are diabetes preventive in the NOD mouse [Ma et al. 2003; Machen et al. 2004; Harnaha et al. 2006] and may involve short-range IL-7 signaling, quite likely inside the pancreatic lymph node of NOD mice, to augment the number of CD4$^+$CD25$^+$ Tregs via suppression of apoptosis of a preexisting pool [Harnaha et al. 2006]. Multiple injections of AS-ODN-treated DCs in NOD mice maintained the animals as diabetes free without affecting the overall T-cell activity against alloantigens. Furthermore, repeated administrations of co-stimulation-deficient DCs reverses hyperglycemia in new-onset diabetes NOD mice. The promising results of this study, together with the low risk of the procedure, demonstrated in numerous anticancer DC-based treatments, have enabled this National Institutes of Health (NIH)-funded protocol to be approved by the

Food and Drug Administration (FDA) office as a phase I clinical trial. Adult (18 years or older) volunteers with a documented evidence of insulin-requiring T1DM of at least five years' duration will be enrolled first, to prove the safety of the procedure. Leukocytes of the patient will be obtained by apheresis, and DCs will be generated in vitro and engineered with the addition of AS-ODN. These DCs, which express low levels of CD80, CD86, and CD40 will then be injected into the patient by intradermal administration at an anatomical site proximal to the pancreas. Attracted to the focus of inflammation, these treated cells will acquire apoptotic cells inside the islets (hence, the antigen specificity) and then will migrate into the pancreas-draining lymph nodes, where they will deliver an anergizing signal to the T cells they encounter and/or induce regulatory immune cells. The vicious cycle that promotes the T-cell-mediated anti-beta-cell-antigen spreading phenomenon will be interrupted this way, enabling recovery of the physiologic endocrine function of the gland with time. The abrogation of the autoimmune diabetogenic insult should be sufficient to promote rescue or regeneration of the insulin-producing beta cells in the host endocrine pancreas, even after onset of the disease (Fig. 16-1). Once safety has been demonstrated, a phase II efficacy trial will start, involving new-onset diabetic patients.

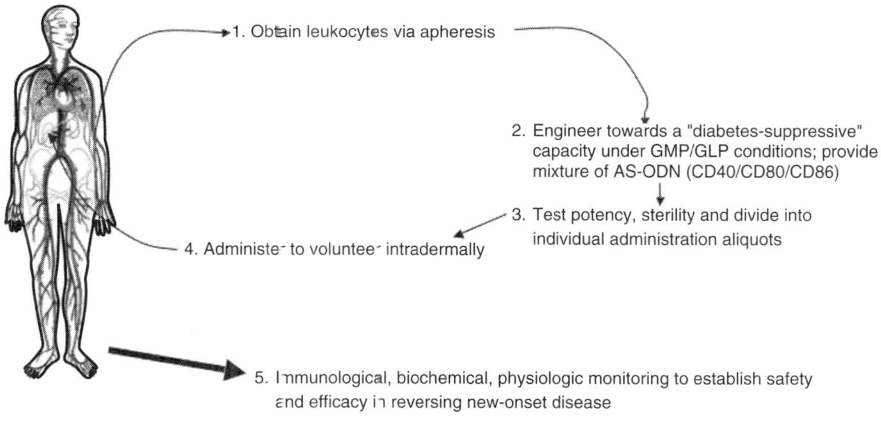

Figure 16-1 Schema of U.S. Food and Drug Administration–approved safety trial administering autologous diabetes-suppressive DCs into established type 1 diabetic volunteers (Pittsburgh Study). The protocol will enroll established type 1 diabetic volunteers between the ages of 18 to 25 who are otherwise healthy. They must be diabetic for more than six years. Autologous DCs will be generated in vitro from apheresis product. Half of the study group will be administered autologous DCs engineered in vitro with a mixture of CD40, CD80, and CD86 antisense oligonucleotides, and the other half will receive untreated autologous DCs. The volunteers will be monitored immunologically, physiologically, and biochemically to determine the safety of the approach. If the engineered DCs are safe, the protocol will be submitted for consideration to enroll new-onset diabetics with the objective of determining the effect of the engineered autologous DCs on residual functional beta-cell mass and markers of autoimmunity.

Multiple alternative methods exist to generate tolerogenic DCs, and the question arises: Are all such DC embodiments equivalent and translatable for clinical use? Some methods converge upon identical cellular and molecular pathways (augmentation of Treg numbers, NF-κB inhibition, co-stimulation blockade). Others are not so obvious. First, it is important to understand that transplantation immunobiology may not be identical to autoimmunity, and vice versa. Indeed, there are numerous instances where a therapeutic regimen achieving long-term allograft survival has failed to abrogate autoimmunity [Markees et al. 1999; Rossini et al. 2001; Pearson et al. 2003a–c; Seung et al. 2003; Rossini 2004; Gordon et al. 2005]. Therefore, DCs that are able to suppress donor-specific antigen alloreactivity may not evoke the appropriate regulatory mechanisms, capable of controlling and reversing autoimmunity. At the same time, although different DC embodiments may exhibit similar cell surface phenotypes and nuclear proteome signatures, by no means can this be a predictor of mechanism of action. Cell viability has rarely been examined in these embodiments, and not all potential mechanisms of action were considered. It is possible that all listed embodiments may intersect at immune regulatory cell levels, but this remains to be determined. Also, the site of action is currently unknown: Although it is generally believed that the DC activity will occur inside the pancreatic lymph nodes, there are equally likely possibilities that the activity of immune tolerance may in fact occur extralymphatically and around the islets. The study by Zinkernagel and colleagues demonstrating a nascent peri-islet lymphoid ultrastructure during diabetes onset is very interesting, instructive, and awaits the discovery of a mechanism [Ludewig et al. 1998b].

Table 16-6 summarizes the few studies that have examined the outcome of diabetes incidence in animals treated with tolerogenic DC embodiments pulsed with putative autoantigens. Although the ongoing insulitis drives the migration of exogenously administered DCs into the islets, where they acquire the antigen specificity to provide beta-cell antigens (from apoptotic/necrotic beta cells) to pancreatic lymph node–resident regulatory immune cells such as $CD25^+Foxp3^+$ T cells, it is currently unknown if ex vivo pulsing with putative autoantigen(s) could stabilize MHC class I to yield more specific Tregs in vivo. Our data, however, indicate that a supply of putative autoantigens may not be necessary, given the endogenous supply acquired by migratory exogenous DCs inside the insulitic lesion. The critical factor is to maintain the DCs in a functionally immature state [Giannoukakis et al. 1999a; Ma et al. 2003; Machen et al. 2004; Giannoukakis and Trucco 2005; Harnaha et al. 2006].

16.5.5 Gene-Based Tolerance Induction Strategies in RA

Similar to T1DM, several different gene and cell therapy approaches have been developed for RA. Initial approaches have focused on transferring therapeutic genes locally to diseased joints to try to block or reverse diseased-associated pathology [Ghivizzani et al. 2001b]. Both ex vivo and in vivo approaches have been used for intraarticular gene transfer. In particular, genetic modification of autologous synovial fibroblasts by retroviral infection followed by intraarticular injection resulted in colonization of the synovial lining and sustained transgene expression in rabbit, murine, and rat models of arthritis [Lechman et al. 1999a]. In addition, in a phase I clinical trial, genetically modified autologous synovial fibroblasts were transplanted successfully into human metacarpaphalangeal joints, where transgene expression was detected without adverse effects [Evans and Robbins 1997; Evans et al. 2000, 2005]. In vivo gene transfer to joints has been demonstrated using adenovirus, adeno-associated virus, herpes simplex virus, and retroviral vectors as well as with nonviral vectors such as liposomes and DNA conjugates [Ghivizzani et al. 2000, 2001b]. Although the viral vectors are able to infect synovial cells in vivo efficiently, the immune response to the different viral vectors currently limits their use clinically. In contrast, the nonviral vectors are far less efficient, but could have potential clinical use if their efficiency was improved, since they appear to be less inflammatory. A clinical trial to deliver a therapeutic agent to human joints by intraarticular injection of naked DNA has already been initiated [Sant et al. 1998].

Similar to other autoimmune diseases, there are a number of different potentially therapeutic genes that could be delivered to human joints to reduce or reverse pathology. In particular, inhibitors of IL-1 and TNF-α, such as IL-1Ra, soluble IL-1 receptors, and sTNF receptors, have shown efficacy in blocking inflammation, synovial cell proliferation, and bone and cartilage erosion in rabbit, rat, and murine models of antigen-induced arthritis [Makarov et al. 1995, 1996; Ghivizzani et al. 1998]. Similarly, intraarticular expression of anti-inflammatory cytokines such IL-10, its viral homolog, vIL-10, IL-4, and IL-13 also appear to be therapeutic following either ex vivo or in vivo intraarticular gene transfer [Ma et al. 1998; Lechman et al. 1999b; Kim et al. 2000]. Gene transfer of NF-κB inhibitors such as IκB or NF-κB decoy oligonucleotides are also able to reduce disease pathology [Miagkov et al. 1998]. In addition to reducing inflammation, several investigators have examined the ability to eliminate the hyperplastic synovial tissue by gene transfer of apoptotic genes such as FasL, TRAIL, p53, or FADD as well as the suicide gene HSV Tk [Okamoto et al. 1998; Yao et al. 2000; Ghivizzani et al. 2001a]. This approach also appears to reduce inflammation either through direct apoptosis of the infiltrating leukocytes or indirectly by down-regulation of resident APCs following phagocytosis of the apoptotic synovial cells. Finally, the ability to stimulate new cartilage synthesis has been demonstrated by intraarticular gene transfer of growth factor genes such as IGF-1 [Somia and Verma 2000].

Several investigators have reported that local intraarticular injection of adenoviral vectors expressing IL-1Ra, sTNF receptor, vIL-10, IL-4, and even FasL resulted in a therapeutic effect in the contralateral or distal untreated joints [Zhang et al. 1997; Ghivizzani et al. 1998, 2001a; Lechman et al. 1999b; Kim et al. 2000]. This effect, first observed in a rabbit knee model of antigen-induced arthritis, was termed the *contralateral effect* [Ghivizzani et al. 1998]. The exact mechanism important for the contralateral effect is unknown. However, it has been demonstrated that intraarticular injection of adenoviral vectors results in infection of resident APCs that are then able to migrate to other sites, such as the contralateral joint space and draining lymph nodes [Lechman et al. 1999b]. These results suggest that the observed suppression of disease in untreated joints following intraarticular gene delivery to a single joint could be mediated by genetically modified APCs. However, it has also been observed in a rabbit knee model that ex vivo gene transfer of IL-1Ra and sTNF receptor using genetically modified synovial fibroblasts results in a similar contralateral effect (unpublished results). This result seems to suggest that direct genetic modification of APCs is not involved in disease.

To examine the mechanism of the contralateral effect in more detail, adoptive transfer studies have been performed in a murine delayed type of hypersensitivity (DTH) model. It has been demonstrated that injection of an adenoviral vector expressing vIL-10 into the hind paw of an immunized mouse is able to block the DTH response to injection of antigen into not only the treated paw but also in the contralateral untreated paw (unpublished results). Injection of APCs isolated from lymph nodes and spleens of Ad.vIL-10-treated animals was also able to confer a protective effect to the treated paw as well as to the contralateral paw. Moreover, injection of DCs, derived from bone marrow of naive mice, infected with Ad.vIL-10 or treated with recombinant IL-10 and then pulsed with antigen, was able to block the DTH response in both treated and untreated paws. Taken together, these results suggest that down-regulation of APC function, either by gene transfer or protein treatment, can confer an anti-inflammatory activity, result, or action in both the treated paw and in the contralateral, untreated paw.

Given the apparent ability of APCs to confer a contralateral effect in animal models of antigen-induced arthritis, Robbins and colleagues have examined the ability of modified DCs to treat established disease. They have shown that intravenous injection of DCs infected with Ad.IL-4 into mice with established collagen-induced arthritis results in disease elimination in over 50% of the treated animals, without recurrence [Kim et al. 2001]. Treatment with DC.IL-4 resulted in a significant reduction in collagen-specific Th1 cells in both lymph node and spleen and a reduction in certain anticollagen Ig isotypes. In addition, they have shown that infection of DCs with Ad.FasL resulted in transient disease regression due to elimination of collagen-reactive T cells (unpublished results). Although it is not yet clear that there is indeed tolerance induction to collagen using genetically modified DCs, these results suggest that it might be possible to reduce or eliminate autoimmunity using modified DCs.

Although whole DCs can be applied toward therapy for autoimmunity, a considerable degree of excitement has recently been generated surrounding the possibility that exosomes derived from tolerogenic DCs are equally as effective as whole DCs in treating autoimmune disorders, with arthritis being the first such disease [Kim et al. 2005, 2006; Taieb et al. 2005; Chaput et al. 2006]. Exosomes are basically DC-derived vesicles that may be of endosomal or secretory vesicle ontogeny. They have been shown to possess MHC classes I and II, along with the major co-stimulation proteins. As such, they have demonstrated efficacy as antitumor vaccines in vitro [Taieb et al. 2005; Chaput et al. 2006]. Although this technology is still in its infancy, once the logistical hurdles are overcome, it promises to add to the ever-expanding varieties of DC-based therapy.

16.6 CONCLUSIONS

Gene modifications of cells are easily achievable today with a variety of vectors, viral and nonviral. It is critical to understand which pathways are involved in promoting the deletion of autoreactive immune cells and to manipulate them in an antigen-restricted manner in autoimmune diseases where the autoantigen is known, or to promote peripheral silencing or deletional mechanisms that will act in a tissue-restricted manner in diseases where there is no known antigen. Manipulation of APCs is one approach, but surrogate APCs other than DCs or macrophages could also be exploited, by conferring inducible antigen presentation and tolerogenic capabilities to tissue-specific progenitor cells that can be infused into a person genetically at risk for autoimmunity. It is anticipated that prevention of autoimmunity altogether will obviate the need for transplantation, systemic immunosuppression, and complications due to toxicities associated with xenobiotic pharmacological interventions.

REFERENCES

Anderson CC and Chan WF. 2004. Mechanisms and models of peripheral CD4T cell self-tolerance. *Front Biosci* 9:2947–2963.

Arnush M, Heitmeier MR, et al. 1998a. IL-1 produced and released endogenously within human islets inhibits beta cell function. *J Clin Invest* 102:516–526.

Arnush M, Scarim AL, et al. 1998b. Potential role of resident islet macrophage activation in the initiation of autoimmune diabetes. *J Immunol* 160:2684–2691.

Ayuso E, Chillon M, et al. 2006. In vivo gene transfer to healthy and diabetic canine pancreas. *Mol Ther* 13:747–755.

Bach JF, Garchon HJ, et al. 2001. Genetics of human type 1 diabetes mellitus. *Curr Dir Autoimmun* 4:1–30.

Baeyens L, De Breuck S, et al. 2005. In vitro generation of insulin-producing beta cells from adult exocrine pancreatic cells. *Diabetologia* 48:49–57.

Balomenos D and Martinez AC. 2000. Cell-cycle regulation in immunity, tolerance and autoimmunity. *Immunol Today* 21:551–555.

Battaglia M, Gregori S, et al. 2006. Tr1 cells: from discovery to their clinical application. *Semin Immunol* 18:120–127.

Beissert S, Schwarz A, et al. 2006. Regulatory T cells. *J Invest Dermatol* 126:15–24.

Bluestone JA. 1996. Costimulation and its role in organ transplantation. *Clin Transplant* 10:104–109.

Bonner-Weir S and Sharma A. 2002. Pancreatic stem cells. *J Pathol* 197:519–526.

Bonner-Weir S, Toschi E, et al. 2004. The pancreatic ductal epithelium serves as a potential pool of progenitor cells. *Pediatr Diabetes* 5(Suppl 2): 16–22.

Bottino R and Trucco M. 2005. Multifaceted therapeutic approaches for a multigenic disease. *Diabetes* 54:S79–S86.

Bottino R, Lemarchand P, et al. 2003. Gene- and cell-based therapeutics for type I diabetes mellitus. *Gene Ther* 10:875–889.

Boudaly S, Morin J, et al. 2002. Altered dendritic cells (DC) might be responsible for regulatory T cell imbalance and autoimmunity in nonobese diabetic (NOD) mice. *Eur Cytokine Netw* 13:29–37.

Brennan PJ, Saouaf SJ, et al. 2003. Anergy and suppression as coexistent mechanisms for the maintenance of peripheral T cell tolerance. *Immunol Res* 27:295–302.

Brinster C and Shevach EM. 2005. Bone marrow–derived dendritic cells reverse the anergic state of $CD4^{+}CD25^{+}$ T cells without reversing their suppressive function. *J Immunol* 175:7332–7340.

Burton EA, Huang S, et al. 2003. Use of the herpes simplex viral genome to construct gene therapy vectors. *Methods Mol Med* 76:1–31.

Chaput N, Flament C, et al. 2006. Dendritic cell derived-exosomes: biology and clinical implementations. *J Leukoc Biol* 80:471–478.

Chen D, Sung R, et al. 2002. Gene therapy in transplantation. *Transpl Immunol* 9: 301–314.

Christen U and von Herrath MG. 2002. Transgenic animal models for type 1 diabetes: linking a tetracycline-inducible promoter with a virus-inducible mouse model. *Transgen Res* 11:587–595.

Christen U and von Herrath MG. 2004a. Induction, acceleration or prevention of autoimmunity by molecular mimicry. *Mol Immunol* 40:1113–1120.

Christen U and von Herrath MG. 2004b. Manipulating the type 1 vs type 2 balance in type 1 diabetes. *Immunol Res* 30:309–325.

Clare-Salzler M and Mullen Y. 1992. Marked dendritic cell-T cell cluster formation in the pancreatic lymph node of the non-obese diabetic mouse. *Immunology* 76:478–484.

Clarkson MR and Sayegh MH. 2005. T-cell costimulatory pathways in allograft rejection and tolerance. *Transplantation* 80:555–563.

Coates PT and Thomson AW. 2002. Dendritic cells, tolerance induction and transplant outcome. *Am J Transplant* 2:299–307.

Concannon P, Gogolin-Ewens KJ, et al. 1998. A second-generation screen of the human genome for susceptibility to insulin-dependent diabetes mellitus. *Nat Genet* 19:292–296.

Conrad B and Trucco M. 1994. Superantigens as etiopathogenetic factors in the development of insulin-dependent diabetes mellitus. *Diabetes Metab Rev* 10:309–338.

Couzin J and Kaiser J. 2005. Gene therapy: As Gelsinger case ends, gene therapy suffers another blow. *Science* 307:1028.

Dahlen E, Dawe K, et al. 1998. Dendritic cells and macrophages are the first and major producers of TNF-alpha in pancreatic islets in the nonobese diabetic mouse. *J Immunol* 160:3585–3593.

Davis ID, Jefford M, et al. 2003. Rational approaches to human cancer immunotherapy. *J Leukoc Biol* 73:3–29.

Dhodapkar MV, Steinman RM, et al. 2001. Antigen-specific inhibition of effector T cell function in humans after injection of immature dendritic cells. *J Exp Med* 193:233–238.

Di Nicola M, Anichini A, et al. 1998. Human dendritic cells: natural adjuvants in antitumor immunotherapy. *Cytokines Cell Mol Ther* 4:265–273.

Ehl S, Hombach J, et al. 1998. Viral and bacterial infections interfere with peripheral tolerance induction and activate CD8+ T cells to cause immunopathology. *J Exp Med* 187:763–774.

Eibl N, Spatz M, et al. 2002. Impaired primary immune response in type-1 diabetes: results from a controlled vaccination study. *Clin Immunol* 103:249–259.

Eisenbarth GS. 2003. Insulin autoimmunity: immunogenetics/immunopathogenesis of type 1A diabetes. *Ann N Y Acad Sci* 1005:109–118.

Eisenbarth GS, Moriyama H, et al. 2002. Insulin autoimmunity: prediction/precipitation/prevention type 1A diabetes. *Autoimmun Rev* 1:139–145.

Enk AH. 2006. DCs and cytokines cooperate for the induction of tregs. *Ernst Schering Res Found Workshop*: 97–106.

Evans C and Robbins P. 1997. Gene therapy for arthritis. *Expert Opin Invest Drugs* 6:837–840.

Evans CH, Robbins PD, et al. 1996. Clinical trial to assess the safety, feasibility, and efficacy of transferring a potentially anti-arthritic cytokine gene to human joints with rheumatoid arthritis. *Hum Gene Ther* 7:1261–1280.

Evans CH, Ghivizzani SC, et al. 2000. Clinical trials in the gene therapy of arthritis. *Clin Orthop Relat Res*: S300–S307.

Evans CH, Robbins PD, et al. 2005. Gene transfer to human joints: progress toward a gene therapy of arthritis. *Proc Natl Acad Sci U S A* 102:8698–8703.

Faideau B, Larger E, et al. 2005. Role of {beta}-cells in type 1 diabetes pathogenesis. *Diabetes* 54(Suppl 2):S87–S96.

Farilla L, Hui H, et al. 2002. Glucagon-like peptide-1 promotes islet cell growth and inhibits apoptosis in Zucker diabetic rats. *Endocrinology* 143:4397–4408.

Feili-Hariri M, Dong X, et al. 1999. Immunotherapy of NOD mice with bone marrow–derived dendritic cells. *Diabetes* 48:2300–2308.

Fugger L and Svejgaard A. 2000. Association of MHC and rheumatoid arthritis. HLA-DR4 and rheumatoid arthritis: studies in mice and men. *Arthritis Res* 2:208–211.

Furlan R, Butti E, et al. 2004. Gene therapy for autoimmune diseases. *Curr Opin Mol Ther* 6:525–536.

Gabay C. 2000. IL-1 inhibitors: novel agents in the treatment of rheumatoid arthritis. *Expert Opin Invest Drugs* 9:113–127.

Gallucci S and Matzinger P. 2001. Danger signals: SOS to the immune system. *Curr Opin Immunol* 13:114–119.

Garcia-Ocana A, Takane KK, et al. 2000. Hepatocyte growth factor overexpression in the islet of transgenic mice increases beta cell proliferation, enhances islet mass, and induces mild hypoglycemia. *J Biol Chem* 275:1226–1232.

George M, Ayuso E, et al. 2002. Beta cell expression of IGF-I leads to recovery from type 1 diabetes. *J Clin Invest* 109:1153–1163.

Ghivizzani SC, Lechman ER, et al. 1998. Direct adenovirus-mediated gene transfer of interleukin 1 and tumor necrosis factor alpha soluble receptors to rabbit knees with experimental arthritis has local and distal anti-arthritic effects. *Proc Natl Acad Sci U S A* 95:4613–4618.

Ghivizzani SC, Oligino TJ, et al. 2000. Gene therapy approaches for treating rheumatoid arthritis. *Clin Orthop Relat Res*: S288–S299.

Ghivizzani SC, Oligino TJ, et al. 2001a. Direct gene delivery strategies for the treatment of rheumatoid arthritis. *Drug Discov Today* 6:259–267.

Ghivizzani SC, Oligino TJ, et al. 2001b. Direct gene delivery strategies for the treatment of rheumatoid arthritis. *Drug Discov Today* 6:259–267.

Giannoukakis N and Trucco M. 2003. Current status and prospects for gene and cell therapeutics for type 1 diabetes mellitus. *Rev Endocr Metab Disord* 4:369–380.

Giannoukakis N and Trucco M. 2005. Gene therapy for type 1 diabetes. *Am J Ther* 12:512–528.

Giannoukakis N, Rudert WA, et al. 1999a. Targeting autoimmune diabetes with gene therapy. *Diabetes* 48:2107–2121.

Giannoukakis N, Thomson A, et al. 1999b. Gene therapy in transplantation. *Gene Ther* 6:1499–1511.

Goins WF, Krisky DM, et al. 2002. Development of replication-defective herpes simplex virus vectors. *Methods Mol Med* 69:481–507.

Goodnow CC, Sprent J, et al. 2005. Cellular and genetic mechanisms of self tolerance and autoimmunity. *Nature* 435:590–597.

Gordon EJ, Wicker LS, et al. 2005. Autoimmune diabetes and resistance to xenograft transplantation tolerance in NOD mice. *Diabetes* 54:107–115.

Green EA, Eynon EE, et al. 1998. Local expression of TNFalpha in neonatal NOD mice promotes diabetes by enhancing presentation of islet antigens. *Immunity* 9:733–743.

Guo Y, Lu Y, et al. 2005. Pancreatic islet-specific expression of an insulin-like growth factor-I transgene compensates islet cell growth in growth hormone receptor gene-deficient mice. *Endocrinology* 146:2602–2609.

Hackstein H, Morelli AE, et al. 2001. Designer dendritic cells for tolerance induction: guided not misguided missiles. *Trends Immunol* 22:437–442.

Hardin JA. 2005. Dendritic cells: potential triggers of autoimmunity and targets for therapy. *Ann Rheum Dis* 64(Suppl 4):iv86–90.

Harnaha J, Machen J, et al. 2006. Interleukin-7 is a survival factor for $CD4^+CD25^+$ T-cells and is expressed by diabetes-suppressive dendritic cells. *Diabetes* 55:158–170.

Heremans Y, Van De Casteele M, et al. 2002. Recapitulation of embryonic neuroendocrine differentiation in adult human pancreatic duct cells expressing neurogenin 3. *J Cell Biol* 159:303–312.

Hoglund P, Mintern J, et al. 1999. Initiation of autoimmune diabetes by developmentally regulated presentation of islet cell antigens in the pancreatic lymph nodes. *J Exp Med* 189:331–339.

Huber S and Schramm C. 2006. TGF-beta and $CD4^+CD25^+$ regulatory T cells. *Front Biosci* 11:1014–1023.

Hugues S, Boissonnas A, et al. 2006. The dynamics of dendritic cell–T cell interactions in priming and tolerance. *Curr Opin Immunol* 18:491–495.

Jansen A, Rosmalen JG, et al. 1996. Effect of prophylactic insulin treatment on the number of $ER\text{-}MP23^+$ macrophages in the pancreas of NOD mice. Is the prevention of diabetes based on beta-cell rest? *J Autoimmun* 9:341–348.

Jindal RM, Karanam M, et al. 2001. Prevention of diabetes in the NOD mouse by intramuscular injection of recombinant adeno-associated virus containing the preproinsulin II gene. *Int J Exp Diabetes Res* 2:129–138.

Jonuleit H, Schmitt E, et al. 2000. Induction of interleukin 10–producing, nonproliferating CD4(+) T cells with regulatory properties by repetitive stimulation with allogeneic immature human dendritic cells. *J Exp Med* 192:1213–1222.

Kim SH, Evans CH, et al. 2000. Gene therapy for established murine collagen-induced arthritis by local and systemic adenovirus-mediated delivery of interleukin-4. *Arthritis Res* 2:293–302.

Kim SH, Kim S, et al. 2001. Effective treatment of established murine collagen-induced arthritis by systemic administration of dendritic cells genetically modified to express IL-4. *J Immunol* 166:3499–3505.

Kim SH, Lechman ER, et al. 2005. Exosomes derived from IL-10-treated dendritic cells can suppress inflammation and collagen-induced arthritis. *J Immunol* 174:6440–6448.

Kim SH, Bianco N, et al. 2006. Exosomes derived from genetically modified DC expressing FasL are anti-inflammatory and immunosuppressive. *Mol Ther* 13:289–300.

Kishimoto K, Dong VM, et al. 2000. The role of costimulatory molecules as targets for new immunosuppressives in transplantation. *Curr Opin Urol* 10:57–62.

Kotzin BL, Falta MT, et al. 2000. Use of soluble peptide-DR4 tetramers to detect synovial T cells specific for cartilage antigens in patients with rheumatoid arthritis. *Proc Natl Acad Sci U S A* 97:291–296.

Kubach J, Becker C, et al. 2005. Dendritic cells: sentinels of immunity and tolerance. *Int J Hematol* 81:197–203.

Lechler R, Chai JG, et al. 2001a. T-cell anergy and peripheral T-cell tolerance. *Philos Trans R Soc London B Biol Sci* 356:625–637.

Lechler R, Chai JG, et al. 2001b. The contributions of T-cell anergy to peripheral T-cell tolerance. *Immunology* 103:262–269.

Lechman ER, Jaffurs D, et al. 1999a. Direct adenoviral gene transfer of viral IL-10 to rabbit knees with experimental arthritis ameliorates disease in both injected and contralateral control knees. *J Immunol* 163:2202–2208.

Lechman ER, Jaffurs D, et al. 1999b. Direct adenoviral gene transfer of viral IL-10 to rabbit knees with experimental arthritis ameliorates disease in both injected and contralateral control knees. *J Immunol* 163:2202–2208.

Lenschow DJ, Walunas TL, et al. 1996. CD28/B7 system of T cell costimulation. *Annu Rev Immunol* 14:233–258.

Liu F and Huang L. 2002. Development of non-viral vectors for systemic gene delivery. *J Control Release* 78:259–266.

Liu YJ. 2001. Dendritic cell subsets and lineages, and their functions in innate and adaptive immunity. *Cell* 106:259–262.

Lo D, Reilly CR, et al. 1993. Antigen-presenting cells in adoptively transferred and spontaneous autoimmune diabetes. *Eur J Immunol* 23:1693–1698.

Lohr J, Knoechel B, et al. 2006. Regulatory T cells in the periphery. *Immunol Rev* 212:149–162.

Ludewig B, Ehl S, et al. 1998a. Dendritic cells efficiently induce protective antiviral immunity. *J Virol* 72:3812–3818.

Ludewig B, Odermatt B, et al. 1998b. Dendritic cells induce autoimmune diabetes and maintain disease via de novo formation of local lymphoid tissue. *J Exp Med* 188:1493–1501.

Ma L, Qian S, et al. 2003. Prevention of diabetes in NOD mice by administration of dendritic cells deficient in nuclear transcription factor-kappaB activity. *Diabetes* 52:1976–1985.

Ma Y, Thornton S, et al. 1998. Inhibition of collagen-induced arthritis in mice by viral IL-10 gene transfer. *J Immunol* 161:1516–1524.

Machen J, Harnaha J, et al. 2004. Antisense oligonucleotides down-regulating costimulation confer diabetes-preventive properties to nonobese diabetic mouse dendritic cells. *J Immunol* 173:4331–4341.

Makarov SS, Olsen JC, et al. 1995. Retrovirus mediated in vivo gene transfer to synovium in bacterial cell wall-induced arthritis in rats. *Gene Ther* 2:424–428.

Makarov SS, Olsen JC, et al. 1996. Suppression of experimental arthritis by gene transfer of interleukin 1 receptor antagonist cDNA. *Proc Natl Acad Sci U S A* 93:402–406.

Manfredi AA, Sabbadini MG, et al. 2005. Dendritic cells and the shadow line between autoimmunity and disease. *Arthritis Rheum* 52:11–15.

Manz MG, Traver D, et al. 2001a. Dendritic cell development from common myeloid progenitors. *Ann N Y Acad Sci* 938:167–173; discussion, 173–174.

Manz MG, Traver D, et al. 2001b. Dendritic cell potentials of early lymphoid and myeloid progenitors. *Blood* 97:3333–3341.

Markees TG, Serreze DV, et al. 1999. NOD mice have a generalized defect in their response to transplantation tolerance induction. *Diabetes* 48:967–974.

Marleau AM and Singh B. 2002. Myeloid dendritic cells in non-obese diabetic mice have elevated costimulatory and T helper-1-inducing abilities. *J Autoimmun* 19:23–35.

Matzinger P. 1994. Tolerance, danger, and the extended family. *Annu Rev Immunol* 12:991–1045.

Matzinger P. 1998. An innate sense of danger. *Semin Immunol* 10:399–415.

Matzinger P. 2001. Essay 1: the danger model in its historical context. *Scand J Immunol* 54:4–9.

Matzinger P. 2002. An innate sense of danger. *Ann N Y Acad Sci* 961:341–342.

McClane SJ, Chirmule N, et al. 1997. Characterization of the immune response after local delivery of recombinant adenovirus in murine pancreas and successful strategies for readministration. *Hum Gene Ther* 8:2207–2216.

McMahon MM and Bistrian BR. 1995. Host defenses and susceptibility to infection in patients with diabetes mellitus. *Infect Dis Clin North Am* 9:1–9.

Mennechet FJ and Uze G. 2006. Interferon-lambda-treated dendritic cells specifically induce proliferation of FOXP3-expressing suppressor T cells. *Blood* 107:4417–4423.

Miagkov AV, Kovalenko DV, et al. 1998. NF-kappaB activation provides the potential link between inflammation and hyperplasia in the arthritic joint. *Proc Natl Acad Sci U S A* 95:13859–13864.

Morelli AE and Thomson AW. 2003. Dendritic cells: regulators of alloimmunity and opportunities for tolerance induction. *Immunol Rev* 196:125–146.

Nikolic T, Bunk M, et al. 2004. Bone marrow precursors of nonobese diabetic mice develop into defective macrophage-like dendritic cells in vitro. *J Immunol* 173:4342–4351.

Nouri-Shirazi M and Thomson AW. 2006. Dendritic cells as promoters of transplant tolerance. *Expert Opin Biol Ther* 6:325–339.

Okamoto K, Asahara H, et al. 1998. Induction of apoptosis in the rheumatoid synovium by Fas ligand gene transfer. *Gene Ther* 5:331–338.

Oldstone MB. 1989. Molecular mimicry as a mechanism for the cause and a probe uncovering etiologic agent(s) of autoimmune disease. *Curr Top Microbiol Immunol* 145:127–135.

Pandya S, Klimatcheva E, et al. 2001. Lentivirus and foamy virus vectors: novel gene therapy tools. *Expert Opin Biol Ther* 1:17–40.

Paul S, Calmels B, et al. 2002. Improvement of adoptive cellular immunotherapy of human cancer using ex-vivo gene transfer. *Curr Gene Ther* 2:91–100.

Pearson T, Markees TG, et al. 2003a. Genetic disassociation of autoimmunity and resistance to costimulation blockade-induced transplantation tolerance in nonobese diabetic mice. *J Immunol* 171:185–195.

Pearson T, Markees TG, et al. 2003b. Islet cell autoimmunity and transplantation tolerance: two distinct mechanisms? *Ann N Y Acad Sci* 1005:148–156.

Pearson T, Markees TG, et al. 2003c. NOD congenic mice genetically protected from autoimmune diabetes remain resistant to transplantation tolerance induction. *Diabetes* 52:321–326.

Peng R, Li Y, et al. 2003. Abnormal peripheral blood dendritic cell populations in type 1 diabetes. *Ann N Y Acad Sci* 1005:222–225.

Raper SE and DeMatteo RP. 1996. Adenovirus-mediated in vivo gene transfer and expression in normal rat pancreas. *Pancreas* 12:401–410.

Rehman KK, Bertera S, et al. 2003. Protection of islets by in situ peptide mediated transduction of the Ikappa B kinase (IKK) inhibitor nemo binding domain (NBD) peptide. *J Biol Chem* 9:9.

Rehman KK, Wang Z, et al. 2005. Efficient gene delivery to human and rodent islets with double-stranded (ds) AAV-based vectors. *Gene Ther* 12:1313–1323.

Robbins PD and Ghivizzani SC. 1998. Viral vectors for gene therapy. *Pharmacol Ther* 80:35–47.

Robbins PD, Tahara H, et al. 1998. Viral vectors for gene therapy. *Trends Biotechnol* 16:35–40.

Roep BO and De Vries RR. 1992. T-lymphocytes and the pathogenesis of type 1 (insulin-dependent) diabetes mellitus. *Eur J Clin Invest* 22:697–711.

Roncarolo MG, Gregori S, et al. 2006. Interleukin-10-secreting type 1 regulatory T cells in rodents and humans. *Immunol Rev* 212:28–50.

Rood PP, Hara H, et al. 2005. Preformed antibodies to alpha1,3-galactosyltransferase gene-knockout (GT-KO) pig cells in humans, baboons, and monkeys: implications for xenotransplantation. *Transplant Proc* 37:3514–3515.

Rossini AA. 2004. Autoimmune diabetes and the circle of tolerance. *Diabetes* 53:267–275.

Rossini AA, Mordes JP, et al. 2001. Islet cell transplantation tolerance. *Transplantation* 72:S43–S46.

Rothstein DM and Sayegh MH. 2003. T-cell costimulatory pathways in allograft rejection and tolerance. *Immunol Rev* 196:85–108.

Rutella S, Bonanno G, et al. 2006. Hepatocyte growth factor favors monocyte differentiation into regulatory interleukin $(IL)^{-}10^{++}IL^{-}12^{low/neg}$ accessory cells with dendritic-cell features. *Blood* 108:218–227.

Sant SM, Suarez TM, et al. 1998. Molecular lysis of synovial lining cells by in vivo herpes simplex virus–thymidine kinase gene transfer. *Hum Gene Ther* 9:2735–2743.

Saouaf SJ, Brennan PJ, et al. 2003. Mechanisms of peripheral immune tolerance: conversion of the immune to the unresponsive phenotype. *Immunol Res* 28:193–199.

Sayegh MH and Turka LA. 1995. T cell costimulatory pathways: promising novel targets for immunosuppression and tolerance induction. *J Am Soc Nephrol* 6:1143–1150.

Seaberg RM, Smukler SR, et al. 2004. Clonal identification of multipotent precursors from adult mouse pancreas that generate neural and pancreatic lineages. *Nat Biotechnol* 22:1115–1124.

Sen P, Bhattacharyya S, et al. 2003. NF-kappa B hyperactivation has differential effects on the APC function of nonobese diabetic mouse macrophages. *J Immunol* 170:1770–1780.

Seung E, Mordes JP, et al. 2003. Induction of tolerance for islet transplantation for type 1 diabetes. *Curr Diabetes Rep* 3:329–335.

Shapiro AM, Geng Hao E, et al. 2002. Defining optimal immunosuppression for islet transplantation based on reduced diabetogenicity in canine islet autografts. *Transplantation* 74:1522–1528.

Shevach EM, DiPaolo RA, et al. 2006. The lifestyle of naturally occurring $CD4^{+}CD25^{+}Foxp3^{+}$ regulatory T cells. *Immunol Rev* 212:60–73.

Shifrin AL, Auricchio A, et al. 2001. Adenoviral vector-mediated insulin gene transfer in the mouse pancreas corrects streptozotocin-induced hyperglycemia. *Gene Ther* 8:1480–1489.

Shimizu J, Carrasco-Marin E, et al. 1995. Relationship between beta cell injury and antigen presentation in NOD mice. *J Immunol* 155:4095–4099.

Singh NJ and Schwartz RH. 2006. Primer: mechanisms of immunologic tolerance. *Nat Clin Pract Rheumatol* 2:44–52.

Smits HH, de Jong EC, et al. 2005a. Different faces of regulatory DCs in homeostasis and immunity. *Trends Immunol* 26:123–129.

Smits HH, Engering A, et al. 2005b. Selective probiotic bacteria induce IL-10-producing regulatory T cells in vitro by modulating dendritic cell function through dendritic cell–specific intercellular adhesion molecule 3-grabbing nonintegrin. *J Allergy Clin Immunol* 115:1260–1267.

Somia N and Verma IM. 2000. Gene therapy: trials and tribulations. *Nat Rev Genet* 1:91–99.

Stassi G, Maria RD, et al. 1997. Nitric oxide primes pancreatic beta cells for Fas-mediated destruction in insulin-dependent diabetes mellitus. *J Exp Med* 186:1193–1200.

Steinman RM and Nussenzweig MC. 2002. Avoiding horror autotoxicus: the importance of dendritic cells in peripheral T cell tolerance. *Proc Natl Acad Sci U S A* 99:351–358.

Steinman RM, Inaba K, et al. 1999. Antigen capture, processing, and presentation by dendritic cells: recent cell biological studies. *Hum Immunol* 60:562–567.

Steinman RM, Turley S, et al. 2000. The induction of tolerance by dendritic cells that have captured apoptotic cells. *J Exp Med* 191:411–416.

Steinman RM, Hawiger D, et al. 2003. Tolerogenic dendritic cells. *Annu Rev Immunol* 21:685–711.

Strid J, Lopes L, et al. 2001. A defect in bone marrow derived dendritic cell maturation in the nonobesediabetic mouse. *Clin Exp Immunol* 123:375–381.

Suarez-Pinzon WL, Yan Y, et al. 2005. Combination therapy with epidermal growth factor and gastrin increases {beta}-cell mass and reverses hyperglycemia in diabetic NOD mice. *Diabetes* 54:2596–2601.

Suciu-Foca N, Manavalan JS, et al. 2005. Molecular characterization of allospecific T suppressor and tolerogenic dendritic cells: review. *Int Immunopharmacol* 5:7–11.

Summers KL, Behme MT, et al. 2003. Characterization of dendritic cells in humans with type 1 diabetes. *Ann N Y Acad Sci* 1005:226–229.

Summers KL, Marleau AM, et al. 2006. Reduced IFN-alpha secretion by blood dendritic cells in human diabetes. *Clin Immunol* 121:81–89.

Suzuki A, Nakauchi H, et al. 2004. Prospective isolation of multipotent pancreatic progenitors using flow-cytometric cell sorting. *Diabetes* 53:2143–2152.

Taieb J, Chaput N, et al. 2005. Dendritic cell-derived exosomes as cell-free peptide-based vaccines. *Crit Rev Immunol* 25:215–223.

Tang Q and Bluestone JA. 2006. Regulatory T-cell physiology and application to treat autoimmunity. *Immunol Rev* 212:217–237.

Tarbell KV, Yamazaki S, et al. 2004. $CD25^+CD4^+$ T cells, expanded with dendritic cells presenting a single autoantigenic peptide, suppress autoimmune diabetes. *J Exp Med* 199:1467–1477.

Tarner IH and Fathman CG. 2002. The potential for gene therapy in the treatment of autoimmune disease. *Clin Immunol* 104:204–216.

Tarner IH, Slavin AJ, et al. 2003. Treatment of autoimmune disease by adoptive cellular gene therapy. *Ann N Y Acad Sci* 998:512–519.

Trucco M. 2005. Regeneration of the pancreatic beta cell. *J Clin Invest* 115:5–12.

Trucco M, Robbins PD, et al. 2002. Gene therapy strategies to prevent autoimmune disorders. *Curr Gene Ther* 2:341–354.

Trudeau JD, Dutz JP, et al. 2000. Neonatal beta-cell apoptosis: a trigger for autoimmune diabetes? *Diabetes* 49:1–7.

Uchizono Y, Iwase M, et al. 2004. Tacrolimus impairment of insulin secretion in isolated rat islets occurs at multiple distal sites in stimulus-secretion coupling. *Endocrinology* 145:2264–2272.

Verhagen J, Blaser K, et al. 2006. Mechanisms of allergen-specific immunotherapy: T-regulatory cells and more. *Immunol Allergy Clin North Am* 26:207–231.

Vigna E and Naldini L. 2000. Lentiviral vectors: excellent tools for experimental gene transfer and promising candidates for gene therapy. *J Gene Med* 2:308–316.

Vigouroux S, Yvon E, et al. 2004. Antigen-induced regulatory T cells. *Blood* 104:26–33.

Vlad G, Cortesini R, et al. 2005. License to heal: bidirectional interaction of antigen-specific regulatory T cells and tolerogenic APC. *J Immunol* 174:5907–5914.

Volpers C and Kochanek S. 2004. Adenoviral vectors for gene transfer and therapy. *J Gene Med* 6(Suppl 1):S164–S171.

Von Herrath MG. 2002. Regulation of virally induced autoimmunity and immunopathology: contribution of LCMV transgenic models to understanding autoimmune insulin-dependent diabetes mellitus. *Curr Top Microbiol Immunol* 263:145–175.

Von Herrath M and Homann D. 2004. Islet regeneration needed for overcoming autoimmune destruction: considerations on the pathogenesis of type 1 diabetes. *Pediatr Diabetes* 5(Suppl 2): 23–28.

Walther W and Stein U. 2000. Viral vectors for gene transfer: a review of their use in the treatment of human diseases. *Drugs* 60:249–271.

Wang Z, Zhu T, et al. 2006. Widespread and stable pancreatic gene transfer by adeno-associated virus vectors via different routes. *Diabetes* 55:875–884.

Watanabe N, Wang YH, et al. 2005. Hassall's corpuscles instruct dendritic cells to induce $CD4^+CD25^+$ regulatory T cells in human thymus. *Nature* 436:1181–1185.

Weaver DJ Jr, Poligone B, et al. 2001. Dendritic cells from nonobese diabetic mice exhibit a defect in NF-kappa B regulation due to a hyperactive I kappa B kinase. *J Immunol* 167:1461–1468.

Weets I, Truyen I, et al. 2006. Sex- and season-dependent differences in C-peptide levels at diagnosis of immune-mediated type 1 diabetes. *Diabetologia* 49:1158–1162.

Wheat LJ. 1980. Infection and diabetes mellitus. *Diabetes Care* 3:187–197.

Wheat W, Kupfer R, et al. 2004. Increased NF-kappa B activity in B cells and bone marrow–derived dendritic cells from NOD mice. *Eur J Immunol* 34:1395–1404.

Yamazaki S, Iyoda T, et al. 2003. Direct expansion of functional $CD25^+CD4^+$ regulatory T cells by antigen-processing dendritic cells. *J Exp Med* 198:235–247.

Yang Z, Chen M, et al. 2002. Suppression of autoimmune diabetes by viral IL-10 gene transfer. *J Immunol* 168:6479–6485.

Yao Q, Glorioso JC, et al. 2000. Adenoviral mediated delivery of Fas ligand to arthritic joints causes extensive apoptosis in the synovial lining. *J Gene Med* 2:210–219.

Yvon ES, Vigouroux S, et al. 2003. Overexpression of the Notch ligand, Jagged-1, induces alloantigen-specific human regulatory T cells. *Blood* 102:3815–3821.

Zaiss AK and Muruve DA. 2005. Immune responses to adeno-associated virus vectors. *Curr Gene Ther* 5:323–331.

Zhang H, Yang Y, et al. 1997. Amelioration of collagen-induced arthritis by CD95 (Apo-1/Fas)-ligand gene transfer. *J Clin Invest* 100:1951–1957.

Zhang L, Yi H, et al. 2006. Transforming growth factor-beta: an important role in $CD4^+CD25^+$ regulatory T cells and immune tolerance. *Autoimmunity* 39:269–276.

Zorina TD, Subbotin VM, et al. 2003. Recovery of the endogenous beta cell function in the NOD model of autoimmune diabetes. *Stem Cells* 21:377–388.

17

ENGINEERING OF VIRAL CAPSIDS TO EVADE THE HOST IMMUNE SYSTEM

LUCA PERABO, PH.D., AND JORGE BOUCAS, M.S.

Clinic I for Internal Medicine, University of Cologne, Cologne, Germany

OLIVER COUTELLE, M.D., PH.D., MICHAEL HALLEK, M.D., AND HILDEGARD BÜNING, PH.D.

Clinic I for Internal Medicine and Center for Molecular Medicine, University of Cologne, Cologne, Germany

Gene Therapy Immunology, Edited by Roland Herzog

17.1 INTRODUCTION

The success of gene therapy applications is highly dependent on the development of efficient gene transfer systems. The currently available vector systems, nonviral as well as viral, are hampered by the induction of innate and adaptive immune responses to vector particles. In addition, viral vectors are targets of preexisting humoral and cellular immunity, which may preclude successful application to patients with exposure to the wild-type virus earlier in life. In this chapter we summarize capsid engineering strategies that have been employed so far to blunt immune responses to viral vectors and to enable efficient cell transduction, regardless of the presence of neutralizing antibodies using adenoviral and adeno-associated viral vectors as examples.

17.2 CHEMICAL MODIFICATIONS OF THE ADENOVIRUS CAPSID

17.2.1 Adenoviral Vectors

Recombinant adenoviral vectors are currently the most popular viral vector system in gene therapy and are used widely in basic research and in vaccine development. Conventionally, adenoviral vectors are based on serotype 2 or 5 (group C adenoviruses). Within the past 20 years of vector technology, three different types of adenoviral vectors have been developed that differ in the amount of viral genes, which remain within the vector genome and thus in their immunotoxicity (Table 17-1): Adenoviral gene products expressed from first-generation vectors limited transgene expression, due to the induction of strong antiviral immune responses, a hurdle that has been overcome with the development of high-capacity third-generation vectors [Volpers and Kochanek 2004; Kreppel and Kochanek 2008]. Nevertheless, even third-generation vectors are immunogenic (Chapter 4). The innate immune system is activated by adenoviral vector–mediated cell transduction (Chapter 4). This occurs extremely rapidly (10 to 20 minutes) [Hartman et al. 2008] and is at least partially dependent on the coxsackie- and adenovirus-receptor (CAR) and integrin receptor binding, in

TABLE 17-1 Comparison of Adenoviral Vector Types

Vector Generation	Deletion	Coding Capacity	Immunotoxicity	Transgene Expression
First	E1 (and optionally E3)	Up to 8 kb	+++	Short-term
Second	E1 (and optionally E3), E2, and/or E4	Up to 12 kb	++	Prolonged in comparison to first-generation vectors
Third	All viral genes	Up to 36 kb	+	Long-term

Source: Volpers and Kochanek [2004].

both immune and nonimmune cells. Furthermore, in naive recipients, delivery of adenoviral vectors induces a strong humoral and cell-mediated immune response to the viral capsid, which limits repeated vector administration. In addition, even the initial vector application may be hampered by preexisting neutralizing antibodies, which directly impair cell transduction after intravenous vector injection. Furthermore, nonneutralizing antiadenovirus antibodies can opsonize vector particles, and reactivated memory T cells may suppress transgene expression from adenoviral vector–transduced cells (Chapter 4). One strategy to avoid preexisting immunity against adenovirus type 5–based vectors is the use of alternate human serotypes. Although this may prevent antibody-mediated clearance, this strategy offers no escape from cellular immunity, since at least one immunodominant epitope recognized by $CD4^+$ and $CD8^+$ T cells is conserved among human adenovirus serotypes. Thus, immunosuppression, or the development of adenoviral vectors based on animal serotypes, have been proposed as alternative strategies (Chapter 4). A totally different approach to overcoming these hurdles is the use of covalent chemical modification of adenoviral vector particles [Kreppel and Kochanek 2008].

17.2.2 Modification of Adenoviral Vectors with Polymers

Currently, two different types of synthetic polymers, polyethylene glycol (PEG) and poly-*N*-(2-hydroxlpropoyl) methacrylamide (polyHPMA), are being used to shield adenoviral vector particles from the immune system [Kreppel and Kochanek 2008]. The first attempt to modify adenoviral vector particles by PEG dates back to 1999 [O'Riordan et al. 1999]. PEG is a linear polymer of repetitive CH_2CH_2O subunits that can be synthesized to varying chain length. It is an uncharged, hydrophilic, and nonimmunogenic molecule that has been shown to reduce antigenicity and immunogenicity of modified proteins. Furthermore, PEG increases solubility of covalently attached proteins and protects them from proteolytic degradation. Thus, PEG shows many properties that are ideally suited to improve adenoviral vector functions and application in vivo [Delgado et al. 1992; Veronese and Pasut 2005; Haag and Kratz 2006; Kumar et al. 2006; Parveen and Sahoo 2006; Kreppel and Kochanek 2008].

Prior to its use, PEG has to be chemically activated since the terminal hydroxyl groups are inactive. Activation involves the attachment of *N*-hydroxysucchinimide (NHS) esters (via a linker) to the terminal hydroxyl groups. NHS esters are highly reactive toward amino groups of lysine residues forming a covalent (amid) bond between PEG and this amino acid upon NHS release (for further details see the references in Kreppel and Kochanek [2008]). O'Riordan and colleagues showed that up to 18,000 amino groups on the surface of adenovirus serotype 5 are accessible for PEGylation. Thus, under optimized conditions, PEGylation results in the formation of a shield that protects the vector particle [O'Riordan et al. 1999]. The viral capsid of adenoviral particles is composed of hexon and penton capsomeres [Volpers and Kochanek 2004; Kreppel and Kochanek 2008]. The hexon capsomeres form the 20 triangular faces of the icosahedron, while the pentons build up fibers that protrude from the 12 vertices. Hexon, penton, and fiber proteins have been described as targets for antibody binding and are also targets for reactive PEGs. However, adenoviral core proteins that are associated with the viral genome remain unmodified [O'Riordan et al. 1999; Volpers and Kochanek 2004]. Thus, PEGylation blocks potential antibody-binding sites but does not interfere with vector particle integrity. The density of the PEG shield is dependent on the number and molecular weight of the activated PEG molecules. As shown by Wortmann and colleagues, a 100-fold excess of PEG molecules to amino groups saturates PEG acceptors (independent of the molecular weight of PEG) on the vector particle, but shielding is almost tenfold more efficient if high (e.g., 20 kDa)- instead of low (2 or 5 kDa)- molecular-weight PEGs are used [Wortmann et al. 2008]. Of note, the PEG shield impairs antiadenovirus antibody binding even when the degree of PEGylation is only 70% [Croyle et al. 2000]. In addition to facilitating escape from preexisting antibodies, the use of PEGylated vectors has been shown to decrease the level of induction of neutralizing antibodies in naive animals [Croyle et al. 2001; Kreppel and Kochanek 2008]. The extent of the decrease in antibody induction, however, seems to be dependent on the linker, which is used for PEGylation [Croyle et al. 2001; Kreppel and Kochanek 2008]. Thus, the linker as such seems to be a target for the immune system, and the success of a repeated administration is dependent on variations of the linker used for PEGylation [Croyle et al. 2001].

Besides a decrease in the induction of humoral immune responses and in binding of preexisting antibodies, PEGylation also effectively reduces the production of several inflammatory cytokines, such as IL-6, IL-12, and TNF-α, as well as adenovirus-induced thrombocytopenia [Kreppel and Kochanek 2008]. These effects may be due to the reduced interaction of adenoviral vectors with Kupffer cells and macrophages [O'Riordan et al. 1999; Croyle et al. 2002, 2005] and/or the detargeting from liver or spleen (systemic application) and draining lymph nodes (local application) [Wortmann et al. 2008].

Adenoviral vectors are used as gene delivery devices in gene addition therapy but are also commonly used for vaccination purposes. Critical for the use of adenoviral vectors in vaccination is the observation of Wortmann and colleagues that PEGylation did not impair cellular and humoral immune responses against the vector-encoded transgene product [Wortmann et al. 2008]. In the respective mouse immunization study, a first-generation adenoviral vector encoding the surface antigen of hepatitis B virus (HbsAg) and PEGylated with a high-molecular-weight PEG was used. In comparison to non-PEGylated vectors, a reduced but detectable cellular immune response with comparable kinetics of induction and a significant humoral immune response against HbsAg was observed for the PEGylated vectors. This, in combination with a lower overall immunotoxicity and a reduced promiscuity, prompted the investigators to propose the use of PEGylated vectors for vaccination approaches. In this context, an important advantage of PEGylation is a significant increase in thermostability (from 42°C to −20°C) [Croyle et al. 2000; Kreppel and Kochanek 2008].

As mentioned, PEGylation with high-molecular-mass PEG results in detargeting from liver, which is probably due to shielding of receptor-binding ligands [Wortmann et al. 2008] As a consequence, PEGylated adenoviral vectors show a reduction in infectivity [Kreppel et al. 2005; Wortmann et al. 2008]. By further targeted modifications, PEGylated vectors can regain infectivity and at the same time increase specificity (vector targeting). One example was presented by Kreppel et al. [2005]. In this work, chemical capsid modification by PEG was combined with the introduction of cysteine residues at the solvent exposed HI-loop (genetic capsid modification), which enabled the coupling of a receptor-specific ligand via thioether bonds. Another option is the use of heterobifunctional PEG molecules in which one end of the molecule is bound to the viral capsid while the other enables the coupling of receptor-specific ligands [Romanczuk et al. 1999; Lanciotti et al. 2003].

HPMA is used as an alternative to PEG (for details, see Kreppel and Kochanek [2008]). It is activated by incorporation of amino-reactive 4-nitrophenoxy groups on the diglycyl side chains. This results in the generation of a multivalent 21-kDa random copolymer with up to 10 reactive groups per 100 monomer units. Due to this composition, one single polymer can attach to multiple sites of the viral capsids, which clearly distinguish HPMA from conventional semitelechelic PEG, which binds univalently. Under appropriate conditions, not all reactive nitrophenoxy groups are covalently linked to the capsid surface, thereby enabling the coupling of receptor-specific ligands to the unoccupied binding sites and the creation of targeting vectors. As demonstrated by Stevenson and colleagues, such modified vectors transduce cells in a receptor-specific manner while inducing less toxicity due to reduced uptake in liver and spleen [Stevenson et al. 2007].

17.3 GENETIC MODIFICATIONS OF THE ADENO-ASSOCIATED VIRAL CAPSID

17.3.1 Adeno-associated Viral Vectors

For historical reasons, most preclinical studies and the vast majority of clinical studies that used adeno-associated virus (AAV) for therapeutic gene transfer have been conducted with vectors based on serotype 2 (AAV2). In comparison to other systems, AAV vectors induce only mild immune responses, but the efficiency of AAV-mediated transduction can be reduced dramatically by the patient's immune system (Chapter 6). While activation of innate immunity by recombinant AAV vectors is debated controversially (for details, see Chapter 6), experimental evidence shows that vector application induces robust humoral immune response and is likely to reactivate memory T cells. These memory T cells are the products of naturally occurring co-infections with AAV and its helper virus, and have been shown to preclude AAV vector application in clinical trials [Mingozzi and High 2007; Mingozzi et al. 2007]. Furthermore, there is a high prevalence of preexisting neutralizing antibodies against AAV2 in the human population (Chapter 6).

Similar to adenovirus vectors, the use of alternative natural serotypes has been proposed as a strategy to overcome the preexisting immunity toward AAV2. However, recent studies have shown that preexisting immunity (antibodies and T cell-mediated) is an issue for some of these serotypes as well (Chapter 6). In addition, alternative serotypes often differ substantially in their tissue tropism, which may be inappropriate for the gene therapy intervention required. For these reasons, much effort has been directed toward identifying immunogenic sites on the viral (AAV2) capsid with the aim of re-engineering virions with a "stealth" phenotype that abolishes or diminishes recognition by neutralizing antibodies while preserving receptor binding, cell entry, or subsequent steps of cell transduction. These studies are summarized below.

17.3.2 Structure of the AAV2 Capsid

Recently, the atomic structure of AAV has been determined at 3 Å resolution by x-ray crystallography [Xie et al. 2003] (Fig. 17-1A). Each viral capsid is composed of 60 subunits arranged with $T = 1$ icosahedral symmetry. The three structural proteins VP1, VP2, and VP3, which share overlapping sequences and differ only at their N-termini, make up the AAV capsid with a relative stoichiometry of about 1:1:8 [Kronenberg et al. 2001]. The central motif of each subunit is an antiparallel β-barrel, which is highly conserved among parvoviruses. This β-barrel motif forms elongated smooth lumps at the inner surface of the capsid at the two-fold symmetry axis [Kronenberg et al. 2001]. Between the strands of the β-barrel core large loop, insertions are found that share only low similarity among the parvovirus family. These loops comprise two-thirds of the capsid surface features that interact with antibodies and cellular receptors. These surface features include a hollow cylinder at the five-fold axis of symmetry, which is surrounded by a circular depression ("canyon") and a depression spanning the two-fold axis ("dimple") (Fig. 17-1A). The most prominent features of the capsid are the three-fold-proximal peaks, which cluster around the three-fold symmetry axis (Fig. 17-1A). These peaks are derived from two adjacent subunits rather than a single capsid subunit. Other interactions between loops of neighboring subunits are found at the five-fold cylinder.

At the three-fold-proximal peaks, in the valleys separating the three peaks of one three-fold axis, clusters of positive charges are located, which are implicated in receptor binding. Mutational analyses have identified these locations as being involved in binding to AAV2's primary receptor HSPG [Kern et al. 2003; Opie et al. 2003] and mutations of the basic amino acids (aa) R484, R487, K532, R585, and R588 have been shown to affect HSPG binding [Kern et al. 2003; Opie et al. 2003].

17.3.3 Identification of Immunogenic Regions on the Viral Capsid

Several studies are aimed at identifying AAV2 capsid regions that are recognized by antibodies. Wobus and colleagues used four different murine monoclonal

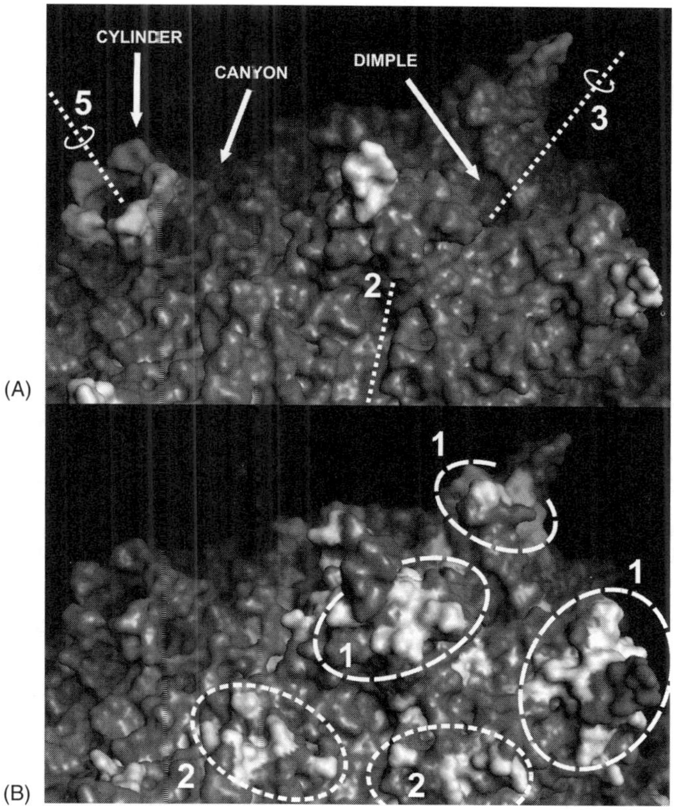

Figure 17-1 (**A**) Detail of the AAV2 capsid structure as determined by x-ray crystallography. The cylinder and the spikes are depicted in white. Lines and numbers indicate the two-, three-, and five-fold symmetry axes. (From Xie et al. [2003].) (B) Immunogenic residues found in the studies discussed in the text are depicted in white. The circles indicate two different major immunogenic regions (1 and 2).

antibodies (A20, C24-B, C37-B, and D3) to identify conformational epitopes of AAV2 by insertional mutagenesis, peptide scanning, and competition experiments [Wobus et al. 2000]. A20, C24-B, and C37-B are examples of neutralizing antibodies. Specifically, A20 precipitates intact AAV2 and AAV3 capsids and impairs viral infection at a postentry step not yet characterized further. For the A20 binding site, three peptide sequences distributed across the linear VP sequence were identified initially (Table 17-2). However, following capsid assembly, these sequences form together a conformational epitope for the antibody.

The monoclonal antibodies C24-B and C37-B interact with intact capsids and single capsid subunits and have been shown to interfere with cell binding. Two different peptide sequences (Table 17-2) are recognized by C37-B, albeit with different affinities (high for SADNNNSEYSWT at aa 492–503 and low for

TABLE 17-2 Amino Acid Sequence of the AAV2 Capsid Subunit (VP1) and Location of Immunogenic Sites Identified So Far

M M

MAADGYLPDWL**E**DTLSEGIRQWWKLKPGPPPPKPAERHKDD**S**RGLVLPGYK

YLGPFNGLDKGEPVNEADAAALEHDKAYDRQLDSGDNPYLKYNHADAEFQE

M

RLKEDTSFGGNLGR**A**VFQAKKRVLEPLGLVEEPVKTAPGKKRPVEHSPVEPD

M M

SSSGTGK**A**GQQPARKRLNFGQTGDA**D**SVPDPQPLGQPPAAPSGLGTNTMA

TGSGAPMADNNEGADGVGNSSGNWHCDSTWMGDRVITTSTRTWALPTYNN

M L L A20

HLY**K**QISS**QS**GASNDNHYFGYSTPWGYFDFNRFHCHFSPRDWQRLINNNW

GFRPKRLNFKLFNIQVKEVTQNDGTTTIANNLTSTVQVFTDSEYQLPYVLGSA

A20 L L

HQGCLPPFPADVFMVPQYGYLTLNNG**SQ**AVGRSSFYCLEYFPSQMLRTGNN

M P

FTFSYTFED**V**PFHSSYAHSQSLDRLMNPLIDQYLYYLSRTNTPSGTTTQS**R**LQ

D3 M C37 L L

FSQAGASDIRDQSRNWLPGPCYRQQRVSKTS**A**DNN**NS**EYSWTGATKYHLN

L L L P

GRDSLVNPGPAMASHKDDE**E**KFFPQSGVLIFGKQGS**E**K**TN**VDIEKVMITDEE

M A20 L M C37

EI**RT**TNPVATEQYGSVSTNLQR**GN**RQAATADVNTQGVLPGMVWQDRDVYLQ

GPIWAKIPHTDGHFHPSPLMGGFGLKHPPPQILIKNTPVPANPSTTFSAAKFAS

L L M M

FITQYSTGQVSVEIEWELQKENSKRWNPEIQYTSNY**N**KS**V**NVDF**T**VD**T**NGVY

SEPRPIGTRYLTRNL

[a]The boxes indicate epitopes recognized by monoclonal antibodies (A20, C-37B, and D3). Residues whose mutation led to decreased antibody binding and/or neutralization are depicted in bold. Letters indicate the study in which they were identified (**L**, Lochrie et al. [2006]; **M**, Maheshri et al. [2006]; **P**, Perabo et al. [2006a]).

LPGMVWQDRD at aa 601–610). These sequences map to either side of the second-highest peak of the AAV2 capsid, which is found at the threefold symmetry axis (Fig. 17-1). Two residues involved in HSPG binding, R585 and R588, are located at the summit of this peak. Therefore, C37-B binding may interfere sterically with HSPG binding, which would explain the neutralizing effect of this antibody. In contrast to C37-B, no specific peptide sequence recognized by C24-B has thus far been identified.

In contrast to the other three antibodies, D3 binds to intact capsids and to single capsid proteins but fails to neutralize viral infection. The epitope recognized by this antibody has been identified as SRNWLPGPCY (aa 483 to 474; Table 17-2). A peptide scan conducted by Moskalenko and colleagues using small (15 aa) overlapping peptides spanning the VP1 protein and human sera identified the same sequence [Moskalenko et al. 2000].

17.3.4 Capsid Engineering and Generation of Immune-Escape Viral Particles

Various mechanisms for antibody-mediated neutralization of viral particles have been described [Smith 2001]: (1) aggregation of viral particles, (2) induction of conformational changes in the capsid, (3) interference with receptor attachment, and (4) inhibition of uncoating due to capsid stabilization. Irrespective of the mechanism responsible for neutralization, all of these mechanisms are dependent on antibody binding to an epitope expressed on the viral capsid surface. Mutations affecting the structural and biochemical properties of these epitopes are likely to alter the affinity for antibody binding. Therefore, capsid engineering could make the generation of virus variants possible that escape neutralizing antibodies.

Capsid Engineering by Rational Design One way to generate immune-escape mutants is to predict putative capsid sites that constitute immunogenic epitopes and disrupt them by targeted mutations. Lochrie and colleagues [2006] sought to identify immunogenic epitopes on the AAV2 capsid by in silico modeling of antibody binding using the following rationale: (a) immunogenic sites are exposed at the external surface of the capsid; (b) the contact surface between antibody and antigen typically encompasses an area of 600 to 900 Å^2; therefore, amino acids that had a solvent-accessible surface area of less than 20 Å^2 were excluded; (c) in silico docking of a murine IgG2a to the AAV2 capsid identified capsid regions that were less likely to be accessible (the canyon region surrounding the cylinder and the "dimple").

Based on these assumptions, Lochrie and colleagues closed in on 64 putative residues, which were modified by amino acid substitutions. Binding affinity and neutralization ability of murine monoclonal antibodies and human polyclonal sera were then measured, comparing the mutants with AAV2 with wild-type capsid (wtAAV2). A20 analysis revealed an involvement of amino acid positions Q263, S264, S384, Q385, E548, and V708 in binding or neutralization

(Table 17-2). These residues are located next to each other, co-localize within the region identified by Wobus and colleagues for A20 binding [Wobus et al. 2000], and with the exception of E548, have counterparts on AAV3, a serotype that cross-reacts with A20 antibodies.

When repeating these experiments with three different human sera containing polyclonal neutralizing antibodies, single mutations were found to decrease antibody-mediated neutralization. However, the sites identified did not map to a distinct epitope, suggesting that a polyclonal antibody mixture can recognize and interact with different epitopes. Interestingly, even though the set of mutations that were found to interfere with neutralization varied when using different sera, two mutations (R471A and N587A) had a significant effect for all three sera tested. In addition, mutations at positions 497, 498, 531, 548, 550, 586, 705, and 708 produced particles that were less efficiently neutralized by at least one of the sera. Two of these positions, 548 and 708, are also involved in A20 binding [Wobus et al. 2000; Lochrie et al. 2006].

When using purified human IgG prepared from thousands of blood donors [intravenous immunoglobulin (IVIG)], the highest reduction in antibody binding was observed for a 708 mutant, but no correlation between mutations affecting binding to IVIG and those affecting neutralization could be observed. Perhaps mutations affecting neutralization do not have a detectable effect on the overall binding capacity of antibodies in a polyclonal serum because neutralizing antibodies represent only a small fraction of the total amount of binding antibodies.

Another "rational design" approach was inspired by the work of Girod and colleagues [1999], in which a 14-amino acid peptide ligand containing an integrin-binding RGD motif (QAGTFALRGDNPQG) was inserted at amino acid positions 261, 381, 447, 534, 573, or 587 of the AAV2 capsid to identify positions that allow the display of the peptide and AAV vector targeting to cellular integrins without disrupting critical viral functions. These positions were selected on the basis of structural alignments with related viruses—canine parvovirus (CPV), B19, and feline panleukopenia virus (FPV)—as being flexible, highly variable, and located on the outer surface of the capsid. Based on these characteristics, these positions were also good candidates for immunogenic regions. Huttner and colleagues [2003] set out to determine the influence of peptide insertions at these sites on the affinity and neutralization capability of human serum antibodies. AAV capsid mutants with an insertion at aa position 534 or 573 were less efficiently bound than wtAAV2 in 66% of the samples analyzed. Although separated by 38 amino acids in the primary sequence, these sites are located in close proximity in the three-dimensional structure of the assembled capsid. These data seem to corroborate those of Wobus and colleagues (for C37-B binding), suggesting the importance of the threefold symmetry axis for antibody binding. However, it remains to be elucidated whether aa positions 543 and 573 are directly involved in antibody binding or if insertion of peptides in these positions induces a structural change in adjacent regions interfering with antibody binding.

Among the various capsid insertion mutants, only one clone (587) produced a good transducing titer and was further characterized [Huttner et al. 2003]. Although the binding of anti-AAV antibodies to the "587-peptide insertion mutants" was reduced only slightly ($\geq$15% in comparison to wtAAV2), these mutants were able to escape neutralizing antibodies in human sera without losing their ability to transduce cells via the inserted peptide. As we stated when discussing the results obtained by Lochrie and colleagues, the discrepancy between binding and neutralizing effects are probably due to the fact that neutralizing antibodies represent only a small fraction of the binding antibodies. In marked contrast, incubations with the same sera significantly reduced (or inhibited) the transduction of wtAAV2. The results of Huttner and colleagues, besides contributing to the mapping of immunogenic capsid sites, demonstrate that it is possible to tailor viral vectors for gene therapy by peptide insertion, modifying both the specific tropism and the ability to escape the humoral immune system.

Using Capsid Engineering by Combinatorial Approaches to Identify Residues Involved in Antibody Binding Although the atomic structure of the AAV2 capsid is known, capsid modification on the basis of educated guesses and rational design is a labor-intensive approach. Our understanding of the structure–phenotype relation is still poor, and even a minor modification of capsid proteins may adversely affect virus particle function, stability, and infectivity. In the study of Lochrie et al. [2006], for example, half of the capsid mutants generated by point mutations (63 out of 127) yielded infectious titers that were 10-fold lower than wtAAV2, and a quarter of the mutants (31) produced titers that were 100-fold lower. An attractive alternative that has recently been proposed is the employment of high-throughput combinatorial technology. This strategy is based on the generation of large libraries of clones with random mutations that can be screened to isolate capsid variants with a desired phenotype.

Two studies have shown the potential of this approach [Maheshri et al. 2006; Perabo et al. 2006a]. In both cases, a library of AAV variants with point mutations scattered throughout the capsid was generated by amplifying the *cap* open reading frame, which encodes the three AAV2 capsid proteins using error-prone polymerase chain reaction (PCR). PCR products were cloned into plasmids containing the viral genome, replacing the wtAAV2 *cap* sequence and yielding a pool of plasmids that was used to package a library of AAV capsid mutants. Since some point mutations impair capsid formation or stability, a first selection—for packaging efficiency and capsid stability—occurs when these viral particles are produced from the plasmid pool. Thereafter, specific selection conditions are applied to isolate clones with a desired phenotype, as, for example, the ability to escape neutralizing antibodies.

Perabo and colleagues preincubated their randomized library with a polyclonal anti-AAV2 neutralizing human serum followed by HeLa cell infection and replication in the presence of adenovirus (Fig. 17-2) [Perabo et al. 2006a]. After three rounds of selection, three-point mutations at two different positions

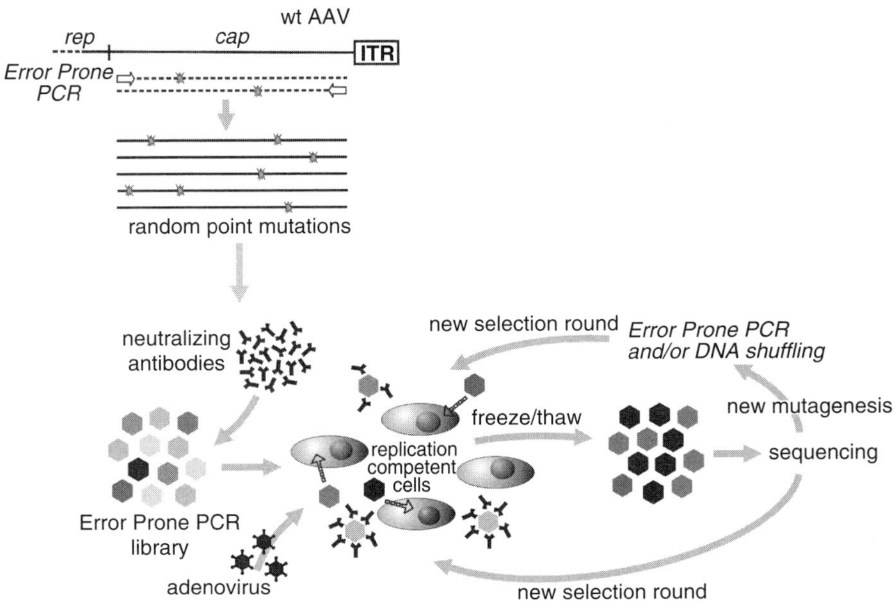

Figure 17-2 Library production and screening procedure for the isolation of capsid variants that escape neutralization.

were strongly selected: R459G, and N551D. The double mutant R459K and N551D was also detected (Table 17-2). Although the two residues 459 and 551 are separated by 92 amino acids in the primary sequence of the capsid protein, in the three-dimensional structure they are located in close proximity at the threefold-symmetry peak. In addition to these strongly selected positions, mutations in 22 other residues appeared in the viral progeny rescued, although less frequently. When all these sites were mapped on the capsid structure, 73% of them clustered in the same capsid region as the two strongly selected positions.

To evaluate whether these mutations allowed escape from antibody neutralization, AAV vectors carrying the strongly selected mutations and the double mutation were generated and compared with wtAAV2 for their ability to transduce HeLa cells in the presence of neutralizing antibodies from human sera obtained from different donors. Although the mutants could still be inactivated by less diluted sera, all of them showed an improved ability to escape neutralization. The double mutant was particularly effective in this regard, suggesting that introduction of multiple mutations is likely to yield further improved phenotypes.

In a similar approach, Masheshri and colleagues incubated their library with an AAV2 neutralizing serum they had generated by injection of wtAAV2 into a rabbit hind limb muscle [Maheshri et al. 2006]. HEK293 were then infected and viral progeny harvested for several selection cycles. In this case, selective pressure was gradually increased, with each round using increased serum concentration.

Additionally, DNA shuffling was introduced to swap mutations between different clones and therefore increase the chance of obtaining variants carrying multiple mutations. With their first round of selection, four AAV variants were selected that packaged at high titers and showed transduction efficiencies comparable to wtAAV2 in the absence of neutralizing sera. In the presence of serum, a three-fold improvement in infection efficiency was observed. Interestingly, all four mutants shared the mutation T716A (Table 17-2). Additional mutations were found in three of the four mutants.

To further improve the results, the library was subjected to another round of mutagenesis and selection. This procedure resulted in the selection of one very promising AAV2 variant, with an improved ability to evade the immune response in comparison to the mutants selected in their first round of selection. In subsequent in vivo experiments, in which recombinant versions of the respective AAV variants were incubated with neutralizing serum prior to muscle injection, 1- to 3-log higher expression levels were determined compared to wtAAV2. The most efficient mutant had five mutations: E12A, K258N, T567S, N587I, and T716A [Maheshri et al. 2006; Kwon and Schaffer 2008]. The identification of positions 567 and 587 marks the threefold-proximal peaks as major antigenic determinants (see Fig. 17-1B) for antibody binding, in agreement with results obtained by other groups using different approaches, as described above [Wobus et al. 2000; Huttner et al. 2003; Lochrie et al. 2006; Perabo et al. 2006a]. Residues T567, K258, and T716 map in a region recognized by the murine monoclonal antibody A20 [Wobus et al. 2000] and by human sera [Moskalenko et al. 2000; Kwon and Schaffer 2008], indicating this area as a second major epitope (Fig. 17-1B). Interestingly, AAV serotype 4, which is able to escape anti-AAV2 antibodies, has an alanine at position 716 [Maheshri et al. 2006].

17.4 CONCLUSIONS

The remarkable advances in understanding mechanisms of viral infection and of innate and adaptive immunity are beginning to enable scientists to generate "stealth" gene therapy vectors that evade immune responses. Two strategies that shield viral capsids from immune recognition have been described in this chapter: covalently linked polymers and substitution of capsid residues involved in immune recognition by genetic modification. While shielding strategies enabled adenoviral vectors to escape neutralization by antibodies and reduce the induction of humoral and cellular immune responses, the potential of genetic engineering of AAV capsids has so far been demonstrated only for blunting preexisting anti-AAV neutralizing antibody responses.

However, it has recently been shown that the exchange of a certain epitope from AAV2 into AAV8 capsids can boost the cellular immune responses against AAV8 [Vandenberghe et al. 2006]. Conversely, other genetic modifications might have an inhibitory effect on the induction of cellular immunity. One strategy to generate such mutations is by vector targeting. To redirect vector tropism, receptor-specific ligands are introduced into the viral capsid (for a review, see Büning et al. [2003], Muzyczka and Warrington [2005], and Kwon and Schaffer [2008]). By optimizing target selectivity and abrogating natural tropism, transduction of nontarget organs such as the spleen can be minimized [Perabo et al. 2006b], thus avoiding the induction of anti-AAV2 cellular immune responses [Vandenberghe et al. 2006]. In addition, by increasing target transduction efficiencies, it will be possible to reduce further the vector doses required for administration to patients, thereby minimizing the risk of adverse immune responses. Technologies such as those described here will soon yield highly efficient and specific viral vectors that offer the possibility to treat patients, including those with preexisting immunity, perhaps without eliciting toxic immune reactions even after repeated application.

REFERENCES

Büning H, Ried MU, et al. 2003. Receptor targeting of adeno-associated virus vectors. *Gene Ther* 10:1142–1151.

Croyle MA, Yu QC, et al. 2000. Development of a rapid method for the PEGylation of adenoviruses with enhanced transduction and improved stability under harsh storage conditions. *Hum Gene Ther* 11:1713–1722.

Croyle MA, Chirmule N, et al. 2001. 'Stealth' adenoviruses blunt cell-mediated and humoral immune responses against the virus and allow for significant gene expression upon readministration in the lung. *J Virol* 75:4792–4801.

Croyle MA, Chirmule N, et al. 2002. PEGylation of E1-deleted adenovirus vectors allows significant gene expression on readministration to liver. *Hum Gene Ther* 13:1887–1900.

Croyle MA, Le HT, et al. 2005. PEGylated helper-dependent adenoviral vectors: highly efficient vectors with an enhanced safety profile. *Gene Ther* 12:579–587.

Delgado C, Francis GE, et al. 1992. The uses and properties of PEG-linked proteins. *Crit Rev Ther Drug Carrier Syst* 9:249–304.

Girod A, Ried M, et al. 1999. Genetic capsid modifications allow efficient re-targeting of adeno-associated virus type 2. *Nat Med* 5:1052–1056.

Haag R and Kratz F. 2006. Polymer therapeutics: concepts and applications. *Angew Chem Int Ed Engl* 45:1198–1215.

Hartman ZC, Appledorn DM, et al. 2008. Adenovirus vector induced innate immune responses: impact upon efficacy and toxicity in gene therapy and vaccine applications. *Virus Res* 32:1–14.

Huttner NA, Girod A, et al. 2003. Genetic modifications of the adeno-associated virus type 2 capsid reduce the affinity and the neutralizing effects of human serum antibodies. *Gene Ther* 10:2139–2147.

Kern A, Schmidt K, et al. 2003. Identification of a heparin-binding motif on adeno-associated virus type 2 capsids. *J Virol* 77:11072–11081.

Kreppel F and Kochanek S. 2008. Modification of adenovirus gene transfer vectors with synthetic polymers: a scientific review and technical guide. *Mol Ther* 16:16–29.

Kreppel F, Gackowski J, et al. 2005. Combined genetic and chemical capsid modifications enable flexible and efficient de- and retargeting of adenovirus vectors. *Mol Ther* 12:107–117.

Kronenberg S, Kleinschmidt JA, et al. 2001. Electron cryo-microscopy and image reconstruction of adeno-associated virus type 2 empty capsids. *EMBO Rep* 2:997–1002.

Kumar TR, Soppimath K, et al. 2006. Novel delivery technologies for protein and peptide therapeutics. *Curr Pharm Biotechnol* 7:261–276.

Kwon I and Schaffer DV. 2008. Designer gene delivery vectors: molecular engineering and evolution of adeno-associated viral vectors for enhanced gene transfer. *Pharm Res* 25:489–499.

Lanciotti J, Song A, et al. 2003. Targeting adenoviral vectors using heterofunctional polyethylene glycol FGF2 conjugates. *Mol Ther* 8:99–107.

Lochrie MA, Tatsuno GP, et al. 2006. Mutations on the external surfaces of adeno-associated virus type 2 capsids that affect transduction and neutralization. *J Virol* 80:821–834.

Maheshri N, Koerber JT, et al. 2006. Directed evolution of adeno-associated virus yields enhanced gene delivery vectors. *Nat Biotechnol* 24:198–204.

Mingozzi F and High KA. 2007. Immune responses to AAV in clinical trials. *Curr Gene Ther* 7:316–324.

Mingozzi F, Maus MV, et al. 2007. CD8(+) T-cell responses to adeno-associated virus capsid in humans. *Nat Med* 13:419–422.

Moskalenko M, Chen L, et al. 2000. Epitope mapping of human anti-adeno-associated virus type 2 neutralizing antibodies: implications for gene therapy and virus structure. *J Virol* 74:1761–1766.

Muzyczka N and Warrington KH Jr. 2005. Custom adeno-associated virus capsids: the next generation of recombinant vectors with novel tropism. *Hum Gene Ther* 16:408–416.

Opie SR, Warrington KH Jr., et al. 2003. Identification of amino acid residues in the capsid proteins of adeno-associated virus type 2 that contribute to heparan sulfate proteoglycan binding. *J Virol* 77:6995–7006.

O'Riordan CR, Lachapelle A, et al. 1999. PEGylation of adenovirus with retention of infectivity and protection from neutralizing antibody in vitro and in vivo. *Hum Gene Ther* 10:1349–1358.

Parveen S and Sahoo SK. 2006. Nanomedicine: clinical applications of polyethylene glycol conjugated proteins and drugs. *Clin Pharmacokinet* 45:965–988.

Perabo L, Endell J, et al. 2006a. Combinatorial engineering of a gene therapy vector: directed evolution of adeno-associated virus. *J Gene Med* 8:155–162.

Perabo L, Goldnau D, et al. 2006b. Heparan sulfate proteoglycan binding properties of adeno-associated virus retargeting mutants and consequences for their in vivo tropism. *J Virol* 80:7265–7269.

Romanczuk H, Galer CE, et al. 1999. Modification of an adenoviral vector with biologically selected peptides: a novel strategy for gene delivery to cells of choice. *Hum Gene Ther* 10:2615–2626.

Smith TJ. 2001. Antibody interactions with rhinovirus: lessons for mechanisms of neutralization and the role of immunity in viral evolution. *Curr Top Microbiol Immunol* 260:1–28.

Stevenson M, Hale AB, et al. 2007. Incorporation of a laminin-derived peptide (SIKVAV) on polymer-modified adenovirus permits tumor-specific targeting via alpha6-integrins. *Cancer Gene Ther* 14:335–345.

Vandenberghe LH, Wang L, et al. 2006. Heparin binding directs activation of T cells against adeno-associated virus serotype 2 capsid. *Nat Med* 12:967–971.

Veronese FM and Pasut G. 2005. PEGylation, successful approach to drug delivery. *Drug Discov Today* 10:1451–1458.

Volpers C and Kochanek S. 2004. Adenoviral vectors for gene transfer and therapy. *J Gene Med* 6(Suppl 1):S164–S171.

Wobus CE, Hugle-Dorr B, et al. 2000. Monoclonal antibodies against the adeno-associated virus type 2 (AAV-2) capsid: epitope mapping and identification of capsid domains involved in AAV-2-cell interaction and neutralization of AAV-2 infection. *J Virol* 74:9281–9293.

Wortmann A, Vohringer S, et al. 2008. Fully detargeted polyethylene glycol–coated adenovirus vectors are potent genetic vaccines and escape from pre-existing anti-adenovirus antibodies. *Mol Ther* 16:154–162.

Xie Q, Somasundaram T, et al. 2003. Structure determination of adeno-associated virus 2: three complete virus particles per asymmetric unit. *Acta Crystallogr D Biol Crystallogr* 59:959–970.

INDEX

Gene Therapy Immunology, Edited by Roland Herzog